Transradial Access

TECHNIQUES FOR
DIAGNOSTIC ANGIOGRAPHY AND
PERCUTANEOUS INTERVENTION

Transradial Access

TECHNIQUES FOR DIAGNOSTIC ANGIOGRAPHY AND PERCUTANEOUS INTERVENTION

■ ■ ■

Howard A. Cohen, MD, FACC, FSCAI
Temple University Health System
Philadelphia, Pennsylvania

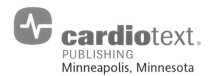

cardiotext.
PUBLISHING
Minneapolis, Minnesota

Cardiotext Publishing, LLC
3405 W. 44th Street
Minneapolis, Minnesota 55410
USA

www.cardiotextpublishing.com

Any updates to this book may be found at: www.cardiotextpublishing.com/titles/detail/
9781935395416

Comments, inquiries, and requests for bulk sales can be directed to the publisher at:
info@cardiotextpublishing.com.

Library of Congress Control Number: 2012955217

ISBN: 978-1-935395-41-6

Printed in the United States of America.

Contents

■ Contributors

About the Editor

Howard A. Cohen, MD, FACC, FSCAI
Professor of Medicine; Director, Temple
Interventional Heart and Vascular Institute;
Director, Cardiac Catheterization Laboratories
and Cardiac Intervention, Temple University
Health System, Philadelphia, Pennsylvania

About the Contributors

Richard P. Abben, MD, FACC, FSCAI
Director, Cardiac Interventions,
Cardiovascular Institute of the South, Houma,
Louisiana; Associate Clinical Professor of
Medicine, Louisiana State University School
of Medicine, New Orleans, Louisiana

Eltigani Abdelaal, MD, MBBS, MRCP (UK), CCST
Cardiology (UK)
Interventional Cardiology Fellow, Clinical
Research & Interventional Cardiology
Laboratories, Quebec Heart-Lung
Institute, Université Laval, Quebec City,
Quebec, Canada

Gérald R. Barbeau, MD, CSPQ, FACC, FRCPC
Cardiologue d'intervention & Imagerie
cardiovasculaire par résonance magnétique,
Institut universitaire de cardiologie et de
pneumologie de Québec, Université Laval,
Quebec City, Quebec, Canada

Hakim Benamer, MD
Institut Cardiovasculaire Paris Sud,
Massy, France

Olivier F. Bertrand, MD, PhD, FSCAI
Interventional Cardiologist, Quebec Heart-
Lung Institute; Associate-Professor, Faculty of
Medicine, Université Laval; Adjunct-Professor,
Department of Mechanical; Engineering,
McGill University; Director, CAIC Transradial
Interventions Working Group; Scientific
Director, Université Laval RADIAL Research &
Education Fund, Quebec City, Quebec, Canada

Ronald P. Caputo, MD, FACC, FSCAI
Director of Cardiac Services, St. Joseph's
Hospital, Clinical Associate Professor of
Medicine, SUNY Upstate Medical School,
Syracuse, New York

Gary Chaisson, RTR, RCSA
Technical Director Cardiac Catheterization
Lab, Cardiovascular Institute of the South,
Houma, Louisiana

John T. Coppola, MD, FACC, FSCAI
Assistant Clinical Professor of Cardiology,
NYU Langone Medical Center, New York,
New York

Jean-Pierre Déry, MD, MSc, FACC, FRCPC
Cardiologue d'intervention, Institut
universitaire de cardiologie et de pneumologie
de Québec, Université Laval, Quebec
City, Quebec, Canada

Aaron M. From, MD
Iowa Heart Center of Mercy Hospital,
Des Moines, Iowa

Kirk N. Garratt, MD, MSc
Lenox Hill Heart and Vascular Institute
of New York; Associate Chair, Quality and
Research; Director, Cardiac Interventions,
Northshore/LIJ Lenox Hill Hospital,
New York, New York

Ian C. Gilchrist, MD, FACC, FSCAI, FCCM
Professor of Medicine, Interventional
Cardiology, Pennsylvania State University,
Penn State Heart and Vascular Institute,
Hershey, Pennsylvania

Rajiv Gulati, MD, PhD, FACC, FSCAI
Associate Professor of Medicine, College
of Medicine: Consultant, Division of
Cardiovascular Diseases Mayo Clinic,
Rochester, Minnesota

Robert W. Harrison, MD
Fellow, Department of Internal Medicine,
Division of Cardiology, Duke University
Medical Center, Durham, North Carolina

Sameer J. Khandhar, MD
Assistant Professor of Medicine, Center for
Quality, Outcomes and Clinical Research,
Heart and Vascular Institute, University
of Pittsburgh Medical Center, Pittsburgh,
Pennsylvania

Thierry Lefèvre, MD, FESC, FSCAI
Institut Cardiovasculaire Paris Sud,
Massy, France

Yves Louvard, MD, FSCAI
Institut Cardiovasculaire Paris Sud,
Massy, France

Tift Mann, MD, FACC
Wake Heart and Vascular Associates, Raleigh,
North Carolina

Oscar C. Marroquin, MD, FACC, FSCAI
Assistant Professor of Medicine and
Epidemiology; Director, UPMC Provider
Analytics, Heart and Vascular Institute,
University of Pittsburgh Medical Center,
Pittsburgh, Pennsylvania

Suresh R. Mulukutla, MD, FACC, FSCAI
Assistant Professor of Medicine and
Epidemiology; Director, Center for Quality,
Outcomes and Clinical Research, Heart and
Vascular Institute, University of Pittsburgh
Medical Center, Pittsburgh, Pennsylvania

Pierre-Louis Nadeau, MD, CSPQ, FRCPC
Interniste, Résident en cardiologie; Institut
universitaire de cardiologie et de pneumologie
de Québec, Université Laval, Quebec
City, Quebec, Canada

Samir B. Pancholy, MD, FACP, FACC, FSCAI
Program Director, Cardiology Fellowship,
The Wright Center for Graduate Medical
Education; Associate Professor of Medicine,
Cardiovascular Diseases, The Commonwealth
Medical College, Scranton, Pennsylvania

Ankitkumar K. Patel, MD, MPH
Cardiology Fellow, Division of Cardiology,
Cooper University Hospital, Cooper Medical
School of Rowan University, Camden,
New Jersey

Tejas Patel, MD, DM, FCSI, FACC, FESC, FSCAI
Chairman and Chief Interventional
Cardiologist, Apex Heart Institute,
Ahmedabad, Gujarat, India

Sunil V. Rao, MD, FACC, FSCAI
Associate Professor of Medicine, Department
of Internal Medicine, Division of Cardiology,
Duke University Medical Center, The
Duke Clinical Research Institute, Durham,
North Carolina

Charanjit S. Rihal, MD, MBA
Professor and Chair, Division of
Cardiovascular Diseases, Mayo Clinic,
Rochester, Minnesota

Sanjay C. Shah, MD, DM
Director of Cardiology, APEX Heart Institute,
Ahmedabad, Gujarat, India

Cezar Staniloae, MD, FACC
Clinical Assistant Professor, Leon Charney
Division of Cardiology, NYU Langone Medical
Center, New York, New York

Zoltan G. Turi, MD
Director, Cooper Vascular Center, Cooper
University Hospital; Professor of Medicine,
Cooper Medical School of Rowan University,
Camden, New Jersey

Foreword

Introduced nearly 25 years ago as an alternative to femoral or brachial artery puncture, transradial cardiac catheterization and percutaneous coronary revascularization has emerged as the dominant vascular access strategy in many clinical practices worldwide. The adoption of this method has been advanced by both observational experience and clinical trials demonstrating reductions in bleeding and vascular access complications, lower resource utilization, and improved patient satisfaction. In particular, recent evidence indicates that the clinical advantages of a transradial approach may be especially evident among patients representing the highest risk for bleeding events, for example, those with acute myocardial infarction.

Despite these unequivocal benefits of a transradial approach, its prevalence relative to femoral arterial access remains varied, in part challenged by uncertainties regarding technical challenges specific to radial catheterization, misperceptions of incapabilities related to complex coronary revascularization, and, until recently, a general lack of operator and staff training. The greatest determinant of whether a patient is treated by femoral or radial artery access is not the comparative evidence but instead the clinician's skill set. At present, however, the learning curve for adoption of transradial catheterization and revascularization has never been more abbreviated due to increasing awareness of patient-oriented benefits, opportunities for practice differentiation, implementation of didactic programs through proctoring, regional training and media, and, more generally, increased attention to this method in interventional conferences and clinical trials. More specifically, reports following institutional and even multicenter adoption of transradial cardiac catheterization and revascularization have demonstrated that following only a modest case volume, reductions in procedural time and resource utilization, increasing procedural success, and even improved patient outcomes may be realized. Furthermore, increasing comparative study of femoral- versus radial-directed percutaneous coronary intervention related to unprotected left main disease, chronic total occlusions, and acute myocardial infarction affirms the capabilities of a transradial approach, reporting similar procedural success and clinical outcome.

In one of the most progressive fields of medicine, the radial approach to cardiac catheterization and coronary intervention is part of the natural evolution of interventional cardiology. As attention to procedural safety, cost containment, and patient-reported satisfaction increases, radial vascular access represents a solution. To this purpose, the chapters in this book were developed to inform the technical, procedural, and evidence-based aspects of transradial catheterization and intervention for both beginning and advanced practitioners.

David E. Kandzari, MD, FACC, FSCAI
Director, Interventional Cardiology
and Chief Scientific Officer
Piedmont Heart Institute
Atlanta, Georgia

■ Abbreviations

ACC   American College of Cardiology
ACS   acute coronary syndromes
ACT   activated clotting time
ACUITY   Acute Catheterization and Urgent Intervention Strategy
AHA   American Heart Association
APR-DRG   All Patient Refined Diagnosis Related Group
ASB   access site bleeding
A-V   anterior-venous
AVF   arteriovenus fistulae
BA   brachial artery
BARC   Bleeding Academic Research Consortium
BMI   body mass index
CA   coronary angiography
CABG   coronary artery bypass graft
CAD   coronary artery disease
CARAFE   Coronary Angiography Through the Radial or Femoral Approach
CHF   congestive heart failure
CMS   Centers for Medicare and Medicaid Services
COPD   chronic obstructive pulmonary disease
CRUSADE   Can Rapid Risk Stratification of Unstable Angina Patients Suppress Adverse Outcomes with Early Implementation of the ACC/AHA Guidelines
CTO   chronic total occlusion
CVA   cerebrovascular accident
DAP   dose area product
DES   drug-eluting stents
DPA   deep palmar arch
D2B   door-to-balloon
EASY   Early Discharge After Transradial Stenting of Coronary Arteries
ECG   electrocardiogram
ECMO   extra-corporeal membrane oxygenation
e-GFR   estimated glomerular filtration rate
EPIC   Evaluation of c7E3 for the Prevention of Ischemic Complications

FARMI   Five French Arterial access with Reopro in Myocardial Infarction
FDA   Food and Drug Administration
Fr   French
GI   gastrointestinal bleeding
GP   glycoprotein
GRACE   Global Registry of Acute Coronary Events
GU   genitourinary bleeding
GUSTO   Global Use of Strategies to Open Occluded Coronary Arteries
Hgb   hemoglobin g/dL
HORIZONS-AMI   Harmonizing Outcomes with Revascularization and Stents in Acute Myocardial Infarction
ICH   intracranial hemorrhage
IIb/IIIa   glycoprotein IIb/IIIa inhibitor
IMA   internal mammary artery
INR   international normalized ratio
IQR   interquartile range
IUCPQ   Institut Universitaire de Cardiologie et de Pneumologie de Québec
IVUS   intravascular ultrasound
LAD   left anterior descending coronary artery
LAO   left anterior oblique
LCX   left circumflex coronary artery
LMCA   left main coronary artery
LMWH   low-molecular-weight heparin
LOS   length of stay
LVEF   left ventricular ejection fraction
MACE   major adverse cardiac events
MI   myocardial infarction
M.O.R.T.A.L   Mortality Benefit of Reduced Transfusion after Percutaneous Coronary Intervention via the Arm or Leg
MRA   magnetic resonance angiography
NCDR   National Cardiovascular Data Registry
NHLBI   National Heart, Lung, and Blood Institute
NPO   nothing by mouth
NR   not randomized

NSTEMI   non-ST-elevation myocardial infarction

OASIS   Organization to Assess Strategies for Ischemic Syndromes

OCTOPLUS   Comparison of Transradial and Transfemoral Approaches for Coronary Angiography and Angioplasty in Octogenarians

OX   pulse oximetry

PAF   paroxysmal atrial fibrillation

PCI   percutaneous coronary intervention

PL   plethysmography

POBA   plain old balloon angioplasty

PPC   potentially preventable complications

PTCA   percutaneous transluminal coronary angioplasty

PURSUIT   Platelet Glycoprotein IIb/IIIa in Unstable Angina: Receptor Suppression Using Integrilin Therapy

PVD   peripheral vascular disease

R   retrospective data collection

RA   radial artery, right atrium/atrial

RADIAL   Radial vs. Femoral Access for Coronary Intervention

RADIAMI   Radial vs. Femoral Approach for Percutaneous Coronary Interventions in Patients with Acute Myocardial Infarction

RAO   radial artery occlusion

RAO   right anterior oblique

RCA   right coronary artery

RCT   randomized clinic trial

REPLACE-2   Randomized Evaluation in PCI Linking Angiomax to Reduced Clinical Events II

RIVAL   Radial vs. Femoral access for coronary intervention

RIVIERA   Registry on Intravenous Anticoagulation In the Elective and Primary Real World of Angioplasty

RP   retroperitoneal bleed

SC   single center

SCAAR   Swedish Coronary Angiography and Angioplasty Register

SCAI   Society for Cardiovascular Angiography and Interventions

SPA   superficial palmar arch

STEMI   ST-elevation myocardial infarction

STRIDE   Same-day Transradial Intervention and Discharge Evaluation

TEMPURA   Test for Myocardial Infarction by Prospective Unicenter Randomization for Access sites

TF   transfemoral

TFA   transfermoral approach

TIMI   thrombolysis in myocardial infarction

TR   transradial

TRA   transradial access, transradial approach

UA   ulnar artery

VCD   vascular closure device

chapter 1

Introduction

Lucien Campeau was the first to describe transradial access for diagnostic angiography.[1] Ferdinand Kiemeneij subsequently reported the use of transradial access for percutaneous transluminal coronary angioplasty (PTCA) and for stent implantation.[2,3] Early on, it became clear that one of the major advantages of transradial access was the elimination of access site complications. Furthermore, patient preference and satisfaction has clearly favored the transradial approach.

In 1997, Kiemeneij reported the results of the ACCESS trial[4] comparing the results of transfemoral versus transbrachial versus transradial access revealing the decreased complications of the transradial approach that have been replicated in virtually all subsequent trials comparing access site and subsequent complication rates, especially if one considers the "expert" high-volume operator. This became particularly apparent in those patients with acute coronary syndromes requiring vigorous anticoagulation. In the most recently reported RIVAL trial, comparing transradial to transfemoral access, there was a difference in access site complications in those patients with acute coronary syndrome who required vigorous anticoagulation. Furthermore, when stratified by radial percutaneous coronary intervention (PCI) volume per center, the high-volume centers had significantly improved outcomes.[5]

Despite the apparent benefits of the transradial approach, the adoption of this technique has been slow, particularly in the United States. There are several reasons for this, not the least of which are the increased technical aspects of this approach because of a smaller artery, a more difficult access

Transradial Access: Techniques for Diagnostic Angiography and Percutaneous Intervention
©2013 Howard A. Cohen (Editor). Cardiotext Publishing, ISBN 978-1-935395-41-6.

to the central circulation, and a more diffi-cult engagement of the coronary arteries compared to the transfemoral approach. In addition, most fellows receive good training in the transfemoral approach with the transra-dial approach being taught in only a very few training programs, although this appears to be changing rapidly. The "learning curve" for the transradial technique is steep, requiring approximately 200 cases for the operator to feel completely comfortable with this approach for diagnostic as well as interven-tional procedures. This will, of course, vary depending on the experience and the skill of the individual operator. The majority of operators in the United States do not perform 200 cases per year, making it difficult for them to attain and to maintain the necessary skills to perform this technique. Conversely, those operators who are performing multiple cases per day may find themselves "too busy" to master the skills necessary for this approach.

Any operator of reasonable talent, however, who is willing to spend the time required to learn the technique can acquire the skills necessary to master the transradial approach. The "learning curve" certainly can be flat-tened by spending time in a busy laboratory with experienced and dedicated transradial operators.

■ HOW TO USE THIS BOOK

The purpose of this textbook is to provide, in one place, the necessary tools for the already experienced transfemoral operator and for the newly minted transradial operator to master this technique. In addition, the textbook is meant to be a resource to learn new techniques for the already experienced transradial operator. We have attempted to make this textbook rich in still frame images and video callouts that can be viewed at www.transradial.cardiotextpublishing.com in an effort to demonstrate the technical issues involved. In this regard, the textbook is avail-able digitally so that the reader can readily access the links to the teaching videos.

As the editor, I have taken the liberty to add *[Editor's notes]* in an effort to emphasize points or to give some additional perspective.

Chapter 2: Rationale for Transradial Access   In this chapter, the authors describe diagnostic angiography and percutaneous coronary interventions and why they play a critical role in treating patients with ischemic heart disease. Over the past 2 decades, advancements in pharmacotherapy, device therapy, and application of PCI have led to significant improvements in outcomes. In light of such advances in efficacy, maximizing the safety of therapies and procedures has become a clinical priority. Bleeding and vascular complications are a significant source of morbidity, mortality, and cost in the invasive treatment of coronary artery disease and acute coronary syndromes in particular. Studies indicate a significant reduction in access site bleeding and vascular complica-tions with the radial approach. These benefits are also associated with reduced mortality in specific clinical settings and among patients treated at experienced radial centers and by experienced operators. In addition, the reduction in procedural complications is associated with decreased length of stay, decreased hospital costs, decreased nursing workload, and increased patient satisfaction. Wider adoption of transradial percutaneous procedures has the potential to significantly affect public health in a positive way.

Chapter 3: Vascular Anatomy of the Arm and Hand   This chapter recognizes that radial access has emerged as an important advance in vascular medicine and, when applied appropriately, it results in improved outcomes and patient satisfaction. To safely, effectively perform this technique, under-standing the vascular anatomy of the arm and hand is essential. With this knowledge, one can alertly identify and avoid potential procedural pitfalls that may result from the presence of vascular anomalies, variances in vascular supply and vessel diameter, and encroachments of tissue integrity. This broad understanding will foster excellent success while maintaining complication rates at a minimal level.

Chapter 4: Preoperative Evaluation of the Potential Patient for Transradial Access This chapter describes some of the issues to be addressed before performing a transradial procedure. Careful evaluation of the patency of hand collateral arteries via the ulnopalmar arch is a fundamental step before radial artery cannulation. Using combined plethysmography (PL) and oximetry (OX) for the evaluation of the hand collateral circulation has the advantage of being fast, simple, and objective while avoiding many of the pitfalls of the modified Allen's test. Although the modified Allen's test could identify a large proportion of patients suitable for transradial approach in the authors' series, PL and OX had a higher sensitivity. Using this method during the last 15 years, including Type A, B, and C patterns, the authors have seen no ischemic hand complications in case of radial artery occlusion after a transradial procedure.

Chapter 5: Obtaining Access Transradial access is technically more difficult than transfemoral access because of the size of the artery, the increased incidence of severe spasm, and anatomic variation such as loops and tortuosity. Nevertheless, the technique can be easily learned and mastered if the operator is committed. This chapter describes the techniques that can be used to successfully obtain radial access as well as access to the central circulation, particularly when there is difficult anatomy.

Chapter 6: Closure and Hemostasis after Transradial Access This chapter explains why hemostasis after radial artery access is a simple, highly successful, cheap, and extremely effective portion of the transradial procedure. Its effect on subsequent radial artery occlusion is frequently unrecognized and needs to be underscored, with special attention paid to maintenance of radial artery flow throughout hemostatic compression in order to prevent radial artery occlusion. Radial artery occlusion, although asymptomatic from an ischemia standpoint, eliminates the use of that radial artery in the future. Radial artery occlusion deprives the patient of a low-risk vascular access site for future percutaneous coronary intervention. Patent hemostasis

is an extremely successful technique that preserves the radial artery as an access site.

Chapter 7: Basic Catheter Techniques for Diagnostic Angiography and PCI This chapter recognizes that patient selection, appropriate use of right as opposed to left radial access, and thoughtful catheter selection are crucial to easing the transition to the radial approach. The benefits of transradial access are well documented but are fully experienced only with its routine use. A commitment to transradial access is essential.

Chapter 8: Sheathless Transradial Intervention Sheathless guides are currently available outside the United States but not yet approved in the United States. This chapter explains how the sheathless technique can be utilized with currently available technology. As the guide's outer diameter is 2-Fr sizes smaller than the sheath, a 7-Fr guide used without a sheath can be exchanged, for example, for a 5-Fr sheath over a long guidewire without upsizing the access site. The advantages and disadvantages of this approach are discussed.

Chapter 9: Transradial Access and Outpatient PCI: State-of-the-Art and Persisting Challenges This chapter explains that same-day-discharge practice after uncomplicated PCI is both safe and extremely effective in selected patients. In this regard, the transradial approach offers a tremendous advantage over the standard femoral approach as hemostasis can be obtained while the patient is already ambulatory. As hemostasis is usually completed within 2 hours of radial access, it remains prudent to have an observation period of 4 to 6 hours to detect any severe complications prior to hospital discharge. Because a recent survey revealed that fewer than 50% of radial operators in the world discharge patients the same day of the procedure, several nonmedical issues and obstacles remain to be resolved in order to promote outpatient practice.

Chapter 10: Transradial Access for PCI in Acute Myocardial Infarction This chapter discusses how treating acute coronary patients with the combination of medical therapy and revascularization has improved mortality in the ACS setting. However, despite these remarkable advances, these patients are among those at highest risk for bleeding complications following interventional procedures. Furthermore, considerable recent evidence suggests that bleeding in the ACS setting increases MACE and death, and reducing bleeding should now be made a priority. As such, the authors recommend that the approach to care of patients with ACS further evolve with efforts to reduce bleeding.

The authors' approach to revascularization in the ACS setting is to consider all patients eligible for TRA and have a thoughtful process behind choosing radial access. Transradial PCI has been shown in multiple trials to achieve equal success rates without prolonging door-to-balloon times in the setting of ST-elevation myocardial infarction. Despite trends toward lower rates of mortality by radial access utilization, further trials are still necessary to precisely define the benefit. Nonetheless, improved patient satisfaction and the potential for decreased bleeding complications are compelling reasons to increase utilization of transradial PCI in this clinical population.

Certainly, several studies have shown that there is a learning curve with TRA, and the authors recommend that operators be proficient with TRA in the elective setting prior to attempting in ACS patients. In addition, the authors advocate for identifying patients at risk of bleeding using the predictive models discussed in this chapter. This will help to identify those patients who are at highest risk for bleeding and those who may benefit the most from bleeding-avoidance strategies such as TRA.

Chapter 11: Transradial Approach to Peripheral Interventions   In this chapter, the authors explain how peripheral vascular interventions can be safely performed using the radial artery as an access point. This approach is particularly beneficial because the patients with severe peripheral arterial disease are at higher risk for access site complications. The main limitation to this approach is the lack of equipment that could easily access every vascular bed, particularly at the level of superficial femoral artery and tibial vessels.

Chapter 12: Right Heart Catheterization and Transradial Access   This chapter focuses

on how central venous access can actually be readily obtained using forearm veins. Whether needed for catheter-based hemodynamic monitoring or diagnosis, for temporary pacing during periods of iatrogenic bradycardia from interventional techniques, or for a trans-venous interventional procedure, forearm venous access can provide a reliable and safe entry site to complement or complete the transradial procedure. Venous access from the forearm can be accomplished efficiently and without compromise by avoiding otherwise riskier anatomical approaches. Understanding venous techniques and recognizing this important adjunct to transradial interventions completes the operator's radial skills and further advances the potential of transradial interventions.

Chapter 13: The Learning Curve for Transradial Access   Use of the transradial route in interventional cardiology procedures may practically eradicate the occurrence of arterial access complications with their subsequent effects on mortality, morbidity, disability, and health care costs. Such improvements may be achieved with a modest increase in x-ray exposure for coronary angiography (decreased with increasing experience), but without any increase in procedural time, patient or operator irradiation for coronary angioplasty, or any differences in terms of efficiency in almost all patients and all clinical and technical settings.

However, these results can only be achieved after completion of a long learning curve. Thanks to the multiple training opportunities available and after appropriate patient selection, a good command of clinical and technical predictors of failure allows trans-radial operators to obtain rapidly acceptable success rates, procedural durations, and x-ray exposure. This may encourage colleagues, coworkers, paramedics, patients, and hospital managers to support widespread use of this vascular approach.

Chapter 14: Transradial Arterial Access: Economic Considerations   Transradial arterial access for coronary and peripheral arterial procedures provides economic advantages compared to transfemoral arterial access. Significant benefit is realized through decreased vascular and bleeding complications that are associated with added expenses related to diagnosis, treatment, and prolonged length of stay. Decreasing vascular complications is especially relevant in today's health care environment, given the emergence of value-related reimbursement. Early and safe mobility following TRA also confers economic advantage by decreasing nursing requirements, improving patient flow efficiency, and facilitating safe outpatient PCI.

Chapter 15: Tips and Tricks for Transradial Access   In this chapter, the authors try to resolve practically all important issues related to TRA. The tips and tricks discussed here shall help both beginners and experienced operators. To become a "committed radialist," a person needs to go through a process known as "a new learning curve" and understand normal vascular anatomy of the region, acquired variations, and congenital anomalies.

Chapter 16: Complications of Transradial Access   As with other aspects of medical practice, awareness of complication possibilities, knowledge of appropriate preventive and corrective actions, and recognition of actual adverse events are the keys to a transradial interventional practice characterized by a minimum of complications.

The principal benefit of radial artery access for angioplasty is the added safety it offers. This chapter describes how the complications are less frequent than with femoral artery access, but they can still occur and can be very serious. Common complications include radial artery spasm, sterile granuloma development, and radial artery occlusion (transient or persistent), which are generally benign in nature; the risk of all these complications can be readily diminished with simple measures easily incorporated into routine practice. More serious vascular complications include the development of a forearm hematoma with compartment syndrome, which stands as the most important to recognize quickly and manage correctly because it can lead quickly to permanent neurologic injury. Surgical decompression of the forearm compartment is the mainstay of therapy for this problem. Radial artery pseudoaneurysms and arteriovenous fistulae are rare but can cause forearm perfusion problems and discomfort and often require surgical intervention for repair.

Chapter 17: How to Start a Transradial Program at Your Hospital   As the chapter title indicates, the authors offer advice on how to start a transradial program at your hospital. Transradial catheterization is increasingly being used throughout the world. Patient satisfaction and lower complication rates have driven the transition for many femoral access laboratories to primarily radial operations. With adequate preparation and perseverance through the learning curve, the radial approach can become the primary means of catheterization for all except large sheath and some limited peripheral access procedures. As newer technologies specifically designed for the transradial approach come to market, radialists will have an even greater range of procedures that they can perform. Careful introduction of the radial technique should make the transition relatively seamless.

We have attempted to present a comprehensive approach and perspective, and I am certain that those who are committed to and have an abiding interest in this technique will continue to learn along the way. We all hope that this textbook will be a valuable resource for the transradial operator, whether a neophyte or an expert.

■ REFERENCES

1. Campeau L. Percutaneous radial artery approach for coronary angiography. *Cathet Cardiovasc Diagn.* 1989;16:3–7.
2. Kiemeneij F, Laarman GJ. Percutaneous transradial artery approach for coronary stent implantation. *Cathet Cardiovasc Diagn.* 1993;2:173–178.
3. Kiemeneij F, Laarman GJ, et al. Transradial artery coronary angioplasty. *Am H J.* 1995;129(1):1–7.
4. Kiemeneij F, Laarman GJ, et al. A randomized comparison of percutaneous transluminal coronary angioplasty by the radial, brachial and femoral approaches: the ACCESS study. *J Am Coll of Cardiol.* 1997;29(6):1269–1275.
5. Jolly SS, Yusuf S, et al. Radial vs. femoral access for coronary angiography and intervention in patients with acute coronary syndromes (RIVAL): a randomized, parallel group, multicentre trial. *The Lancet.* 2011;377(9775):1409–1420.

chapter 2

Rationale for Transradial Access

Robert W. Harrison, MD
Sunil V. Rao, MD

■ INTRODUCTION

Diagnostic angiography and percutaneous coronary interventions (PCIs) are the most commonly performed invasive cardiac procedures and have an integral role in diagnosing and treating the entire spectrum of coronary artery disease—from stable refractory angina to acute myocardial infarction. Since the 1950s, there have been significant advances in catheter design, interventional devices, and adjunctive pharmacotherapy such that procedures are routinely performed on higher-risk patients with low rates of complications.[1,2] Evolution in the use of potent adjunctive antiplatelet and antithrombotic therapies has played an important role in improving outcomes after PCI. However, the widespread application of PCI to high-risk patients such as those with acute myocardial infarction has highlighted concerns about safety, particularly with regard to periprocedural bleeding. Post-PCI bleeding has emerged in recent years as a significant clinical concern due to its strong and consistent association with death, (re)infarction, stroke, and stent thrombosis.[3–5] Bleeding complications after PCI can occur both at the vascular access site and remote from the access site. Implementing specific therapeutic strategies can reduce the risk for both types of bleeding. The focus of this chapter is to outline the role of radial artery access for PCI in reducing bleeding risk. By virtually eliminating access site bleeding, transradial PCI is associated with markedly reduced procedural complications and, in some clinical settings, reduced mortality.

Transradial Access: Techniques for Diagnostic Angiography and Percutaneous Intervention
©2013 Howard A. Cohen (Editor). Cardiotext Publishing, ISBN 978-1-935395-41-6.

■ DEFINING BLEEDING AND VASCULAR COMPLICATIONS

A discussion of bleeding and vascular complications is not complete without summarizing how these events are defined. Definitions have a significant effect on the measured incidence of complications. For example, an extremely conservative definition of bleeding—one that includes data elements that reflect severe blood loss—can lead to very low rates of reported bleeding because severe blood loss is relatively rare in current clinical practice. On the other hand, a liberal definition of bleeding—one that includes data elements reflecting mild or modest blood loss—can result in higher rates of reported bleeding. Table 2.1 lists the definitions of bleeding used in several clinical trials. Therefore, standardizing bleeding definitions has become a priority.[6] Standardization efforts have focused on the fact that bleeding occurs in several different settings—access site, non-access site, coronary artery bypass graft (CABG)-related, and so on.

Although the definition of a vascular complication is likely to have a similar effect on the reported incidence, this area has not been the subject of as much scrutiny. Although most operators are likely to agree that arteriovenous fistulae or pseudoaneurysms are clinically important vascular complications, whether an access site hematoma is considered a "clinically significant" vascular complication would likely be debatable. As will be detailed later in this chapter, specific types of vascular complications are associated with an increased risk for short- and long-term adverse outcomes.

■ INCIDENCE OF ACCESS SITE BLEEDING AND VASCULAR COMPLICATIONS

Despite the influence of definition on the reported rates of bleeding and vascular complications, one can look to both clinical trials and observational studies to determine the incidence of these events. Vascular complications are obviously related directly to the access site, whereas bleeding complications can be either access site related or non-access site related. Based on the available data, bleeding complications are more common than vascular complications, but they are not mutually exclusive events and often occur together.

Access site bleeding accounts for a significant proportion of the bleeding events associated with elective PCI (Figure 2.1). Kinnaird et al performed a retrospective analysis of 10,974 patients who underwent elective or urgent PCI at a single center between 1991 and 2000. In this analysis, major bleeding was based on the thrombolysis in myocardial infarction (TIMI) criteria. They found that 588 (5.4%) patients had major bleeding, and 1,394 (12.7%) had minor bleeding. Four hundred (68%) of the major bleeds (370 hematomas and 30 retroperitoneal bleeds) and 834 (60%) of the minor bleeds (823 hematomas and 11 retroperitoneal bleeds) were related to the arterial access site.[7] Verheugt et al[8] performed a pooled analysis of 17,393 patients enrolled in the REPLACE-2, ACUITY, and HORIZONS-AMI trials. All of these trials assessed bleeding using the TIMI major and minor criteria (in addition to other criteria). Overall, there were 357 episodes (2.1%) of access site bleeding and another 145 episodes of combined access and non-access site bleeding (0.8%). Results from similar pooled analyses from PCI trials are shown graphically in Figure 2.1. This demonstrates that the proportion of access site-related and non-access site-related bleeds are dependent on the baseline risk of the patient population. That is, in the elective PCI setting where upstream antithrombotic therapy is rarely used, access site bleeds are predominant; in contrast, in the setting of acute coronary syndrome, non-access site bleeding accounts for a greater proportion of overall bleeding events (see Table 2.1).

Data on vascular complications are more difficult to come by because they are not systematically captured in clinical trial databases. However, some clinical trials and

Table 2.1 Bleeding Definitions Used in Acute Coronary Syndrome Clinical Trials.

TIMI[34]	
Major	Intracranial hemorrhage Bleeding resulting in a ≥ 5 g/dL decrease in the hemoglobin concentration or in a ≥ 15% absolute decrease in the hematocrit
Minor	Observed blood loss: ≥ 3 g/dL decrease in the hemoglobin concentration or ≥ 10% decrease in the hematocrit No observed blood loss: ≥ 4 g/dL decrease in the hemoglobin concentration or a ≥ 12% decrease in the hematocrit
Minimal	Any clinical overt sign of hemorrhage (including imaging) associated with a < 3 g/dL decrease in the hemoglobin concentration or a < 9% decrease in the hematocrit
GUSTO[34]	
Severe or Life-Threatening	Intracranial hemorrhage Bleeding that causes hemodynamic compromise and requires intervention
Moderate	Bleeding that requires blood transfusion but does not result in hemodynamic compromise
Mild	Bleeding that does not meet criteria for either severe or moderate bleeding
ACUITY and HORIZONS-AMI[6]	
Major	Intracranial or intraocular hemorrhage Access site hemorrhage requiring intervention Hematoma ≥ 5 cm in size Retroperitoneal hemorrhage Reduction in hemoglobin concentration ≥ 4 g/dL without overt source Reduction in hemoglobin concentration ≥ 3 g/dL with overt source Reoperation for bleeding Use of any blood product transfusion
OASIS-2[35]	
Major	Fatal bleeding Intracranial hemorrhage Bleeding requiring surgical intervention Bleeding that requires ≥ 4 units of blood or plasma expanders Bleeding judged to be disabling or requiring 2 or 3 units of blood
Minor	All other bleeding events
CURRENT-OASIS 7[6,36]	
Severe	Requiring transfusion ≥ 4 units of PRBC or equivalent whole blood Resulting in hemoglobin decrease ≥ 5 g/dL Leading to hypotension requiring inotropes Requiring surgery Symptomatic intracranial hemorrhage Fatal bleeding
Other Major	Requiring transfusion of 2–3 units of blood
Minor	Other bleeding that leads to modification of drug regimen
Other	Bleeding not meeting criteria for major or minor

Continued

Table 2.1 *Continued*

RIVAL[10]	
Major	Fatal bleeding Intracranial and symptomatic or intraocular with significant vision loss Resulting in transfusion of ≥ 2 units of PRBC or whole blood Causing substantial hypotension requiring inotropes Requiring surgical intervention (surgical access site repair qualifies if associated with substantial hypotension or transfusion of ≥ 2 units of blood) Resulting in severely disabling sequelae Resulting in ≥ 5 g/dL decrease in hemoglobin concentration
ACUITY N on-CABG Major	RIVAL major bleeding Large hematoma (per investigator's clinical judgment) Pseudoaneurysm requiring intervention
Minor	Bleeding not meeting definition for major bleeding and requiring transfusion of 1 unit of blood or modification of drug regimen

several large regional and national quality improvement registries do capture PCI-related vascular complications. For example, Rao et al reported on the incidence of vascular complications (defined as arterial occlusion, peripheral embolization, arterial dissection, arterial pseudoaneurysm, or arteriovenous fistula formation) from the National Cardiovascular Data Registry (NCDR), which collects outcomes in PCI procedures from more than 600 sites across the United States. In their analysis of 585,290 transfemoral cases, the combined incidence of vascular complications with a transfemoral approach was 0.7%. The incidence of complications was highest in the elderly (> 74 years old, 1.0%), women (1.1%), and ST-elevation myocardial infarction (STEMI) patients (0.8%).[9] The RIVAL study comparing the radial and femoral approaches to angiography and intervention among acute coronary syndrome (ACS) patients captured vascular complications in detail.[10] In this trial, 3.7% of patients had major vascular complications—defined as a large hematoma, development of a pseudoaneurysm or atrreriovenous fistula, or an ischemic limb requiring surgery. However, the majority of these complications were hematomas. Excluding these, there was a vascular complication rate of 0.7%—similar to the results described in the NCDR. It should be noted, however, that a large hematoma, particularly one that requires transfusion, is not without serious consequence and is predictive of adverse procedural outcome and mortality.[13]

■ NON-ACCESS SITE-RELATED BLEEDING

Bleeding that is unrelated to arteriotomy occurs primarily due to the use of adjunctive antithrombotic and antiplatelet agents in a population at risk for bleeding, such as the elderly, females, and those with ACS. Verheugt et al, in their analysis of the REPLACE-2, ACUITY, and HORIZONS-AMI clinical trials, report that 61% of bleeding events were not related to the access site—an overall incidence of 3.3%.[8] Approximately half of the non-access site bleeding could not be localized to a specific site. Of those events that could be localized, genitourinary bleeding occurred in 18%, followed by gastrointestinal in 15%, head and neck in 10%, and pulmonary in 1%.[8] The RIVAL trial showed a similar proportion of access site to non-access site major bleeding. Non-CABG major bleeding was defined as per Table 2.1. Overall, the non-CABG major bleeding rate was 0.8%, with 70% of these occurring distant from the access site. Specifically, gastrointestinal bleeds accounted for 27%, followed by intracranial and pericardial bleeding.[10]

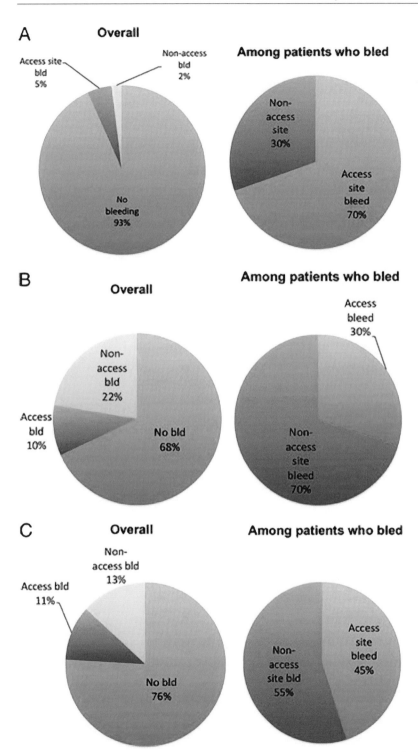

Figure 2.1 Rates of access site and non-access site bleeding in PCI and ACS clinical trials. Rates of overall and access site-related bleeding in a sample of PCI trials (REPLACE-2 and ESPRIT) (**A**); non-ST-segment elevation acute coronary syndrome trials (PARAGON A, PARAGON B, GUSTO IIb non-ST-segment elevation cohort, PURSUIT, and SYNERGY) (**B**); and ST-segment elevation myocardial infarction clinical trials (GUSTO I, GUSTO IIb ST-segment elevation cohort, GUSTO 3, HERO-2, and ASSENT-2) (**C**). *Source*: Rao SV, Cohen MG, Kandzari DE, Bertrand OF, Gilchrist IC. The transradial approach to percutaneous coronary intervention: historical perspective, current concepts, and future directions. *J Am Coll Cardiol*. May 18 2010;55(20):2187–2195.

■ ASSOCIATION BETWEEN BLEEDING AND OUTCOMES

Mortality

Multiple registry and clinical trial analyses have demonstrated bleeding to be associated with short- and long-term morbidity and mortality. In a retrospective "real world" sample of 10,974 patients undergoing PCI, Kinnaird and colleagues found that major bleeding was associated with increased in-hospital mortality (odds ratio 3.5), and blood transfusion was associated with increased 1-year mortality (odds ratio 1.9).[7] Rao et al demonstrated similar associations in a clinical trial population consisting of ACS patients.[11] In this study, patients were pooled from 4 large acute coronary syndrome trials—GUSTO IIb, PARAGON A and B, and PURSUIT. A total of 26,452 patients were

included in these trials. At least one bleeding event occurred in 27.6% of the patients. Mild bleeding occurred in 16.6%, with moderate and severe bleeding occurring in 9.8% and 1.2%, respectively. After multivariate analysis, bleeding was associated with increased risk of death at 30 days, death or myocardial infarction (MI) at 30 days, and 6-month mortality with a "dose response" increase in the risk from mild to severe bleeding. Figure 2.2 shows the relationship between mortality and the various levels of GUSTO bleeding. Bleeding is not only associated with increased risk of death after MI, but the level of risk has been shown to be equivalent to that associated with having a recurrent MI.[12] Furthermore, the risk associated with bleeding appears persistent beyond 30 days after the event, unlike the risk associated with MI, which is manifest only within the 30 days after the event.[12]

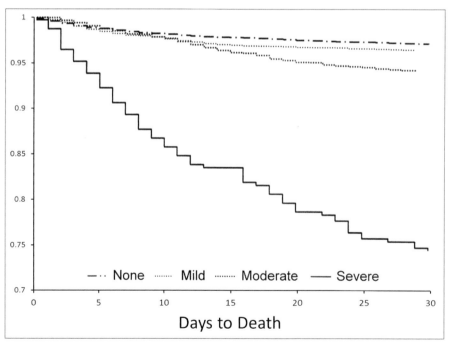

Figure 2.2 Effect of bleeding severity on mortality. Kaplan-Meier estimates of 30-day survival among patients enrolled in the GUSTO IIb, PURSUIT, PARAGON A, and PARAGON B clinical trials. Survival curves are stratified by GUSTO bleeding category. Log-rank *P* values are < .0001 for all 4 categories, .20 for no bleeding versus mild bleeding, < .0001 for mild versus moderate bleeding, and < .001 for moderate versus severe bleeding. *Source*: Rao SV, O'Grady K, Pieper KS, et al. Impact of bleeding severity on clinical outcomes among patients with acute coronary syndromes. *Am J Cardiol*. 2005;96:1200–1206.

Access site and non-access site bleeding are both associated with increased mortality, with the latter portending a worse prognosis. Verheugt et al discriminated between the outcomes associated with access and non-access site bleeding. As mentioned previously, 61% of the bleeding events in this study were not related to the access site. The adjusted mortality risk was elevated with both access site-only bleeding (hazard ratio 1.8) and non-access site bleeding (hazard ratio 3.9), although the risk attributable to non-access site bleeding was significantly higher.[8] Similarly, data from the National Heart, Lung, and Blood Institute (NHLBI) Dynamic Registry supports the association between access site complications and mortality.[13] After adjusting for multiple variables, hematomas requiring transfusion emerged as an independent predictor of death at 30 days (odds ratio 3.6) and 1 year (odds ratio 1.7). Retroperitoneal hematomas resulting from transfemoral access have also been implicated in worsened clinical outcomes.[14]

Nonmortal Clinical Outcomes

Aside from mortality, hemorrhagic complications are also associated with myocardial infarction, stroke, and stent thrombosis. Eikelboom et al evaluated 34,416 patients with acute coronary syndromes from the OASIS registry, OASIS-2 trial, and CURE trial. Major bleeding occurred in 2% of patients. Similar to other studies, mortality was higher in the group who had major bleeding both at 30 days and at 6 months. However, they also showed an increase in the rates of stroke and myocardial infarction at 30 days (hazard ratios 6.5 and 4.5, respectively).[4] Manoukian et al, in an analysis of the ACUITY trial, demonstrated that bleeding is also associated with an approximate 5-fold increase in stent thrombosis in patients undergoing an invasive strategy for acute coronary syndromes.[5]

Putative Mechanisms

The mechanism by which bleeding may contribute to these adverse outcomes is complex and multifactorial. Frank

exsanguination, which is exceedingly rare after PCI, can lead to adverse outcomes simply through blood loss. Similarly, bleeding in closed spaces such as the cranium or pericardial space can lead directly to mortality through either neurological compromise or hemodynamic embarrassment. Other, more common types of bleeding are associated with worse outcomes likely through secondary mechanisms. As such, they may not be directly causing the outcome. For example, evidence-based antiplatelet and antithrombotic therapies are commonly discontinued in the setting of bleeding, and patients are less likely to leave the hospital on guideline-based antiplatelet therapy if they experienced in-hospital bleeding.[15] Patients with bleeding, depending on the definition used, are also more likely to receive blood transfusions. There is mounting evidence of the harm associated with transfused blood, which may be related to impaired nitric oxide bioactivity and oxygen delivery in banked blood.[16]

■ EFFECT OF TRANSRADIAL ACCESS ON BLEEDING AND CARDIOVASCULAR OUTCOMES

Radial Access and Bleeding

Utilizing the radial artery for PCI is associated with a marked reduction in access site bleeding due to its superficial location, lack of adjacent vascular structures, and ease of compressibility. A significant amount of evidence has accumulated from observational and randomized clinical trials to support a decrease in bleeding with the transradial approach. Rao et al analyzed the NCDR and compared rates of procedural success and bleeding events between 7,804 transradial and 585,290 transfemoral cases.[9] After adjusting for NCDR risk score, gender, antithrombotic use, and glycoprotein IIb/IIIa use, they found that the transradial approach was associated with a 62% reduction in the risk for postprocedural bleeding compared with the transfemoral approach. Procedural success was similar between the 2 cohorts. The association between the transradial approach and decreased bleeding was more pronounced in younger (age < 75) patients, women, and patients with non-ST-elevation myocardial infarction (NSTEMI). Interestingly, among the 241 STEMI cases who had transradial catheterizations, there were no bleeding events or vascular complications, compared with rates of 3% and 0.8%, respectively, in the transfemoral cohort. A meta-analysis of 23 randomized clinical trials comparing the radial and femoral approaches to PCI showed similar findings with a 73% decrease in bleeding among patients assigned to the radial approach.[17] In addition, the absolute risk reduction in bleeding with transradial access was highest for primary or rescue PCI for STEMI (3.1% absolute risk reduction). The rates of vascular complications in the RIVAL trial, which randomized more than 7,000 ACS patients undergoing angiography or intervention to transradial versus transfemoral access, were significantly lower in transradial patients (1.4% vs. 3.7%)—one major vascular complication was prevented for every 43 transradial cases performed.[10] Together, these analyses suggest that procedural success rates are similar for transradial and transfemoral cases, but the radial approach is associated with significantly lower access site bleeds and vascular complications, and this benefit increases as the risk for bleeding increases.

Radial Access and Nonbleeding Clinical Outcomes

Given the well-established association between bleeding and adverse clinical events, it is reasonable to hypothesize that the transradial approach may be associated with reduction in nonbleeding clinical outcomes. Two large contemporary registry analyses have supported this hypothesis. The M.O.R.T.A.L (Mortality benefit Of Reduced Transfusion after percutaneous coronary intervention via the Arm or Leg) study linked a prospective PCI registry with transfusion records and outcomes including 30-day and 1-year mortality. Of the 38,872 cases identified, 20% were performed via the radial approach. Approximately three-quarters were urgent or emergent cases. Mortality at 30 days

was 1.7% and 1.0% for transfemoral and transradial cases, respectively. Similarly, 1-year mortality was 3.9% and 2.8%, respectively. After adjustment for potential confounders, transradial access was associated with a significant 17% reduction in 1-year mortality. Interestingly, blood transfusion emerged as the most powerful predictor of mortality at 1 year.[18] After accounting for transfusion, the association between radial approach and mortality was significantly attenuated, suggesting that the reduction in transfusion was the mechanism that explained the mortality reduction. The RIVIERA (Registry on IntraVenous anticoagulation In the Elective and primary Real world of Angioplasty) study evaluated patients enrolled in a multinational registry of PCI, with a focus on the effect of anticoagulant use on outcomes. The study enrolled 7,962 patients, and 11% of the procedures were performed via the radial approach. Independent variables associated with a decrease in the primary endpoint of in-hospital death or myocardial infarction included the use of enoxaparin, PCI of the left anterior descending artery (LAD), use of nitrates, pretreatment with thienopyridines, and radial access. Of these, radial access was associated with the most significant reduction with an adjusted 84% reduction in in-hospital death or MI. Notably, radial access was also the only variable independently associated with a reduction in bleeding events.[19] The consistency of these analyses strongly suggests that, in certain populations, radial access is associated with a significant reduction in mortality, primarily driven by a reduction in periprocedural bleeding. However, given the observational nature of the studies, causality should not be inferred.

Prior to 2009, there were approximately 23 small, randomized controlled trials investigating the benefits of transradial access, with 12 of these reporting mortality, stroke, or MI as a clinical endpoint. Jolly et al performed a meta-analysis of these trials and showed a trend toward reduction in the combined endpoint of death, MI, or stroke with the radial approach compared with the femoral approach, but this did not reach statistical significance.[17] The overall odds ratio was

0.71 (CI 0.49 – 1.01, $P = 0.058$). There was also a trend toward improvement in mortality alone, but this also did not reach statistical significance with an odds ratio of 0.74 (CI 0.42 – 1.30, $P = 0.29$). The trials included in this meta-analysis were relatively small, often performed at a single center, and therefore underpowered to detect differences in major adverse cardiac events.

The RIVAL trial was conducted to address these deficiencies by enrolling 7,021 ACS patients from 158 hospitals in 32 countries with a composite of death, MI, stroke, or non-CABG-related major bleeding at 30 days as the primary endpoint.[10] Major bleeding was defined as bleeding that was fatal, resulted in transfusion of 2 or more units of blood, caused substantial hypotension with need for inotropes, needed surgical intervention, caused severe sequelae, was intracranial or intraocular, or led to a hemoglobin decrease of at least 50 g/L (see Table 2.1). Prespecified subgroups were designated based on age, sex, body mass index, STEMI versus NSTEMI, each operator's self-reported annual radial volume, and each center's self-reported radial volume. Approximately 27% of the patients were enrolled for STEMI, 27% for NSTEMI, and 45% for unstable angina, and 99.8% underwent angiography with 66% receiving PCI. Overall, there was no significant difference in the primary endpoint, which occurred in 3.7% of the radial group, and 4.0% of the femoral group. Individual components of the composite endpoint were also similar at 30 days, with death occurring in 1.3% and 1.5% of the radial and femoral patients, respectively. Major bleeding, as defined above, was rare in both groups at 0.7% and 0.9%, respectively. There were similar rates of procedure success in both arms, but there was a higher rate of access site crossover from radial to femoral compared with femoral to radial (7.6% vs. 2.0%).

Although it failed to show a benefit for transradial access in the primary endpoint, the results warrant further discussion based on findings in a post hoc analysis using a different definition of bleeding, and in the prespecified subgroups. First, the overall bleeding rates in the trial were quite low relative to those found in other ACS trials. In a post hoc analysis using an alternative definition of bleeding, the study found that the rate of bleeding by the ACUITY definition (RIVAL major bleeding, large hematomas, and pseudoaneurysms requiring intervention) was significantly lower in the transradial group (1.9%) compared to the femoral group (4.5%). This also led to a significant reduction in the composite of death, MI, stroke, or ACUITY bleeding (4.8% vs. 7.3%). Second, as summarized above, two-thirds of the bleeding events in the RIVAL trial were non-access site-related, and therefore would not have been significantly effected by radial access. Third, 2 of the 6 prespecified subgroups showed a significant benefit favoring the transradial group. After stratifying by radial PCI center volume, the investigators found that those patients enrolled at high-volume radial centers (> 146 radial PCI per operator, per year) had a benefit with regard to the primary endpoint, which favored transradial access (1.6% compared to 3.2%). Furthermore, there was lower mortality (0.8% transradial vs. 1.5% transfemoral) and there were fewer vascular complications (0.4% transradial vs. 4.0% transfemoral) at high-volume radial centers. Patients identified as having STEMI as their presenting syndrome also had a significant benefit with transradial access over transfemoral access with regard to the primary outcome (3.7% vs. 4.0%), death (1.3% vs. 3.2%), and vascular complications (1.3% vs. 3.5%).

Jolly et al performed a revised meta-analysis of clinical trials comparing radial with femoral access, which included results of the RIVAL trial.[10] This included a total of approximately 13,000 patients. Similar to the RIVAL trial itself, transradial access was a reduction in major bleeding (0.5% transradial vs. 1.0% transfemoral) and vascular complications (1.0% transradial vs. 3.1% transfemoral), but there was no difference in major cardiovascular outcomes of death, MI, or stroke. However, when stratifying by radial expertise, there was a significant benefit in the composite of death, MI, or stroke among expert radial operators (2.3% transradial vs. 3.5% transfemoral).

■ TRANSRADIAL APPROACH IN STEMI

One of the most interesting subgroups from the RIVAL trial is the group of patients presenting with STEMI. Traditionally, operators avoid the radial approach for primary PCI due to concerns over procedural failure, delays in time to reperfusion, and the necessity for femoral crossover in the middle of the PCI procedure. Studies indicate that access site crossover is more frequent when the primary approach is radial; however, this is counterbalanced by a consistent finding of reduced mortality with transradial primary PCI. In the RIVAL trial, the rate of access site crossover in STEMI patients was 5.3%, compared to 2.0% in the transfemoral group.[10] Similar results were obtained in a meta-analysis of 12 randomized controlled trials, not including the RIVAL trial, investigating transradial access in primary PCI. The odds of access site crossover were 7-fold higher for the transradial approach relative to the transfemoral with individual trials showing rates ranging from 0% to 12%.[20] Operator experience with the transradial approach can have a significant effect on the need for access site crossover. In the RIVAL trial, the rates of access site crossover in the overall trial population decreased from 8% in centers in the lowest tertile of radial volume to 4.4% in centers in the highest tertile.[10]

Despite a higher rate of access site crossover with transradial access, this does not appear to have translated into prolonged door-to-balloon times or PCI failure. As mentioned above, PCI was successful in 95% of both the transfemoral and transradial groups in the RIVAL trial. Similarly, most trials of transradial access in primary PCI published to date have shown statistically equivalent, if not faster, door-to-balloon times with transradial access. The TEMPURA trial was one of the first transradial primary PCI trials conducted and showed needle-to-balloon times of 44 minutes versus 51 minutes in the transradial and transfemoral groups, respectively.[21] Conversely, the RADIAL-AMI trial showed slightly longer times with the transradial approach (32 minutes vs. 26 minutes), but transradial times were still well under the 90-minute standard.[22] The meta-analysis described above, which includes these trials, showed no difference in procedural time or door-to-balloon time between transradial and transfemoral approaches. Pancholy et al published a registry analysis that also suggests equivalent door-to-balloon times in 313 patients undergoing transradial PCI for STEMI.[23]

Similar to the subgroup analysis in the RIVAL trial, the meta-analysis[20] of primary PCI trials also suggests that transradial access confers a significant 46% reduction in mortality and a 70% reduction in major bleeding—benefits that are more pronounced than those observed in patients who do not have STEMI. Thus, despite the risk of access site crossover, using the transradial approach in patients with STEMI is associated with reduced mortality and bleeding without sacrificing door-to-balloon times. Although these benefits are compelling, only centers and operators with significant radial experience should perform transradial primary PCI.

■ NONCLINICAL BENEFITS OF TRANSRADIAL ACCESS

The sections above detail how the transradial PCI is associated with significant reductions in procedural complications and, in some clinical situations, reduced mortality. Studies indicate that the benefits of the radial approach extend beyond bleeding and cardiovascular outcomes and perhaps even beyond the patient receiving the intervention. Transradial PCI has the potential to reduce health care costs, reduce length of stay, improve patient satisfaction, and decrease nursing workload.

There are numerous reasons why a patient may consider a cardiac catheterization to be an uncomfortable procedure—nothing by mouth (NPO) status, arteriotomy pain, discomfort while supine during the procedure and subsequent bed rest after the procedure, anxiety over potential complications, complications or residual pain at the access site, experiencing the manual pressure necessary for hemostasis, time spent in the medical facility and associated loss of productivity, and numerous other factors. Although no modality of cardiac catheterization has the potential to ameliorate all these issues, the transradial approach can improve many. Following a transradial procedure, patients are immediately able to sit upright and can ambulate immediately provided there are no residual effects from procedural sedation. Furthermore, hemostasis can often be obtained with radial compression devices, obviating the need for manual compression and eliminating many of the bleeding and vascular complications described previously. This can translate into greater patient satisfaction and improved quality of life. Cooper et al investigated the effect of transradial access on quality of life and cost of cardiac catheterization.[24] Patients were randomized to transfemoral (99) or transradial (101) access and underwent quality-of-life assessment at 1 day and 1 week postprocedure. They found that patients who had transradial procedures had less back and body pain and improved walking ability at 1 day. At 1 week, transradial patients had improved perception of physical function, bodily pain, social function, and mental health. The RIVAL trial also assessed patient preference and found that 90% of transradial patients preferred to have a transradial approach for their next procedure, compared with only 51% of transfemoral patients.[10]

Vascular access complications and bleeding events may not only contribute to adverse clinical outcomes for the patient, but also pose a significant financial burden on the patient and the medical system. Kugelmass et al performed an analysis of all Medicare beneficiaries who received PCI as part of a hospitalization during fiscal year 2002.[25] In their analysis, they defined complications as in-hospital death, emergency CABG, postoperative stroke, acute renal failure, and vascular complications (hemorrhage, transfusion, and/or surgical repairs). In the absence of any complication, the cost of PCI was $13,861 ± $9,635. Vascular complications, which included hemorrhage and blood transfusion, added an incremental cost of $9,023. Rao et al also investigated the costs of bleeding during treatment for ACS.[26] They found that bleeding resulted in a stepwise

increase in the overall hospital costs ranging from $14,282 in patients with no bleeding, to $21,674 in patients with minor bleeding, to $45,798 in patients with moderate bleeding, to $66,564 in patients with severe bleeding. Adjusted analysis showed that each moderate to severe bleeding event resulted in an incremental cost of $3,770.

Several studies have investigated the health care cost benefits of transradial access. The CARAFE study randomized 210 patients to femoral, right radial, and left radial coronary angiography, and found that hospitalization costs were reduced by approximately 20% in the left radial and right radial groups compared to the femoral group.[27] This was balanced, however, by an increase in equipment and medication costs for the radial group, leading to statistically similar costs between the radial and femoral approaches. Cooper et al investigated hospitalization costs in their trial randomizing 200 patients to transradial or transfemoral diagnostic cardiac catheterization.[24] Although catheterization laboratory costs were the same between the 2 groups, bed and pharmacy costs were significantly lower after transradial catheterization. The median total hospital costs were $2,010 in the transradial group and $2,299 in the transfemoral group. Roussanov et al compared hospital costs in a series of patients undergoing coronary angiography via the radial or femoral approach.[28] A third series of patients in their study received femoral closure devices. In this analysis, average total hospital costs were $370 and $447 for the transradial and transfemoral approaches, respectively. Average costs for femoral cases when a closure device was used totaled $553. The savings observed in the radial group were primarily due to shortened recovery periods as the costs attributable to access equipment ($93 vs. $41) and hemostasis equipment ($61 vs. $36) were higher in the transradial group. Similar savings were found by Mann et al in the setting of PCI.[29] In this study, the radial approach was compared to the femoral approach with use of a closure device.

Expected costs, accounting for supplies, complications, and delayed discharges, were $1,590 in the femoral/closure device group and $1,314 in the radial group. Of their savings, 40% was from reduced supply costs and 60% was attributable to fewer complications and subsequent discharge delays. Together, these studies suggest that the transradial approach can lead to significant savings, primarily by reducing costly complications.

Hospitalizations are prolonged by complications associated with cardiac catheterization, and these extra days spent in the hospital not only have a monetary cost to the patient and medical system, but they also have a significant opportunity cost to both parties. Patients have lost productivity, and hospitals have beds that may otherwise be able to serve other patients. Vascular complications, as captured in the Medicare database described above, resulted in an average length-of-stay increase of 3.4 days if a vascular complication occurred.[25] Similarly, Rao et al demonstrated in the GUSTO IIb trial that the average length of stay for patients with NSTEMI was 5.4 days if no bleeding occurred. This increased to 6.9, 15, and 16.4 days if there was mild, moderate, or severe bleeding, respectively.[26] Several small trials have demonstrated that transradial access is associated with shortened lengths of stay in ACS patients.[30] Mann et al showed that, in ACS patients randomized to either transradial or transfemoral PCI, postprocedural days in the hospital were reduced from 2.3 days to 1.4 days in the transradial group. Total duration of hospitalization was also decreased in the transradial group—3.0 versus 4.5 days.[31] Yan et al showed that, in octogenarian patients undergoing primary PCI for STEMI, total hospital length of stay was reduced from 10.1 to 7.2 days when the transradial approach was used.[32] Conversely, duration of hospitalization was unchanged in the RIVAL trial of patients with ACS, likely due to the lack of difference in bleeding complications between the radial and femoral groups.

Nursing workload has an important effect on the direct and indirect costs imposed on a hospital, and decreasing the demands placed on nursing staff in the periprocedural period may lead to significant savings. Amoroso et al investigated the benefits of transradial access with regard to the demands placed on nursing

staff.[33] Using a self-developed model of nurse workload, they assessed the demands on nurses in the procedural lab as well as on the ward for 52 transradial and 208 transfemoral diagnostic and interventional procedures. They found that procedural nurses committed an average of 174 minutes to the care of transfemoral patients, and 86 minutes to the care of transradial patients. Ward nurses also spent less time caring for transradial patients (386 minutes vs. 720 minutes). After adjusted analysis, transradial approach remained a significant predictor of decreased nurse workload.

Together these data support a conclusion that the transradial approach can improve patient satisfaction, decrease costs, shorten hospitalizations, and improve nurse workflow, all without sacrificing procedural efficacy.

◼ SUMMARY

Diagnostic angiography and percutaneous coronary interventions play a critical role in treating patients with ischemic heart disease. Over the past 2 decades, advancements in pharmacotherapy, device therapy, and application of PCI have led to significant improvements in outcomes. In light of such advances in efficacy, maximizing the safety of therapies and procedures has become a clinical priority. Bleeding and vascular complications are a significant source of morbidity, mortality, and cost in the invasive treatment of coronary artery disease and acute coronary syndromes in particular. Studies indicate a significant reduction in access site bleeding and vascular complications with the radial approach. These benefits are also associated with reduced mortality in specific clinical settings and among patients treated at experienced radial centers and by experienced operators. In addition, the reduction in procedural complications is associated with decreased length of stay, decreased hospital costs, decreased nursing workload, and increased patient satisfaction. Wider adoption of transradial percutaneous procedures has the potential to significantly affect public health in a positive way.

■ REFERENCES

1. Singh M, Rihal CS, Gersh BJ, et al. Twenty-five-year trends in in-hospital and long-term outcome after percutaneous coronary intervention: a single-institution experience. *Circulation*. Jun 5 2007;115(22):2835–2841.

2. Batchelor WB, Anstrom KJ, Muhlbaier LH, et al. Contemporary outcome trends in the elderly undergoing percutaneous coronary interventions: results in 7,472 octogenarians. National Cardiovascular Network Collaboration. *J Am Coll Cardiol*. Sep 2000;36(3):723–730.

3. Rao SV, Eikelboom JA, Granger CB, Harrington RA, Califf RM, Bassand JP. Bleeding and blood transfusion issues in patients with non-ST-segment elevation acute coronary syndromes. *Eur Heart J*. May 2007;28(10):1193–1204.

4. Eikelboom JW, Mehta SR, Anand SS, Xie C, Fox KA, Yusuf S. Adverse impact of bleeding on prognosis in patients with acute coronary syndromes. *Circulation*. Aug 22 2006;114(8):774–782.

5. Manoukian SV, Feit F, Mehran R, et al. Impact of major bleeding on 30-day mortality and clinical outcomes in patients with acute coronary syndromes: an analysis from the ACUITY trial. *J Am Coll Cardiol*. Mar 27 2007;49(12):1362–1368.

6. Mehran R, Rao SV, Bhatt DL, et al. Standardized bleeding definitions for cardiovascular clinical trials: a consensus report from the Bleeding Academic Research Consortium. *Circulation*. Jun 14 2011;123(23):2736–2747.

7. Kinnaird TD, Stabile E, Mintz GS, et al. Incidence, predictors, and prognostic implications of bleeding and blood transfusion following percutaneous coronary interventions. *Am J Cardiol*. 2003;92(8): 930–935.

8. Verheugt FW, Steinhubl SR, Hamon M, et al. Incidence, prognostic impact, and influence of antithrombotic therapy on access and nonaccess site bleeding in percutaneous coronary intervention. *JACC Cardiovasc Interv*. Feb 2011;4(2):191–197.

9. Rao SV, Ou FS, Wang TY, et al. Trends in the prevalence and outcomes of radial and femoral approaches to percutaneous coronary intervention: a report from the National Cardiovascular Data Registry. *JACC Cardiovasc Interv*. Aug 2008;1(4):379–386.

10. Jolly SS, Yusuf S, Cairns J, et al. Radial versus femoral access for coronary angiography and intervention in patients with acute coronary syndromes (RIVAL): a randomised, parallel group, multicentre trial. *Lancet*. Apr 23 2011;377(9775):1409–1420.

11. Rao SV, O'Grady K, Pieper KS, et al. Impact of bleeding severity on clinical outcomes among patients with acute coronary syndromes. *Am J Cardiol*. 2005;96:1200–1206.

12. Mehran R, Pocock SJ, Stone GW, et al. Associations of major bleeding and myocardial infarction with the incidence and timing of mortality in patients presenting with non-ST-elevation acute coronary syndromes: a risk model from the ACUITY trial. *Eur Heart J*. Jun 2009;30(12):1457–1466.

13. Yatskar L, Selzer F, Feit F, et al. Access site hematoma requiring blood transfusion predicts mortality in patients undergoing percutaneous coronary intervention: data from the National Heart, Lung, and Blood Institute Dynamic Registry. *Catheter Cardiovasc Interv*. Jun 1 2007;69(7):961–966.

14. Ellis SG, Bhatt D, Kapadia S, Lee D, Yen M, Whitlow PL. Correlates and outcomes of retroperitoneal hemorrhage complicating percutaneous coronary intervention. *Catheter Cardiovasc Interv*. Apr 2006;67(4):541–545.

15. Wang TY, Xiao L, Alexander KP, et al. Antiplatelet therapy use after discharge among acute myocardial infarction patients with in-hospital bleeding. *Circulation*. Nov 18 2008;118(21):2139–2145.

16. Reynolds JD, Ahearn GS, Angelo M, Zhang J, Cobb F, Stamler JS. S-nitrosohemoglobin deficiency: a mechanism for loss of physiological activity in banked blood. *Proc Natl Acad Sci USA*. Oct 23 2007;104(43):17058–17062.

17. Jolly SS, Amlani S, Hamon M, Yusuf S, Mehta SR. Radial versus femoral access for coronary angiography or intervention and the impact on major bleeding and ischemic events: a systematic review and meta-analysis of randomized trials. *Am Heart J*. Jan 2009;157(1):132–140.

18. Chase AJ, Fretz EB, Warburton WP, et al. Association of the arterial access site at angioplasty with transfusion and mortality: the M.O.R.T.A.L study (Mortality benefit Of Reduced Transfusion after percutaneous coronary intervention via the Arm or Leg). *Heart*. Aug 2008;94(8):1019–1025.

19. Montalescot G, Ongen Z, Guindy R, et al. Predictors of outcome in patients undergoing PCI: results of the RIVIERA study. *Int J Cardiol*. Oct 13 2008;129(3):379–387.

20. Vorobcsuk A, Konyi A, Aradi D, et al. Transradial versus transfemoral percutaneous coronary intervention in acute myocardial infarction: systematic overview and meta-analysis. *Am Heart J*. Nov 2009;158(5):814–821.

21. Saito S, Tanaka S, Hiroe Y, et al. Comparative study on transradial approach vs. transfemoral approach in primary stent implantation for patients with acute myocardial infarction: results of the test for myocardial infarction by prospective unicenter randomization for access sites (TEMPURA) trial. *Catheter Cardiovasc Interv*. May 2003;59(1):26–33.

22. Cantor WJ, Puley G, Natarajan MK, et al. Radial versus femoral access for emergent percutaneous coronary intervention with adjunct glycoprotein IIb/IIIa inhibition in acute myocardial infarction—the RADIAL-AMI pilot randomized trial. *Am Heart J*. Sep 2005;150(3):543–549.

23. Pancholy S, Patel T, Sanghvi K, Thomas M. Comparison of door-to-balloon times for primary PCI using transradial versus transfemoral approach. *Catheter Cardiovasc Interv*. Jun 1 2010;75(7): 991–995.

24. Cooper CJ, El-Shiekh RA, Cohen DJ, et al. Effect of transradial access on quality of life and cost of cardiac catheterization: a randomized comparison. *Am Heart J.* Sep 1999;138(3 Pt 1):430–436.

25. Kugelmass AD, Cohen DJ, Brown PP, Simon AW, Becker ER, Culler SD. Hospital resources consumed in treating complications associated with percutaneous coronary interventions. *Am J Cardiol.* Feb 1 2006;97(3):322-327.

26. Rao SV, Kaul PR, Liao L, et al. Association between bleeding, blood transfusion, and costs among patients with non-ST-segment elevation acute coronary syndromes. *Am Heart J.* Feb 2008;155(2): 369–374.

27. Louvard Y, Lefevre T, Allain A, Morice M. Coronary angiography through the radial or the femoral approach: the CARAFE study. *Catheter Cardiovasc Interv.* Feb 2001;52(2):181–187.

28. Roussanov O, Wilson SJ, Henley K, et al. Cost-effectiveness of the radial versus femoral artery approach to diagnostic cardiac catheterization. *J Invasive Cardiol.* Aug 2007;19(8):349–353.

29. Mann T, Cowper PA, Peterson ED, et al. Transradial coronary stenting: comparison with femoral access closed with an arterial suture device. *Catheterization & Cardiovascular Interventions.* 2000;49(2):150–156.

30. Subherwal S, Rao SV. Economic benefits of the transradial approach. *Cardiac Interventions Today.* Sep 2009:1–5.

31. Mann T, Cubeddu G, Bowen J, et al. Stenting in acute coronary syndromes: a comparison of radial versus femoral access sites. *J Am Coll Cardiol.* Sep 1998;32(3):572–576.

32. Yan ZX, Zhou YJ, Zhao YX, et al. Safety and feasibility of transradial approach for primary percutaneous coronary intervention in elderly patients with acute myocardial infarction. *Chin Med J (Engl).* May 5 2008;121(9):782–786.

33. Amoroso G, Sarti M, Bellucci R, et al. Clinical and procedural predictors of nurse workload during and after invasive coronary procedures: the potential benefit of a systematic radial access. *Eur J Cardiovasc Nurs.* Sep 2005;4(3):234–241.

34. Rao SV, O'Grady K, Pieper KS, et al. A comparison of the clinical impact of bleeding measured by two different classifications among patients with acute coronary syndromes. *J Am Coll Cardiol.* 2006;47(4):809–816.

35. OASIS-2 investigators: effects of recombinant hirudin (lepirudin) compared with heparin on death, myocardial infarction, refractory angina, and revascularisation procedures in patients with acute myocardial ischaemia without ST elevation: a randomised trial. Organization to Assess Strategies for Ischemic Syndromes (OASIS-2) Investigators. *Lancet.* Feb 6 1999;353(9151):429–438.

36. Steinhubl SR, Kastrati A, Berger PB. Variation in the definitions of bleeding in clinical trials of patients with acute coronary syndromes and undergoing percutaneous coronary interventions and its impact on the apparent safety of antithrombotic drugs. *Am Heart J.* Jul 2007;154(1):3–11.

chapter 3

Vascular Anatomy of the Arm and Hand

Richard P. Abben, MD
Gary Chaisson, RTR, RCSA

■ INTRODUCTION

For the practitioner to safely and effectively perform catheter procedures utilizing radial artery access, understanding the nuances of the hand and arm's vascular anatomy is essential. Components of this knowledge base include learning the vascular course of the brachioradial arterial system and its tributaries, identifying anatomic variations that may influence catheter and guidewire direction to reach the central aorta, and understanding key elements of the dual vascular supply to the hand from the radial and ulnar arteries. Indeed, credence for this notion is supported by clinical trials that have correlated procedural outcome data and success rates with vascular patterns and anomalies that occur in the brachioradial arteries.[1–7] Additional valuable parameters whose identification and understanding are worthwhile include recognizing the variety of luminal diameters that the radial artery exhibits and comprehending the anatomic compartments that the vascular segments of the arm reside in, features that may be important should access or bleeding complications occur.[8–10] Clearly grasping these anatomic concepts permits the operator to quickly and safely navigate the arterial tree, thus enabling successful, efficient vascular procedures.

■ ANATOMIC BACKGROUND

Brachial Artery System

The brachial artery forms at the lower margin of the teres major muscle as the continuation of the axillary artery in the upper arm.[11–12] Its course is relatively superficial as it passes through the upper arm, covered by integument and superficial and deep fasciae (Figure 3.1). During its passage, the brachial artery supplies branches to the upper arm musculature, including several collateral branches, that terminates in the radial and ulnar arterial systems. At the base of the elbow, it descends into the antecubital fossae and remains deep prior to its division into the radial and ulnar branches. In terms of radial artery access procedures, once entered, the brachial artery is generally traversed with guidewires and catheters in a relatively straightforward manner. There are some potential anatomic variations, including high origin of the brachial artery and high separation into 2 trunks in the upper arm that usually rejoin to re-form the brachial artery in the lower arm (Figure 3.2), but these variations do not generally create obstacles to catheter-based procedures.[13–15]

Radial Artery System

The radial artery itself originates after the bifurcation of the brachial artery into the radial and ulnar branches.[7,11,12] The bifurcation generally occurs just below the bend of the elbow (Figures 3.3, 3.4) with the radial artery passing on the radial aspect of the forearm with continuation to the wrist (Figure 3.5). Initially, the radial artery is relatively deep, passing between the brachioradialis and pronator teres muscles, and then becomes more superficial between the ligaments of the brachioradialis and flexor carpalis radialis. The upper part of the artery is covered by muscle, but the lower part is covered only by ligamentous tissue and fascia, thus allowing easy palpation and vascular access as it nears the wrist. After reaching the carpus, it winds along the lateral aspect of the wrist near the navicular and greater multiangular bones passing to the dorsal aspect of the hand (see Figure 3.5). A proximal radial

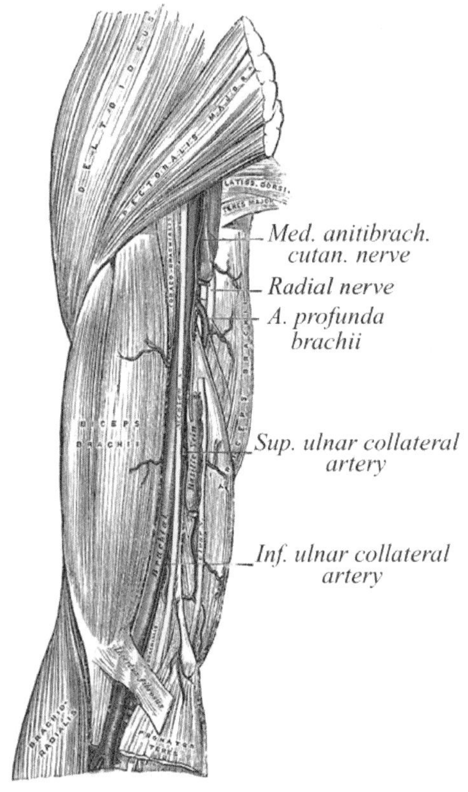

Figure 3.1 Anatomic course of the brachial artery in the upper arm with its major tributaries. *Source:* Reprinted, with permission, from Gray H, Lewis W. *Anatomy of the Human Body.* New York: Bartleby.com, 2000;VI,4.b.2.-3.

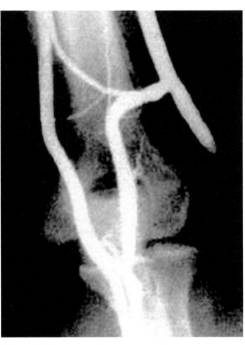

Figure 3.2 Retrograde angiogram demonstrating a double brachial artery anomaly. *Source:* Reprinted, with permission, from Yoo BS, Yoon J, Ko JY, Kim JY, Lee SH, Hwang SO, Choe KH. Anatomic consideration of the radial artery for transradial coronary procedures: arterial diameter, branching anomaly, and vessel tortuosity. *Int J Cardiol.* 2005;101:421–427.

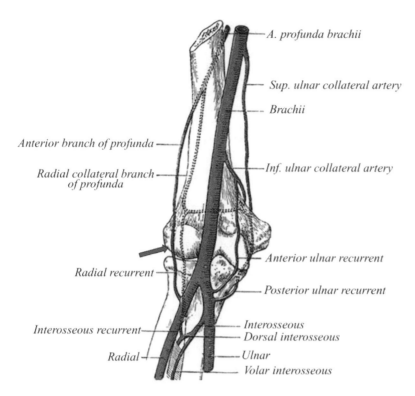

— A. profunda brachii

— Sup. ulnar collateral artery

— Brachii

Anterior branch of profunda —

Radial collateral branch —
of profunda

— Inf. ulnar collateral artery

— Anterior ulnar recurrent

Radial recurrent —

— Posterior ulnar recurrent

Interosseous recurrent—

— Interosseous
— Dorsal interosseous

Radial —

— Ulnar
— Volar interosseous

Figure 3.3 Anatomic illustration of the bifurcation of the brachial artery into radial and ulnar branches near the elbow. Arrow indicates origin of the recurrent radial artery with radiation from the forearm origin to the arm. *Source:* Adapted, with permission, from Gray H, Lewis W. *Anatomy of the Human Body.* New York: Bartleby.com, 2000;VI,4.b.2.-3.

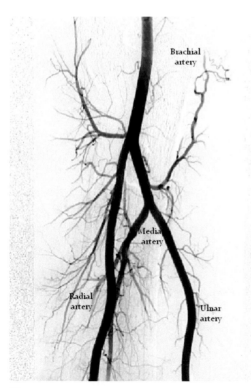

Brachial artery

Media artery

Radial artery

Ulnar artery

Figure 3.4 Angiogram demonstrating the normal vascular anatomy of the right lower arm and upper forearm in the region of the brachial artery bifurcation.

tributary in the hand is the superficial volar branch, and this may join with a superficial branch of the ulnar artery, giving rise to the superficial palmar arch. Dorsal meta-carpal and digital tributaries originate from this arch. The ongoing radial artery then descends to the palmar aspect of the hand, disappearing between the heads of the first interosseus dorsalis with continuation into the palm. Several smaller tributaries originate during its course though the wrist and hand, but the terminal portion or deep volar branch joins with the terminal aspect of the ulnar artery to form the deep palmar arch. The arch gives rise to essential tributaries serving the volar aspect of the hand and fingers. The radial artery contribution to the deep palmar arch is more predictable than its contribution to the superficial arch with its contribution to this arch generally smaller. At times, this superficial radial branch dissipates in size and terminates in the thumb. In this scenario, the ulnar artery would usually supply the bulk of the flow to the superficial arch. As will be discussed later, the anatomic integrity of the superficial and palmar arches of the hand is

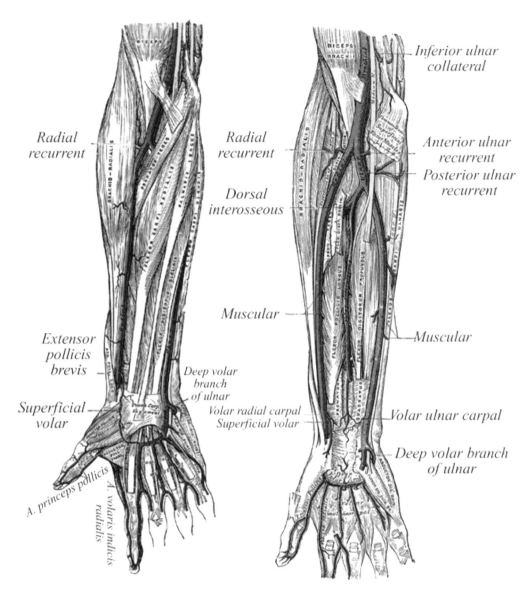

Figure 3.5 Anatomic course of the radial and ulnar arteries in the forearm, wrist, and hand (**left panel**: superficial view; **right panel**: deep view). *Source:* Reprinted, with permission, from Gray H, Lewis W. *Anatomy of the Human Body.* New York: Bartleby.com, 2000;VI,4.b.2.-3.

generally assessed clinically prior to radial access procedure.

Radial Artery Branches

Multiple tributaries originate from the radial artery as it courses from the elbow to the hand, and some of these do affect the retrograde course of vascular equipment as it passes retrograde toward the central aorta.

Recurrent Radial Artery. The recurrent radial artery originates just below the origin of the radial artery near the elbow and passes superiorly toward the upper arm between the brachioradialis and brachialis muscles (see Figure 3.3). It supplies these upper arm muscles and the elbow and anastomoses with collateral branches originating from the deep brachial artery. Because of its anatomic location, guidewires (particularly hydrophilic types) and very small-diameter catheters passed in a retrograde manner through the radial artery may be directed straight into this branch. If it is of sufficient size, it may allow passage directly into the brachial artery through the collateral branches, although significant vasospasm or perforation may occur. Recognition of this anatomic deviation is important because this branch is generally not of sufficient size to accommodate diagnostic catheters, and thus recognition of this aberrant location and appropriate redirection of the guidewire to the true brachioradialis system is required to allow central aortic access.

Muscular Branches. Multiple muscular branches originate from the radial artery supplying the radial aspect of the forearm musculature. Guidewires occasionally may enter into their origins impeding forward progress. Resistance to guidewire passage should signal deviation from the fairly straight-line course to the brachial artery and prompt fluoroscopic examination that could demonstrate branch misdirection in a line perpendicular to the normal radial artery course. [*Editor's note*: A small J-tipped hydrophilic guidewire will usually avoid the small branches (muscular and recurrent radial) and is, therefore, very useful once the sheath has been inserted.]

Wrist and Hand Branches. Additional branches originate near the wrist distal to sites of radial artery entrance for vascular procedures including the volar carpal branch that supplies the wrist and carpal articulations and the superficial volar branch that terminates in the thumb musculature. As the radial artery passes to the hand, additional branches supply the metacarpal and finger regions with the continued vessel anastomosing with the terminal portion of the ulnar artery forming the deep volar arch as described above.

■ VASCULAR ANOMALIES

To achieve safe access to the central aorta, the guidewire and catheters must pass through the brachioradialis system and then the axillary, subclavian, and brachiocephalic vessels. Although some tortuosity may impede progress in the latter group of vascular systems, the radial artery itself must be traversed first, and this can be challenging due to a variety of vascular anomalies one may encounter.[1-6,16,22] Valsecchi and colleagues analyzed the effect of vascular abnormalities on procedural success in 2,200 radial access patients. A vascular anatomic variation was identified in 22.4% of the patients, and in these patients, the procedural success rate was reduced from 98% to 93%.[7] A recent report by Lo et al similarly highlighted this concept by assessing the procedural consequences of vascular anomalies in radial access procedures in 1,540 patients.[1] Radial artery puncture was unsuccessful in 7 patients, and the analysis evaluated the effects of vascular anomalies in the remaining 1,533 patients. Vascular anomalies were present in 13.8% of the patients, and these patients exhibited a higher rate of procedural failure (14.2%) versus patients with normal anatomy (0.9%; $p = 0.0001$). In addition to several rarely occurring vascular abnormalities, both studies identified 3 major vascular anomalies as most common including high radial artery takeoff, radial artery loop, and extreme radial artery tortuosity, with the latter 2 accounting for most of the procedural failures. Because these anomalies may create access difficulties, some investigators have advocated the use of preprocedure vessel analysis with ultrasonography.[16] The present discussion describes potential anatomic variations that may be encountered in radial access procedures. It is the present authors' and others' experience that by effectively identifying these vascular challenges and gaining experience circumventing the pitfalls associated with them, the risk of procedural failure can be reduced to a minimal level.

High Radial Artery Takeoff

Although the brachial artery usually bifurcates near the elbow, the most common vascular anomaly involving the radial artery occurs when the bifurcation is present at a higher level, generally in the region of the middle to upper humerus (Figure 3.6). An anatomic study performed in the 1950s in 750 cadavers identified this occurrence in 14.5% of the

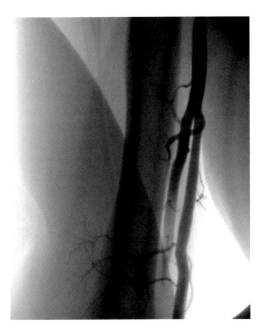

Figure 3.6 High bifurcation of the brachial artery with the radial artery originating in the region of the middle third of the humerus. *Source:* Reprinted, with permission, from Lo TS, Nolan J, Fountzopoulos E, Behan M, Butler R, Hetherton SL, Vijayalakshmi K, Rajagopal R, Fraser D, Zamen A, Hildick-Smith D. Radial artery anomaly and its influence on transradial coronary procedural outcome. *Heart.* 2009;95:410–415.

specimens, 2.1% of which originated directly from the axillary artery itself.[13] Additional reports have emphasized this relatively common occurrence with one anatomic study demonstrating that the proximal origin of the radial artery may result in a fairly superficial anatomic course as it passes toward the elbow.[21,22] In the Lo et al radial access study, the high takeoff occurred in 7% of the patients, and these anomalous vessels were often of small caliber (< 3 mm in diameter). Although procedural failure occurred in only 4.6% of the high bifurcation patients, their smaller caliber did result in a predisposition to vascular spasm and need for smaller French size catheters to complete the procedures. In general, however, as the high bifurcation does not generally create a tortuous, difficult-to-navigate segment, a high success rate for vascular procedures in these patients should be expected when the dimensions of

the vessel are adequate to accept vascular catheters.

Radial Artery Loop

A radial artery loop generally originates just below the bifurcation of the brachial artery in the proximal segment of the radial artery.[1,2,5–7,16,18] The loop may be modest or extreme in angulation and may impede successful guidewire and catheter passage (Figure 3.7). Another pitfall encountered with this vascular anomaly is that the previously described recurrent radial artery branch often originates from the apex of the loop and extends proximally into the upper arm, often with severe diminution in size. Occasionally, 2 recurrent radial arterial branches may originate in this manner from this apical site. The apical location of this branch may be commonly entered with a guidewire after it passes through the distal segments of the loop as the recurrent radial branch offers straight-line access. Previous reports have described a loop incidence ranging from 0.8% to 2.1% with attendant reduction in procedural success. After proper identification, these loops can be carefully and safely crossed with guidewires, particularly the hydrophilic-coated instruments.[6] Our preference in all radial access cases is to start with a 0.035-in hydrophilic guidewire with a soft J-tip (Terumo Medical Corporation, Elkton, Maryland), and this usually can traverse radial loops if necessary. It effectively navigates tortuous brachioradial segments in an atraumatic manner and in our experience is more useful and less traumatic as an initial strategy than a hydrophilic guidewire with an angle tip commonly utilized by many operators (Figure 3.8), but this latter guidewire is an excellent second option when used carefully. In extreme cases, utilization of smaller-diameter (0.014-in) coronary guidewires may be necessary to traverse these segments. Careful guidewire manipulation is essential to avoid dissection and vasospasm, but once they are crossed, the loops often become anatomically straight and allow easy catheter passage (Figure 3.9).

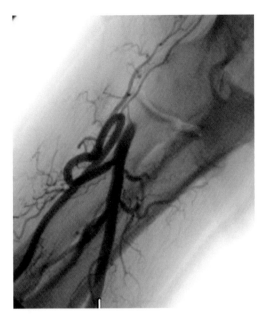

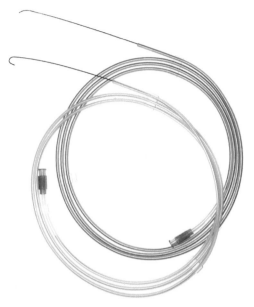

Figure 3.7 Complex radial artery loop with 2 recurrent radial arteries originating from the apex of the loop and extending to the upper arm. *Source:* Reprinted, with permission, from Lo TS, Nolan J, Fountzopoulos E, Behan M, Butler R, Hetherton SL, Vijayalakshmi K, Rajagopal R, Fraser D, Zamen A, Hildick-Smith D. Radial artery anomaly and its influence on transradial coronary procedural outcome. *Heart.* 2009;95:410–415.

Figure 3.8 J-tipped (inferior) and angle-tipped (superior) 0.035-in hydrophilic-coated guidewires (Terumo Medical Corporation, Elkton, Maryland) commonly utilized in radial access procedures.

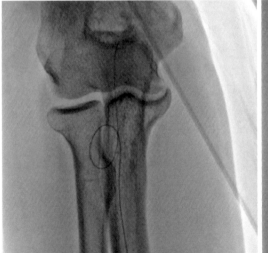

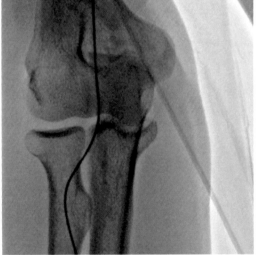

Figure 3.9 Crossing of a radial artery loop with a 0.014-in hydrophilic guidewire (**left panel**). After larger guidewire and catheter exchanged for smaller-diameter guidewire, the loop becomes straightened (**right panel**). *Source:* **Right panel** is reproduced, with permission, from Lo TS, Nolan J, Fountzopoulos E, Behan M, Butler R, Hetherton SL, Vijayalakshmi K, Rajagopal R, Fraser D, Zamen A, Hildick-Smith D. Radial artery anomaly and its influence on transradial coronary procedural outcome. *Heart.* 2009;95:410–415.

Radial Artery Tortuosity

Tortuosity of the radial artery may occur at any location along its course, but most commonly is encountered in the proximal third of the vessel similar to radial loops.[6,7] The reported incidence in the literature is as high as 15.3%[5] with one report describing alpha (α), omega (Ω), Z-, and S-shaped deformities of the radial artery (Figure 3.10). An atraumatic technique similar to the approach utilized with radial loops can be employed to avoid vessel injury and vasospasm while maintaining high procedural success (Figure 3.11). Although one report described prolongation of procedure times with this anomaly, in general the success rates have not been significantly reduced.

Additional Vascular Anomalies

Another less common vascular abnormality is hypoplasia of the radial artery itself. Although rarely described, a report by Yokoyama et al did identify this anomaly in 2 patients (1.7% of their series) prior to the procedure utilizing ultrasonography[16] (Figure 3.12). A femoral approach was used in both cases, and selective angiography confirmed the marked diminution in vessel size that would not have accommodated vascular catheters of sufficient size to perform coronary angiography. Other abnormalities that have been rarely reported include sites of focal stenosis, presence of radial artery atherosclerosis (Figure 3.13), minor abnormalities in bifurcations, and occasional unusual branch vessels. Except for focal stenosis, a finding that can affect procedural success when severe, the other abnormalities are generally not associated with reduction in success rates.

■ VESSEL DIMENSION CONSIDERATIONS

The radial artery has been proven to be a reliable conduit for central vascular procedures, and this has been in part related to its sufficient diameter to accommodate catheter equipment.[2,24] Several studies have evaluated the size of the radial artery in both cadaveric and live subject settings, demonstrating that although the radial artery exhibits fairly large variation in terms of vascular dimensions, in general the radial artery is large enough in most patients to accept catheters of 6-Fr size or less.[8,12,25] In selected patients, particularly larger males, some vessels are able to accept equipment with even larger dimensions.

Pathologic Analysis

In 1996, Shima et al reported findings from a pathologic study of the forearm vessels taken from 52 cadavers.[12] Mean radial artery diameter was 2.3 ± 0.5 mm, and the mean radial artery length was 18.1 ± 1.7 cm. The diameter values are slightly lower than those reported in live subjects utilizing ultrasonography and angiography and may reflect some constriction of the vessels in their anatomic preparation setting.

Dimensional Analysis in Physiologic Setting

Several reports have evaluated the dimensions of the radial artery in living subjects with both ultrasonographic and angiographic techniques. A study by Yoo and associates evaluated radial artery dimensions with this approach in 1,191 radial access patients.[2] Measurements of the radial artery were made 1–2 cm proximal to the styloid process. The mean measured dimension was larger than in the pathologic setting, measuring 2.60 ± 0.4 mm in men and 2.43 ± 0.38 mm in women, with a range of 1.15 to 3.95 mm. The dimensional distribution graph presented in their report is shown in Figure 3.14. In addition, there was good correlation between body surface area and measured radial artery dimension ($r = 0.305$; $p = 0.0001$). The proportion of patients with a measured diameter < 2.3 mm (outer dimension [OD] of a 5-Fr sheath) was 17.3%, < 2.52 mm (OD of 6-Fr sheath) was 31.7%, and < 2.85 mm (OD of 7-Fr sheath) was 74.4%. The patients in the study underwent either coronary angiography with 5-Fr sheaths or coronary interventions with 6-, 7-, or 8-Fr sheaths with 5,000 to 10,000 units of heparin given to all patients in addition to

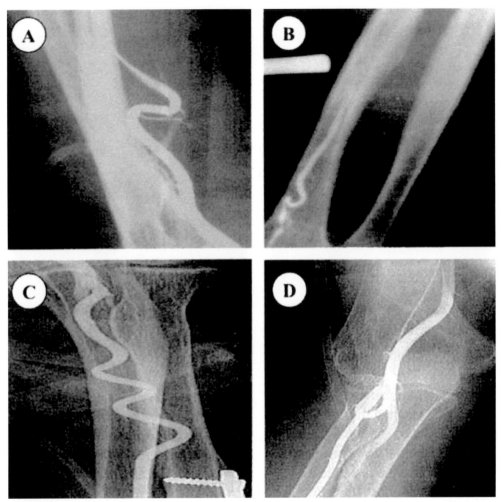

Figure 3.10 Radial artery tortuosity patterns; **Panel A:** α pattern; **Panel B:** Ω pattern; **Panel C:** Z pattern; **Panel D:** S pattern. *Source*: Reproduced, with permission, from Yoo BS, Yoon J, Ko JY, Kim JY, Lee SH, Hwang SO, Choe KH. Anatomic consideration of the radial artery for transradial coronary procedures: arterial diameter, branching anomaly, and vessel tortuosity. *Int J Cardiol*. 2005;101:421–427.

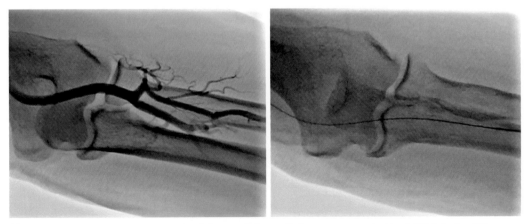

Figure 3.11 Tortuosity in the proximal radial artery (**left panel**) that was traversed with a 0.035-in hydrophilic guidewire with subsequent straightening of the vessel similar to the radial loop.

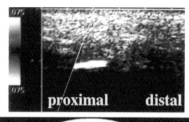

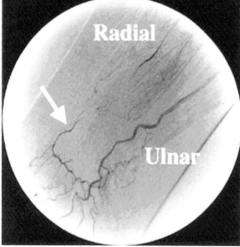

Figure 3.12 Preprocedure Doppler study (**top panel**) demonstrating no radial artery signal in distal vessel with subsequent angiography (**bottom panel**) via the femoral approach confirming radial artery hypoplasia. *Source:* Reproduced, with permission, from Yokoyama N, Takeshita S, Ochiai M, Koyama Y, Hoshino S, Isshiki T, Sato T. Anatomic variations of the radial artery in patients undergoing transradial coronary intervention. *Catheter Cardiovasc Intervent.* 2000;49:357–362.

standard vasodilator agents. It is of note that the smaller-sized vessels did not preclude the use of oversized sheaths. The incidence of postprocedure radial artery occlusion was quite low, 0.8%, and this occurrence bore no relationship to measured radial artery dimension. Although the authors of this report did not tailor their procedures based on dimensional findings, this has been advocated by others utilizing ultrasonographic size analysis.[26] Considering the high success rate of radial artery access procedures with corresponding low occlusion rates, this approach appears unnecessary as a routine. Application does seem reasonable in selected patients, however, particularly in small-framed female patients in whom the use of larger French sheaths is anticipated.

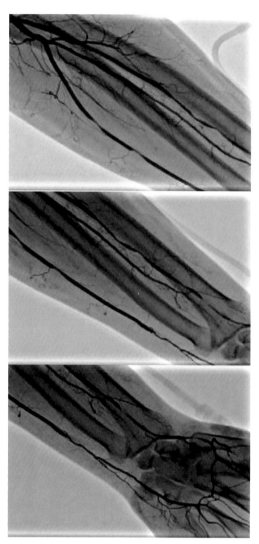

Figure 3.13 Serial views (**top to bottom**) taken from angiography conducted from the femoral approach in a 54-year-old man with history of coronary artery disease and heavy smoking. Allen's test was normal, and the radial artery was entered with a thin-walled needle, but a guidewire could not be advanced. Multiple atherosclerotic obstructions are present in the radial and ulnar arteries.

■ UNDERSTANDING AND ASSESSING THE VASCULAR ANATOMY OF THE HAND

Both the radial and ulnar arteries congruently form the blood supply to the hand, and understanding their relationship to the hand's vascular anatomy is paramount to

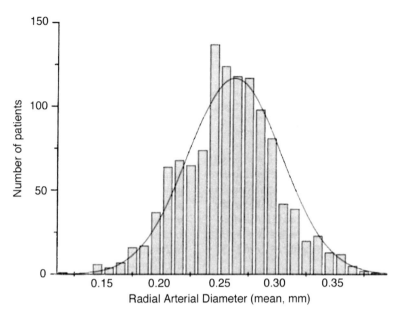

Figure 3.14 Distribution of radial artery diameters measured in 1,191 radial access patients. *Source:* Reproduced, with permission, from Yoo BS, Yoon J, Ko JY, Kim JY, Lee SH, Hwang SO, Choe KH. Anatomic consideration of the radial artery for transradial coronary procedures: arterial diameter, branching anomaly, and vessel tortuosity. *Int J Cardiol.* 2005;101: 421–427.

performing safe and successful radial access procedures. It is generally felt that this dual blood supply offers a high degree of safety in preventing ischemia of the hand in the event of radial artery occlusion. However, there may be anatomic variability in some patients, and assessment of these variances is an important aspect of a successful radial access program. Considering the reported postprocedure occlusion rates ranging from 1.8% to 19%, most experienced operators critically assess the anatomy prior to proceeding with a radial access case.[26–39]

Vascular Anatomy of the Hand

The radial and ulnar arteries enter the wrist in lateral and medial locations, respectively, with branches supplying the carpus and wrist articulations.[11,12,41,42] In rare cases (< 8%), the median artery, a remnant of the embryonic arterial axis of the forearm, is present and generally becomes atretic before it reaches the wrist, running central to the radial and ulnar arteries. In rare situations, it may contribute to the vascular supply to the palm. Several smaller branches originate from both the radial and ulnar arteries as they enter the hand, with one branch from each usually joining to form the superficial volar or palmar

arch. The ongoing continuation of the radial and ulnar arteries later joins in a deeper location to form the larger deep volar or palmar arch (Figure 3.15). Important branches from both the superficial and deep arches supply the hand and the digits. There are significant variations in the relative contributions of the radial and ulnar vessels to these arches. In almost all patients, however, these arches receive some type of dual blood supply from both the radial and ulnar systems, thus ensuring preservation of excellent blood supply to the hand should one of the vessels occlude.

Anatomic Variations of the Palmar Arches

Multiple detailed pathologic studies have carefully evaluated the anatomic variations in the dual blood supply to the hand.[41–45] Although there may be considerable variability in their relative contributions, these studies have demonstrated that in the absence of local atherosclerotic disease, in almost everyone there is some degree of collateral connection between these 2 vascular sources. A large pathologic study reported in 1961 included anatomic vascular evaluation in 650 hands.[41] A complete superficial palmar arch was present in 78.5% of the specimens,

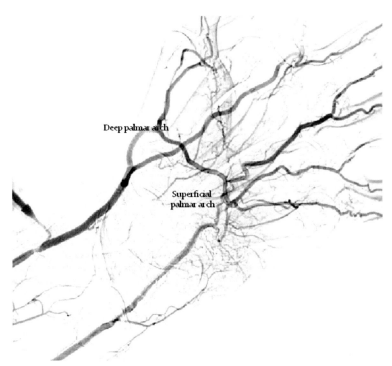

Figure 3.15 Angiogram demonstrating the anatomic course of the terminal portions of the radial and ulnar arteries with resulting formation of the superficial and deep palmar arches in the hand.

including 34.5% that demonstrated the classic complete superficial arch with dual blood supply and 43% in which the ulnar distribution reached the forefinger and thumb. A more recent study analyzing data from 50 hands demonstrated the classic superficial arch only 10% of the time. In contrast, there was a greater reproducibility of data in the analysis of the deep palmar arch with these 2 studies demonstrating the presence of a classic deep palmar arch in 97% and 90% of their specimens, respectively. However, in both studies there was great variability in the relative sizes of both arches.[44] Figure 3.16 displays the anatomic variations that were identified in the study by Ruengsakulrach et al. In addition, these investigators could find no specimen that demonstrated the presence of incomplete superficial and deep palmar arches in the same patients, thus providing reassurance that when an arch is incomplete, the other arch provides collateral support (Figure 3.17). This concept offers some reassurance and confirmation to the reported experience that radial artery access procedures are associated with a very, very low incidence of hand ischemia despite the occasional occurrence of radial artery occlusion. [*Editor's note*: See also chapter on preoperative evaluation.]

Diagnostic Evaluation of the Palmar Arches

Prevention of significant hand ischemia in the setting of radial artery occlusion is paramount. Simple palpation of the ulnar and radial arteries has been felt to be inadequate. A purportedly more accurate method of evaluating the integrity of the palmar arches has been described for more than 80 years.[45,46] The modified Allen's test is commonly utilized in this regard. The Allen's test as it was originally described involved compression of the radial artery and then comparison of the hand color with the opposite hand, a difference in the degree of rubor indicative of inadequate ulnar artery contribution. In the modified test, the ipsilateral fist is clenched, and then the radial and ulnar arteries are compressed simultaneously. Blanching of the palm is observed, and resolution of this blanching in less than 10 seconds after release of ulnar artery compression only is felt to indicate palmar arch integrity.

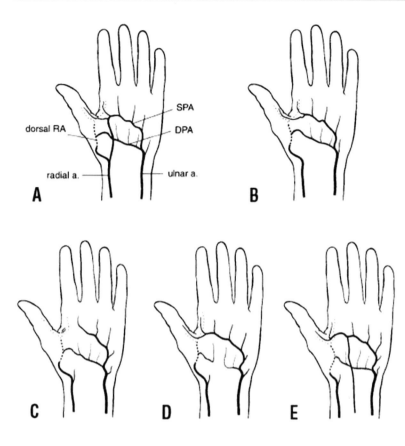

Figure 3.16 Variations of hand circulation, palmar aspect of the left hand (RA: radial artery; SPA: superficial palmar arch; DPA: deep palmar arch). **A** represents the classic or complete arches. In the other variation examples (**B–E**), note that connections are present in each between the superficial and deep arches. *Source:* Reprinted, with permission, from Ruengsakulrach P, Eizenberg N, Fahrer C, Fahrer M, Buxton B. Surgical implications of variations in hand collateral circulation: anatomy revisited. *J Thorac Cardiovasc Surg.* 2001;122:682–686.

Use of the modified Allen's test has been recommended prior to arterial line placement, harvesting of the radial artery for cardiac bypass procedures, and more recently radial access catheterization.[34,47,48] The intent of this approach is to prevent ischemic complications involving the hand, although the incidence of this is quite low, even with indwelling radial artery catheters.[49-51] Although intuitively the preprocedure modified Allen's test makes sense, no conducted study has confirmed its effectiveness in preventing hand ischemia. However, most experienced radial access operators utilize this test routinely prior to each procedure, with an abnormal test resulting in an alternate access approach.

With the advent of radial artery access procedures, utilization of the modified Allen's test has increased significantly. In 1996, a time when the radial approach was gaining acceptance, Nagin et al performed a study, applying the test in 1,000 patients prior to catheterization, and found abnormal findings

(> 10-second cutoff utilized) in 27% of the subjects.[52] As this number may represent an overestimation of the number of abnormal arches, refinements of the modified Allen's test have been made, including the addition of oximetry and plethysmography to further analyze the pattern of ischemia in the hand. In one series, the addition of these techniques demonstrated adequate collateral perfusion in 80% of patients demonstrating an abnormal standard modified Allen's test at baseline.[53] Most commonly, an oximetry module is placed on the thumb. With bilateral compression, a significant change in the pressure waveform and oxygen saturation is observed, with improvement observed upon release of the ulnar artery. It is of note that a delayed phenomenon is occasionally observed with the saturation and waveform returning to baseline 15–30 seconds after release. This probably results from recruitment of the previously described ulnar collaterals and has been felt to represent an acceptable result.

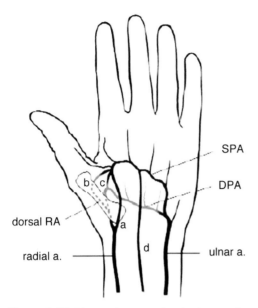

Figure 3.17 Diagram demonstrating the 4 types of communication between the superficial palmar arch of the ulnar artery (UA) and the radial artery (RA) that were observed in the hands studied by Ruengsakulrach et al that manifested connections between the distal superficial palmar arch and the RA (34% of patients evaluated). **a:** through superficial palmar arch of the UA and the RA (10%); **b:** through deep palmar arch (4%); **c:** through digital branch of the dorsal RA (18%); **d:** through the median artery and digital branch of the dorsal RA (2%). *Source:* Reprinted, with permission, from Ruengsakulrach P, Eizenberg N, Fahrer C, Fahrer M, Buxton B. Surgical implications of variations in hand collateral circulation: anatomy revisited. *J Thorac Cardiovasc Surg.* 2001;122:682–686.

The different types of saturation and waveform responses that may be exhibited were described in the study by Barbeau et al.[53]

Controversy Concerning Preprocedural Vascular Assessment

Although the modified Allen's test has been touted as an effective safety measure to avoid ischemic complications with radial access, no study has confirmed its effectiveness, and it is conceivable that reasonable candidates for radial artery access are excluded on the basis of an abnormal test only. However, the general consensus of experienced operators encourages routine utilization of the test to ensure safety. This is not a unanimous viewpoint,

however, and some authors have expressed the opinion that the modified Allen's test is unnecessary, noting the resilient nature of the vascular supply to the hand.[54,55] The pathologic study by Ruengsakulrach et al, described above, offers some anatomic support for this viewpoint.[48] An article by Ghuran et al also supports this approach as it describes the excellent outcomes in a series of radial access patients who received no preprocedure Allen's test screening.[56]

A letter to the editor published in 2011 indicates that based on more recent experience, this viewpoint has remained quite constant.[57] The application of the modified Allen's test issue remains unresolved at present, although conducting the test preprocedure in all patients has very little downside. How abnormal results are applied clinically is a more difficult issue, but in these patients the risks of an alternate site approach should be balanced with the uncertain but probably very low risk (considering the low incidence of radial artery occlusion when appropriate anticoagulation is administered and the resilient nature of the hand's circulation) of proceeding with the radial approach on the ipsilateral side.[2,36]

■ UPPER EXTREMITY COMPARTMENTS: BASIC ANATOMY AND POTENTIAL ROLE IN COMPLICATIONS

The anatomic components of the hand and arm are separated by fascial envelopes into closed spaces or compartments.[11] This collagen-based fascia is relatively inelastic and designed to protect the individual anatomic elements where they reside in the upper arm, forearm, and hand. Although protective, these compartments may promote ischemic injury to the residing tissues when interstitial tissue pressure rises in these closed spaces due to extrinsic compression or tissue edema due to bleeding or inflammation.[10,58,59] Patients undergoing radial access procedures may develop bleeding at the access site or perforations of the brachial or radial arteries and their side branches along the course to the thorax.[60,61] A less common complication associated with these procedures is vessel occlusion with resulting ischemia and inflammation. The incidence of compartment syndrome associated with radial access procedures reported in the literature ranges from 0.4% to a most recently reported value of 0.004%.[10,63] In general, the compartments of the forearm have the greatest potential to be affected by these complications. Understanding the pathoanatomic relationships of the compartments enables the practitioner to recognize and prevent the associated compartment syndromes with their attendant potential to severely compromise upper extremity function. When compartment syndrome develops, neuromuscular function is compromised. There are 3 patterns of clinical findings affecting the arm and the hand depending on which compartment is involved.

Compartment Anatomy

Anatomy. The brachium, or upper arm, comprises 3 anatomic compartments: anterior, posterior, and deltoid. The anterior compartment is bounded by the humerus posteriorly, an intermuscular septum both laterally and medially, and the brachial fascia anteriorly. The deltoid muscle has a thick membrane that can be described as a compartment within a compartment. The deltoid muscle epimysium is not as inelastic as the fascia but is inelastic enough to increase interstitial pressure.[58]

Forearm. The antebrachium, or forearm, is the most common site of compartment syndrome as a result of radial access procedures.[58] The mobile wad, volar compartment, and dorsal compartment make up the 3 general fascial enclosures of the antebrachium. Anatomic interconnections between these compartments exist, and because of these interconnections, a single fasciotomy can oftentimes be performed to decompress the entire forearm.

Hand. The muscular compartments of the hand can be characterized into 5 general groupings including the thenar compartment, hypothenar compartment, adductor compartment, interosseous compartment, and carpal canal.

Compartment Syndrome

In 1881, Volkmann[63] first described the clinical findings of myonecrosis and contracture due to prolonged muscle ischemia. He hypothesized that splints led to diminished arterial inflow, which in turn caused muscle and nerve damage. Jepson,[64] 45 years later, demonstrated that constricting bandages could lead to Volkmann's ischemic contracture, but if the limbs were surgically explored and drained, the animals would avoid permanent muscle damage. Compartment syndrome is a condition that occurs when interstitial tissue pressures rise in an enclosed facial space, preventing adequate tissue oxygenation and ultimately causing cellular necrosis of the compartment contents.

Background. Compartment syndrome results from either intracompartmental swelling or external compression, and both processes can lead to elevated tissue pressures. As interstitial pressure increases, local blood flow decreases. Transmural pressure, the difference between intramural and extraluminal pressure, is the determining factor in local blood flow within a compartment. As elevated intracompartmental pressures rise, local blood flow is diminished due to a decrease in transmural pressure, vessel radius, and arteriovenous gradient. The cells are then subjected to a hypoxic environment, resulting in cell death and subsequent tissue necrosis. Both muscular and neural functions may be severely affected as a result of this cascade of events. Although cooling the affected region may slow this process by reducing the metabolic demands, in general, reversal of severely affected limbs can only be achieved by surgical decompression with a fasciotomy procedure.[58,59,66]

Recognition and Management of Compartment Syndromes. Although the specific hand and arm regions affected are determined by the compartment compromised, in general, compartment syndrome results in both neurologic and muscular symptoms, including the presence of hypothesias and parathesias and localized muscular weakness involving the forearm, wrist, and fingers. When the antebrachium region is involved, there is often localized pain and tenderness in the region of the event, generally out of proportion to the physical findings. Passive motion of the wrist and fingers will often result in painful sensations over the forearm. If vessel occlusion is not present and the syndrome is the result of access site bleeding or perforation, the radial pulse may be intact and full with good capillary refill.

Prompt recognition of access site bleeding and perforations is paramount in the prevention of compartment syndromes. Reversal of anticoagulation and localized compression at bleeding sites can be effective in halting the cascade of events that result in tissue injury and death.[10] An acceptable early treatment includes the technique of inflating a blood pressure cuff to 15 mm Hg below systolic blood pressure for 15-minute intervals.[5] [*Editor's note*: A pressure bag used for blood administration is helpful in this regard when the forearm compartment is involved.] If physical signs of neuromuscular compromise are evident, however, prompt surgical evaluation is mandatory. Percutaneous assessment of local tissue pressures is also useful in determining the degree of compromise.[58,66] Ultimately, however, fasciotomy can be extremely effective in preventing tissue injury and disability when the diagnosis is recognized early in the course of events.

Importance of Prevention and Appropriate Management. Because the diagnosis is difficult with sometimes only obscure physical findings present prior to the onset of tissue compromise, the results of delayed treatment can be poor. A suboptimal outcome may often result in significant disability of the affected limb, and thus it is not surprising that compartment syndrome is one of the most common causes of litigation against physicians in the United States.[67] Therefore, it is essential that practitioners performing radial access procedures are cognizant of preventive measures and understand the

important relationships between the compartments, the anatomic components, and the physiologic events that may become evident when compartment syndrome occurs.

■ SUMMARY

Radial access has emerged as an important advance in vascular medicine and, when applied appropriately, results in improved outcomes and patient satisfaction. To safely, effectively perform this technique, understanding the vascular anatomy of the arm and hand is essential. With this knowledge, one can alertly identify and avoid potential procedural pitfalls that may result from the presence of vascular anomalies, variances in vascular supply and vessel diameter, and encroachments of tissue integrity. This broad understanding will foster excellent success while maintaining complication rates at a minimal level.

■ REFERENCES

1. Lo TS, Nolan J, Fountzopoulos E, Behan M, Butler R, Hetherington SL, Vijayalakshmi K, Rajagopal R, Fraser D, Zamen A, Hildick-Smith D. Radial artery anomaly and its influence on transradial coronary procedural outcome. *Heart*. 2009;95:410–415.
2. Yoo B-S, Yoon J, Ko J-Y, Kim J-Y, Lee S-H, Hwang S-O, Choe K-H. Anatomic consideration of the radial artery for transradial coronary procedures: arterial diameter, branching anomaly, and vessel tortuosity. *Int J Cardiol*. 2005;101:421–427.
3. Yokoyama N, Takeshita S, Ochiai M, Koyama Y, Hoshino S, Isshiki T, Sato T. Anatomic variations of the radial artery in patients undergoing transradial coronary intervention. *Catheter Cardiovasc Intervent*. 2000;49:357–362.
4. Louvard Y, Lefevre T, Morice MC. Radial approach: what about the learning curve? *Catheter Cardiovasc Diagn*. 1997;42:467–468.
5. Bazemore E, Mann JT. Problems and complications of the transradial approach for coronary interventions: a review. *J Invasive Cardiol*. 2005;17:156–159.
6. Barbeau GR. Radial loop and extreme vessel tortuosity in the transradial approach: advantage of hydrophilic-coated guidewires and catheters. *Catheter Cardiovasc Intervent*. 2003;59:442–450.
7. Valsecchi O, Vassileva A, Musumeci G, Rossini R, Tespili M, Guagliumi G, Mihalcsik L, Gavazzi A, Ferrazzi P. Failure of transradial approach during coronary interventions: anatomic considerations. *Catheter Cardiovasc Intervent*. 2006;67:870–878.

8. Saito S, Iker H, Hosokarwa G, Tanaka S. Influence of the ratio between radial artery inner diameter and sheath diameter on radial artery flow after transradial coronary intervention. *Catheter Cardiovasc Interv.* 1999;46:173–178.

9. Wallach S. Cannulation injury of the radial artery: diagnosis and treatment algorithm. *Am J Crit Care.* 2004;13:315–319.

10. Tizon-Marco H, Barbeau GR. Incidence of compartment syndrome of the arm in a large series of transradial approach for coronary procedures. *J Intervent Cardiol.* 2008;21:380–384.

11. Gray H, Lewis W. *Anatomy of the Human Body.* New York: Bartleby.com, 2000;VI,4.b.2.-3.

12. Shima H, Ohno K, Michi K, Egawa K, Takiguchi R. An anatomical study on the forearm vascular system. *J Cran-Maxillofac Surg.* 1996;24:293–299.

13. McCormick TJ, Caudwell EV, Anson BJ. Brachial and antecubital arterial patterns: a study of 750 specimens. *Surg Gynecol Obstet.* 1953;96:44–54.

14. Rodriguez-Niedenfuhr M, Vazquez T, Nearn L, et al. Variations of the arterial pattern in the upper limb revisited: a morphological and statistical study, with a review of the literature. *J Anat.* 2001;199 (Pt 5):547–566.

15. Rodriguez-Niedenfuhr M, Sanudo JR, Vazquez T, et al. Anastomosis at the level of the elbow joint connecting the deep, or normal, brachial artery with major arterial variations of the upper limb. *J Anat.* 2000;196(Pt 1):115–119.

16. Yokoyama N, Takeshita S, Ochiai M, Koyama Y, Hoshino S, Isshiki T, et al. Anatomic variations of the radial artery in patients undergoing transradial coronary intervention. *Catheter Cardiovasc Intervent.* 2000;49:357–362.

17. Drizenco A, Maynou C, Mestdagh H, Mauroy B, Bailleul JP. Variations in the radial artery in man. *Surg Radiol Arch.* 2000;22:299–303.

18. Louvard Y, Lefevre T. Loops and transradial approach in coronary diagnosis and intervention. *Catheter Cardiovasc Interv.* 2000;51:250–252.

19. Fujii T, Masuda N, Tamiya S, Shima M, Toda E, Ito G, Nakazawa T, Matsukage N, Morino N, Tanabe Y, Ikari Y. Angiographic evaluation of right upper-limb arterial anomalies: implications for transradial coronary interventions. *J Inv Cardiol.* 2010:536–540.

20. Chong C, deSouza A. Significance of radial artery anomalies in coronary artery bypass graft surgery. *J Thorac Cardiovasc Surg.* 2008;135:1389–1390.

21. Farman MT, Khan NU, Nadeem S, Rizvi H. Successful transradial percutaneous coronary intervention with radial artery anomaly. *J Pak Med Assoc.* 2010;60:593–595.

22. Keller F, Rosch J, Dotter C, Porter J. Proximal origin of radial artery: potential pitfall in hand angiography. *Am J Roentg.* 1980;134:169–170.

23. Gonzalez-Compta X. Origin of the radial artery from the axillary artery and associated hand vascular anomalies. *J Hand Surg.* [Br] 1991;16A:293–296.

24. Horning B, Arakawa N, Kohler C, Drexler H. Vitamin C improves endothelial function of conduit arteries in patients with chronic heart failure. *Circulation.* 1998;97:363–368.

25. Saito S, Ikei H, Hosokawa G, Tanaka S. Influence of the ratio between radial artery inner diameter and sheath outer diameter on radial artery flow after transradial coronary intervention. *Catheter Cardiovasc Interv.* 1999;46:173–178.

26. Nagai S, Abe S, Sato T, Hozawa K, Yuki K, Hanashima K, Tomoike H. Ultrasonic assessment of vascular complications in coronary angiography and angioplasty after transradial approach. *Am J Cardiol.* 1999;83:180–186.

27. Wu S, Galani R, Bahro A, Moore JA, Burket MW, Cooper CJ. 8 French transradial coronary interventions: clinical outcomes and late effects on the radial artery and hand function. *J Invasive Cardiol.* 2000;12:605–609.

28. Hall J, Arnold A, Valentine R, McCready R, Mick M. Ultrasound imaging of the radial artery following its use for cardiac catheterization. *Am J Cardiol.* 1996;77:108–109.

29. Saito S, Miyake S, Hosokawa G, et al. Transradial coronary intervention in Japanese patients. *Catheter Cardiovasc Interv.* 1999;46:37–41.

30. Stella PR, Kiemeneij F, Laarman GJ, Odekerken D, Slagboom T, vander Wieken R. Incidence and outcome of radial artery occlusion following transradial artery coronary angioplasty. *Catheter Cardiovasc Diagn.* 1997;40:156–158.

31. Nagai S, Abe S, Sato T, et al. Ultrasonic assessment of vascular complications in coronary angiography and angioplasty after transradial approach. *Am J Cardiol.* 1999;83:180–186.

32. Dahm JB, Vogelgesang D, Hummel A, Staudt A, Volzke H, Felix SB. A randomized trial of 5 vs. 6 French transradial percutaneous coronary interventions. *Catheter Cardiovasc Interv.* 2002;57: 172–176.

33. Lee KL, Miller JG, Laitung G. Hand ischaemia following radial artery cannulation. *J Hand Surg.* [Br] 1995;20:493–495.

34. Greenwood MJ, Della-Siega AJ, Fretz EB, Kinloch D, Klinke P, Mildenberger R, Williams MB, Hilton D. Vascular communications of the hand in patients being considered for transradial coronary angiography: is the Allen's test accurate? *J Am Coll Cardiol.* 2005;46:2013–2017.

35. Yoo BS, Lee SH, Ko JY, Kim SN, Lee MO, et al. Procedural outcomes of repeated transradial coronary procedures. *Catheter Cardiovasc Interv.* 2003;58:301–304.

36. Pancholy SB. Comparison of the effect of intra-arterial versus intravenous heparin on radial artery occlusion after transradial catheterization. *Am J Cardiol.* 2009;104:1083–1085.

37. He GW, Yang CQ. Characteristics of adenoreceptors in the human radial artery: clinical implications. *J Thorac Cardiovasc Surg.* 1998;115:1136–1141.

38. Spaulding C, Lefevre T, Funck F, et al. Left radial approach for coronary angiography: results of a prospective study. *Cathet Cardiovasc Diagn.* 1996;39:365–370.

39. Stella PR, Kiemeneij F, Laarman GJ, Odekerken D, Slagboom T, van der Wieken R. Incidence and outcome of radial artery occlusion following transradial artery coronary angioplasty. *Catheter Cardiovasc Diagn.* 1997;40:156–158.

40. Karlsson S, Niechajev IA. Arterial anatomy of the upper extremity. *Acta Radiol Diagn.* 1982;23: 115–121.

41. Coleman SS, Anson BJ. Arterial patterns in the hand based upon study of 650 specimens. *Surg Gynecol Obstet.* 1961;113:409–424.

42. Ikeda A, Ugawa A, Kazihara Y, Hamada N. Arterial patterns in the hand based on a three-dimensional analysis of 220 cadaver hands. *J Hand Surg.* 1988;13:501–509.

43. Mezzogiorno A, Passiatore C, Mezzogiorno V. Anatomic variations of the deep palmar arteries in man. *Acta Anat.* 1994;149:221–224.

44. Ruengsakulrach P, Eizenberg N, Fahrer C, Fahrer M, Buxton B. Surgical implications of variations in hand collateral circulation: anatomy revisited. *J Thorac Cardiovasc Surg.* 2001;122:682–686.

45. Allen E. Thromboangiitis obliterans: methods of diagnosis of chronic occlusive arterial lesions distal to the wrist with illustrative cases. *Am J Med Sci.* 1929;178:237–244.

46. Cable DG, Mullany CJ, Schaff HV. The Allen test. *Ann Thorac Sur.* 1999;67:876–877.

47. Starnes SL, Wolk SW, Lampman RM, Shanley CJ, Prager RL, Kong BK, et al. Noninvasive evaluation of hand circulation before radial artery harvest for coronary artery bypass grafting. *J Thorac Cardiovasc Surg.* 1999;117:261–266.

48. Ruengsakulrach P, Brooks M, Hare DL, Gordon I, Buxton B. Preoperative assessment of hand circulation by means of Doppler ultrasonography and the modified Allen test. *J Thorac Cardiovasc Surg.* 2001;121:526–531.

49. Weiss BM, Gattiker RI. Complications during and following radial artery cannulation: a prospective study. *Intensive Care Med.* 1986;12:424–428.

50. Wilkins RG. Radial artery cannulation and ischaemic damage: a review. *Anaesthesia.* 1985;40: 896–899.

51. Falor WH, Hansel JR, Williams GB. Gangrene of the hand: complication of radial artery cannulation. *J Trauma.* 1976;16:713–716.

52. Benit E, Vranckx P, Jaspers L, Jackmaert R, Poelmans C, Coninx R. Frequency of a positive modified Allen's test in 1,000 consecutive patients undergoing cardiac catheterization. *Cathet Cardiovasc Diag.* 1996;38:352–354.

53. Barbeau GR, Arsenault F, Dugas L, Simard S, Larivere MM. Evaluation of the ulnopalmar arterial arches with pulse oximetry and plethysmography: comparison with the Allen's test in 1010 patients. *Am Heart J.* 2004;147:489–493.

54. Gilchrist IC. Is the Allen's test accurate for patients considered for transradial coronary angiography? *J Am Coll Cardiol.* 2006;48:1247.

55. Saito S. A big challenge to radialists. *Catheter Cardiovasc Interv.* 2010;76:387.

56. Ghuran A, Dixon G, Holmberg S, de Belder A, Hildick-Smith D. Transradial coronary intervention without pre-screening for a dual palmar blood supply. *Int J Cardiol.* 2007;121:320–322.

57. Biondi-Zocccai G, Moretti C, Zuffi A, Agostini P, Romagnoli E, Sangiorgi G. Transradial access without preliminary Allen test: letter of comment on Rhyne et al. *Catheter Cardiovasc Interv.* 2011;78:662–663.

58. Halpern AA, Nagel DA. Compartment syndromes of the forearm: early recognition using pressure measurements. *J Hand Surg Am.* 1978;4:258–263.

59. Gelberman RH, Zakaib GS, et al. Decompression of forearm compartment syndrome. *Clin Ortho.* 1978;134:225–229.

60. Lin YJ, Chu CC, Tsai CW. Acute compartment syndrome after transradial coronary angioplasty. *Int J Cardiol.* 2004;97:311.

61. Wang PJ, Tian X, Zhang Q. Acute compartment syndrome in a patient after transradial access for percutaneous cardiac intervention. *Zhonghua Xin Xue Guan Bing Za Zhi.* 2007;35:496.

62. Caputo R. Avoiding and managing forearm hematomas. *Card Interv Tod.* 2011;5:55–58.

63. Volkmann R. Die ischaemischen muskellahungen und knotrakturn. *Centralbl Chir Leipz.* 1881;8: 801–803.

64. Jepson PN. Ischaemic contracture: experimental study. *Ann Surg.* 1926;84:785–795.

65. Qvist J, Peterfreund RA, Perlmutter GS. Transient compartment syndrome of the forearm after attempted radial artery cannulation. *Anesth Analg.* 1996;83:183–185.

66. Mubarak SJ, Owen CA, et al. Acute compartment syndrome: diagnosis and treatment with the aid of the Wick catheter. *J Bone Joint Surg Am.* 1978;60:1091–1095.

67. Bourne RB, Rorabeck CH. Compartment syndrome of the lower leg. *Clin Ortho.* 1989;240:97–104.

chapter 4

Preoperative Evaluation of the Potential Patient for Transradial Access

Pierre-Louis Nadeau, MD

Jean-Pierre Déry, MD, MSc

Gérald R. Barbeau, MD

Since its first description in 1989 by Campeau et al, percutaneous transradial approach for coronary angiography and interventions has seen a constant and progressive increase in many countries around the world, with the exception of the United States, where it represents less than 5% of coronary procedures.[1,2]

At the Quebec Heart and Lung Institute, the transradial program began in 1994 and since, we have performed more than 75,000 transradial procedures. This chapter will highlight the usual patient evaluation for transradial procedure in our institution.

■ PATIENT SELECTION FOR THE TRANSRADIAL ACCESS

At the Quebec Heart and Lung Institute, the transradial access is the primary approach in all patients referred for coronary angiography and interventions. Preoperative patient evaluation is a fundamental step in order to maximize the rate of successful transradial procedures and prevent potential complications. If the radial approach is seeing an exponential increase in interest, it is partly because there are only few contraindications to its use, as shown in Table 4.1. Specific evaluation before transradial access includes evaluation of hand collateral circulation, previous bypass graft location, previous difficulties during radial or femoral access, and so on. Crossover to the same-side ulnar artery in case of puncture failure or, more frequently, to the contralateral limb in the event of access failure can often be performed. Table 4.2 summarizes right- and left-side advantages. Overall, in our experience, these contraindications represent less than 5% of patients.

Rationale for Evaluation of Hand Collateral Circulation

The most frequent complication associated with the transradial approach is the radial artery occlusion, which occurs in 1% to 12% of cases.[3–12] Higher occlusion rates have been described in patients with blood pressure monitoring in intensive care units, with catheters left in place for prolonged periods in patients without systemic anticoagulation.[13] Rates as low as 1% have been obtained in small series by avoiding intensive postprocedure compression techniques to achieve hemostasis and when using smaller catheters.[3,11,13] Recanalization of the radial artery may also occur in some patients in the first month after the intervention.[5]

Although usually asymptomatic, radial artery occlusion following transradial approach has the potential to induce subsequent hand ischemia. The incidence remains very low because the hand is perfused primarily from both the radial and ulnar arteries through the palmar arterial arches.

This is why careful evaluation of the patency of hand collateral arteries via the ulnopalmar arch is a fundamental step before radial artery cannulation. Serious ischemic damage after prolonged invasive blood pressure monitoring has been estimated to occur in less than 0.1% of cases.[13] The first case of hand ischemia following transradial access for angiography was reported in late 2010.[14] Given the low risk of radial artery occlusion and the extremely low morbidity rate, some authors have advocated that the evaluation of collateral blood supply to the hand was an unnecessary step in the preoperative evaluation.[15] In fact, there is no evidence in the literature of a direct relationship between abnormal hand collateral circulation and subsequent ischemic complication. Some authors have also reported ischemic complications after radial artery occlusion despite normal modified Allen's test results before radial artery cannulation, but this could be explained in part by embolization from prolonged blood pressure monitoring. Approximately 80% of cardiologists worldwide proceed with the evaluation, however, agreeing that patients with an incomplete palmar arch might be at a higher risk of hand ischemia in the event of radial artery occlusion.[23] This might also be influenced by the medical-legal environment. Exceptionally, the transradial approach may be attempted in a patient with incomplete hand collateralization when the risk from a femoral approach is excessive. In these patients, consideration should be given to lower the incidence of radial artery occlusion. See Table 4.3.

Table 4.1 Absolute and Relative Contraindications to the Transradial Access.

Absolute contraindications	Relative contraindications
1. Inefficient hand collateral arterial supply[†]	1. Intended use of the radial artery for arteriovenous fistula or coronary artery bypass grafting
2. Long occlusion of radial artery	2. Contraindication to the use of heparin or other anticoagulation[†††]
3. Arteriovenous fistulas for hemodialysis	3. Patient preference (eg, profession requiring fine manual dexterity)
4. Upper extremity lymphedema	4. Previous failure in transradial approach
5. Intra-aortic balloon pump insertion[††]	

† Tested by modified Allen's test, oximetry, plethysmography, or Doppler ultrasonography.
†† However, in these patients, the radial approach may be used for the coronarography and intervention.
††† Radial approach requires the use of heparin or other anticoagulant to prevent radial artery thrombosis.

Table 4.2 Choice of Right- or Left-Side Approach.

Favors right-side transradial approach	Favors left-side transradial approach
a. Puncture easier for operator	a. Advantages for right-handed patient
b. Use of selected catheters (multipurpose, Barbeau's curve, XB, etc)	b. Use of selected catheters (Judkin's curves, LIMA, etc)
c. In very obese patient	c. In selected patients (long history of hypertension, the very old, etc)
d. In patient with bilateral internal mammary artery (IMA) grafts	d. In patient with only LIMA graft, postpneumonectomy
e. In patient with left-side anatomical anomaly or contraindication	e. Patient with *arteria lusoria* anomaly, known right-side vascular anomaly (arterial loop, etc)
f. In patients with planned harvest of radial artery for graft	f. In patient with right-side contraindications
g. Less x-ray exposure to the operator	g. With right-side transradial approach for contralateral coronary angiography in chronic total occlusion (CTO)

Methods for the Evaluation of Hand Collateral Circulation

A variety of methods have been described for assessing the presence of a functional palmar arterial arch before a transradial heart catheterization. The modified Allen's test and the pulse oximetry and plethysmography (OX and PL) are the first choices given their low cost and high feasibility. The duplex Doppler ultrasonography may also be performed if available. Although numerous other tests have been suggested, including measurement of the thumb pressure and magnetic resonance angiography, they appear less practical and will not be discussed.

Modified Allen's Test. In 1929, Allen was the first to describe a simple bedside test to assess the patency of the ulnopalmar arches in patients with thromboangiitis

Table 4.3 Steps to Decrease the Likelihood of Radial Thrombosis.

a. Proximal artery puncture (larger size)
b. Anticoagulation (> 70 U/kg of unfractionated heparin)
c. Prevention of arterial spasm with a calcium channel blocker
d. Use of smaller catheter
e. Avoiding prolonged and intensive hemostatic pressure

obliterans.[16] The test was modified by Wright in 1952 to evaluate the patency of collateral circulation through the ulnar artery. The modified Allen's test consists of the following steps, as summarized in Figure 4.1. The modified Allen's test is abnormal or negative if palmar blanching persists for ≥ 10 seconds and must be considered as a contraindication for the transradial procedure. The modified Allen's test results can be altered by multiple factors, including overextension of the wrist, contralateral ulnar compression by skin stretching, an examiner error, or inadequate patient cooperation. Subjective interpretation of the change in hand color also limits the diagnostic usefulness of the test. As a result, an appreciable number of false-positive and false-negative results have been reported. This is reflected by the highly variable reported incidence for an abnormal Allen's test in the available literature (1% to 27%).[17,18] However, if the modified Allen's test is abnormal in one hand, it may be normal in the other hand, thus reducing the number of patients with a negative modified Allen's test in both arms to less than 10%.

The inverse modified Allen's test can also be performed to assess the patency of the radial artery. In contrast, occlusion of the ulnar artery is maintained while pressure on the radial artery is released. The criteria for a normal or positive test are the same. The test is helpful to exclude a radial artery occlusion

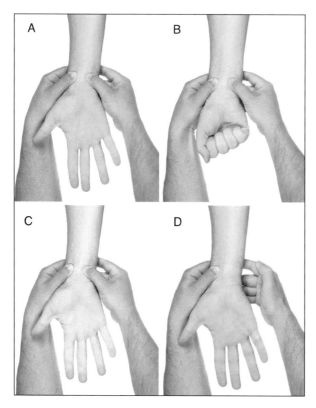

Figure 4.1 Modified Allen's test.

Panel A With the patient in a supine position in a well-lighted room, the examiner feels both the ulnar and the radial pulses.

Panel B The patient repeatedly clenches the hand to expel blood from the hand, causing the hand to blench, and the examiner vigorously compresses both the ulnar and the radial arteries.

Panel C The patient opens the hand, avoiding hyperextension of the wrist and fingers.

Panel D The examiner releases the pressure from the ulnar artery. The test is considered normal if blushing of the palm reappears within 10 seconds, indicating a patent ulnopalmar arch. (The same step can be used to evaluate the radiopalmar arch when the examiner releases the pressure from the radial artery only.)

in a patient who has already had a cannulation or in whom an ulnar approach is considered. It is also helpful for assessment of postprocedure radial artery occlusion.

The relationship between an abnormal modified Allen's test and subsequent ischemic symptoms of the hand was indirectly demonstrated in a study dosing capillary lactate in the thumb after radial artery occlusion. The patients with abnormal modified Allen's test results had a significantly higher level of lactate.[19] The literature also suggests that a normal modified Allen's test safely selects patients for radial artery harvest to serve as a conduit in coronary artery bypass graft. Indeed, most investigators evaluating hand perfusion days or months after surgery using various methods have reported no significant decline in hand perfusion relative to the nonoperated hand.[20] Based on these findings, radial artery catheterization is usually not performed in patients with an abnormal modified Allen's test. However, the clinician must weigh the benefits and risks in a patient for whom the femoral approach should be avoided.

Plethysmography and Pulse Oximetry. As an alternative to the modified Allen's test, the use of plethysmography and pulse oximetry (PL and OX) has been proposed for a more direct assessment of collateral circulation before cannulation of the radial artery.[17] This technique is also more objective, and can thus improve diagnostic accuracy. The equipment required is available in most catheterization laboratories.

The sensor of the pulse oximeter is applied to the fingernail of the patient's thumb. While recording the pulse tracing and oxygen saturation data, the radial artery is compressed for as long as 2 minutes. The 4 different responses of flow wave on monitor are described in Figure 4.2.

During radial artery compression, OX results (SpO2) are either positive (reading present and constant) or negative. The occlusion of the radial artery is occasionally seen with a Type A pattern; in such a case, radial artery compression does not reduce pulsatile blood flow to the thumb. Radial artery occlusion can then be suspected when ulnar artery

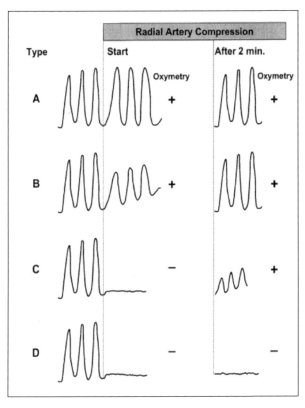

Figure 4.2 Drawing representing the 4 types of ulnopalmar arch patency findings with plethysmography and pulse oximetry.

Panel A No change in the amplitude of the pulse tracing immediately after radial artery compression.

Panel B Reduction in amplitude with compression.

Panel C Loss of pulse tracing and oximetry with initial compression, followed by recovery within 2 minutes (suggesting collateral recruitment induced by relative hand ischemia).

Panel D Loss of pulse tracing and oximetry with no recovery within 2 minutes.

Source: Reproduced with permission from *Am Heart J*. Mar 2004;147(3):489–493.

compression produces a Type D reading. In Type C, pulsatile blood flow, as well as OX, is abolished temporarily by radial artery compression but reappears within 2 minutes, suggesting collateral recruitment induced by relative hand ischemia. This phenomenon cannot be easily evaluated with the modified Allen's test.

Because pulsatile blood flow has been correlated with wound healing and the absence of ischemic necrosis, the Type D pattern is considered to be inadequate for the transradial approach.[21] Patients in the first 3 categories (A, B, and C) are considered to have a patent ulnopalmar arch and can safely be selected for the transradial procedure.[22] The primary advantage of this technique over the modified Allen's test is the improved sensitivity, which decreases rejection rates of potential candidates for a transradial approach.[17] Moreover, excellent correlation was found between the assessment of collateral circulation obtained by OX and the Doppler ultrasound.[23] In the paper by Barbeau et al, the PL and OX Type A, B, or C pattern

was seen in 96%, 95%, 92.3%, and 98.5% of patients on the right side, left side, both sides, or any side, respectively, with only 1.5% of patients (2.0% in men and 0.3% in women; $P < .05$) excluded from either the right or left transradial approach. Multivariate analysis, including the same variables as with the modified Allen's test, also showed increasing age and male sex to be predictors of failure to achieve PL and OX Type A, B, or C.[17]

At the Quebec Heart and Lung Institute, the transradial approach being the primary entry site, all patients are evaluated by the nurse personnel with OX and PL on both arms to evaluate both patency and collaterals of the ulnoradial system. The information is then written in the patient's cath lab report. It is then easier to proceed immediately to the contralateral limb, without extra testing, in case of access failure on one side.

Doppler Ultrasonography. The Doppler ultrasonography is an alternative to the modified Allen's test or PL and OX to assess the collateral circulation of the hand. Various techniques have been described, and the definition for abnormal hand collateral circulation is not standardized.[24] Echographic assessment of palmar circulation provides more accurate information than the modified Allen's test, and like PL and OX, it does not require patient cooperation.[25] It has been used to predict safe radial artery harvest in the majority of patients with an abnormal Allen's test.[26]

In addition to the assessment of collateral circulation, Doppler ultrasonography allows a comprehensive evaluation of the anatomy of the hand, for example:

1. Direct arterial visualization in patients with hypotension, edema, and obesity, in whom palpation of radial artery can be difficult.

2. Detection of anatomical abnormalities (eg, thrombosis, stenosis, hypoplasia, tortuosity, anomalous branching, and radial-ulnar artery loop).

3. Measurement of diameter of the radial and ulnar arteries.

Using echography to measure the radial artery diameter and to detect anatomical abnormalities may help the cardiologist to select suitable patients and interventional devices. Indeed, a radial artery diameter of less than 2 mm and anatomical abnormalities have both been associated with longer procedure time, more puncture failures, and a higher rate of thrombosis.[27] However, complete echographic evaluation is more expensive and more time-consuming than the modified Allen's test or PL and OX. Figure 4.3 shows an example of echographic evaluation of radial and ulnar arteries in a normal subject. [*Editor's note*: Doppler of the palmar arches can also be evaluated and is not subjective as well. The deep or superficial palmar arch is located by the Doppler signal. If the signal persists

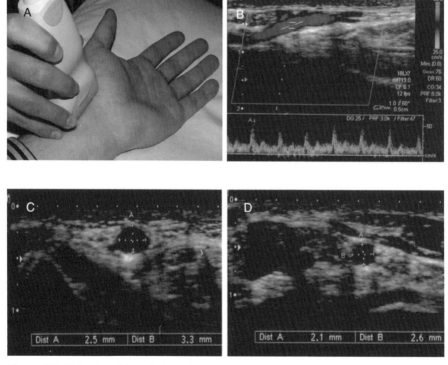

Figure 4.3 Evaluation of the radial and ulnar arteries with Doppler ultrasonography.

Panel A: The Doppler probe is placed over the radial artery.

Panel B: Longitudinal view of a normal radial artery.

Panel C: Axial view of the radial artery. The diameter of the artery is 3.3 × 2.5 mm.

Panel D: Axial view of the ulnar artery. The diameter of the artery is 2.6 × 2.1 mm.

despite the manual occlusion of the radial artery, this confirms an intact palmar arch with ulnar collaterals.]

■ SUMMARY

There are few issues to be addressed before performing a transradial procedure. We believe that careful evaluation of the patency of hand collateral arteries via the ulnopalmar arch is a fundamental step before radial artery cannulation. We described in 1994 a new method using combined PL and OX for the evaluation of the hand collateral circulation. This technique has the advantage of being fast, simple, and objective while avoiding many of the pitfalls of the modified Allen's test. Although the modified Allen's test could identify a large proportion of patients suitable for transradial approach in our series, PL and OX had a higher sensitivity. Using this method during the last 15 years, including Type A, B, and C patterns, we have seen no ischemic hand complications in case of radial artery occlusion after a transradial procedure.

■ REFERENCES

1. Campeau L. Percutaneous radial artery approach for coronary angiography. *Cathet Cardiovasc Diagn.* Jan 1989;16(1):3–7.
2. Rao SV, Ou FS, Wang TY, et al. Trends in the prevalence and outcomes of radial and femoral approaches to percutaneous coronary intervention: a report from the National Cardiovascular Data Registry. *JACC Cardiovasc Interv.* Aug 2008;1(4):379–386.
3. Pancholy S, Coppola J, Patel T, Roke-Thomas M. Prevention of radial artery occlusion-patent hemostasis evaluation trial (PROPHET study): a randomized comparison of traditional versus patency documented hemostasis after transradial catheterization. *Catheter Cardiovasc Interv.* Sep 1 2008;72(3):335–340.
4. Sanmartin M, Gomez M, Rumoroso JR, et al. Interruption of blood flow during compression and radial artery occlusion after transradial catheterization. *Catheter Cardiovasc Interv.* Aug 1 2007;70(2):185–189.
5. Zankl AR, Andrassy M, Volz C, et al. Radial artery thrombosis following transradial coronary angiography: incidence and rationale for treatment of symptomatic patients with low-molecular-weight heparins. *Clin Res Cardiol.* Dec 2010;99(12):841–847.
6. Stella PR, Kiemeneij F, Laarman GJ, Odekerken D, Slagboom T, van der Wieken R. Incidence and outcome of radial artery occlusion following transradial artery coronary angioplasty. *Cathet Cardiovasc Diagn.* Feb 1997;40(2):156–158.
7. Kiemeneij F, Laarman GJ. Percutaneous transradial artery approach for coronary stent implantation. *Cathet Cardiovasc Diagn.* Oct 1993;30(2):173–178.
8. Mann T, Cubeddu G, Bowen J, et al. Stenting in acute coronary syndromes: a comparison of radial versus femoral access sites. *J Am Coll Cardiol.* Sep 1998;32(3):572–576.
9. Wu SS, Galani RJ, Bahro A, Moore JA, Burket MW, Cooper CJ. 8 French transradial coronary interventions: clinical outcome and late effects on the radial artery and hand function. *J Invasive Cardiol.* Dec 2000;12(12):605–609.
10. Nagai S, Abe S, Sato T, et al. Ultrasonic assessment of vascular complications in coronary angiography and angioplasty after transradial approach. *Am J Cardiol.* Jan 15 1999;83(2):180–186.
11. Dahm JB, Vogelgesang D, Hummel A, Staudt A, Volzke H, Felix SB. A randomized trial of 5 vs. 6 French transradial percutaneous coronary interventions. *Catheter Cardiovasc Interv.* Oct 2002;57(2):172–176.
12. Cubero JM, Lombardo J, Pedrosa C, et al. Radial compression guided by mean artery pressure versus standard compression with a pneumatic device (RACOMAP). *Catheter Cardiovasc Interv.* Mar 1 2009;73(4):467–472.
13. Scheer B, Perel A, Pfeiffer UJ. Clinical review: complications and risk factors of peripheral arterial catheters used for haemodynamic monitoring in anaesthesia and intensive care medicine. *Crit Care.* Jun 2002;6(3):199–204.
14. Rhyne D, Mann T. Hand ischemia resulting from a transradial intervention: successful management with radial artery angioplasty. *Catheter Cardiovasc Interv.* Sep 1 2010;76(3):383–386.
15. Ghuran AV, Dixon G, Holmberg S, de Belder A, Hildick-Smith D. Transradial coronary intervention without pre-screening for a dual palmar blood supply. *Int J Cardiol.* Oct 18 2007;121(3):320–322.
16. Allen EV. Thromboangiitis obliterans: methods of diagnosis of chronic occlusive arterial lesions distal to the wrist with illustrative cases. *Am J Med Sci.* 1929;178:237–244.
17. Barbeau GR, Arsenault F, Dugas L, Simard S, Lariviere MM. Evaluation of the ulnopalmar arterial arches with pulse oximetry and plethysmography: comparison with the Allen's test in 1010 patients. *Am Heart J.* Mar 2004;147(3):489–493.
18. Benit E, Vranckx P, Jaspers L, Jackmaert R, Poelmans C, Coninx R. Frequency of a positive modified Allen's test in 1,000 consecutive patients undergoing cardiac catheterization. *Cathet Cardiovasc Diagn.* Aug 1996;38(4):352–354.
19. Greenwood MJ, Della-Siega AJ, Fretz EB, et al. Vascular communications of the hand in patients being considered for transradial coronary angiogra-

phy: is the Allen's test accurate? *J Am Coll Cardiol.* Dec 6 2005;46(11):2013–2017.

20. Slogoff S, Keats AS, Arlund C. On the safety of radial artery cannulation. *Anesthesiology.* Jul 1983;59(1):42–47.

21. Gibbons GW, Wheelock FC Jr, Hoar CS Jr, Rowbotham JL, Siembieda C. Predicting success of forefoot amputations in diabetics by noninvasive testing. *Arch Surg.* Sep 1979;114(9):1034–1036.

22. Barbeau GR, Gleeton O, Roy L. Transradial approach for coronary interventions: procedural results and vascular complications of a series of 7049 procedures [abstract]. *Circulation.* 1999; 100:1–306.

23. Pillow K, Herrick IA. Pulse oximetry compared with Doppler ultrasound for assessment of collateral blood flow to the hand. *Anaesthesia.* May 1991;46(5):388–390.

24. Agrifoglio M, Dainese L, Pasotti S, et al. Preoperative assessment of the radial artery for coronary artery bypass grafting: is the clinical Allen test adequate? *Ann Thorac Surg.* Feb 2005;79(2):570–572.

25. Yokoyama N, Takeshita S, Ochiai M, et al. Direct assessment of palmar circulation before transradial coronary intervention by color Doppler ultrasonography. *Am J Cardiol.* Jul 15 2000;86(2):218–221.

26. Abu-Omar Y, Mussa S, Anastasiadis K, Steel S, Hands L, Taggart DP. Duplex ultrasonography predicts safety of radial artery harvest in the presence of an abnormal Allen test. *Ann Thorac Surg.* Jan 2004;77(1):116–119.

27. Yan ZX, Zhou YJ, Zhao YX, Zhou ZM, Yang SW, Wang ZJ. Anatomical study of forearm arteries with ultrasound for percutaneous coronary procedures. *Circ J.* Apr 2010;74(4):686–692.

chapter 5

Obtaining Access

Howard A. Cohen, MD

Just as with femoral access, there is no single correct way to obtain radial access. Every operator develops a technique that he or she finds to be efficient and safe. Nonetheless, over the past 2 decades, the transradial technique has evolved and continues to evolve, and there are several principles that apply to all operators. In this chapter, we will discuss (1) preparation and positioning of the patient, (2) accessing the artery, (3) preventing spasm and hypotension, and (4) accessing the central aorta from the right as well as the left radial artery. Accessing the coronary arteries for diagnostic angiography as well as for intervention will be discussed in a separate chapter (see Chapter 7).

■ PREPARATION AND POSITIONING OF THE PATIENT

Radial access may be obtained from either the right or the left radial artery, assuming that both are acceptable in terms of the Allen's test. Although the Allen's test has been abandoned in many European centers, for medical-legal reasons, it is still widely accepted and utilized in the United States. For some operators, the left radial is preferable because the catheter manipulation is similar to femoral access. Others prefer right radial access because most catheterization laboratories are conventionally set up for access from the right side of the patient. In either case, the arm may

Transradial Access: Techniques for Diagnostic Angiography and Percutaneous Intervention
©2013 Howard A. Cohen (Editor). Cardiotext Publishing, ISBN 978-1-935395-41-6.

be abducted approximately 60–90 degrees and placed on an inexpensively constructed plywood or metal board (Figure 5.1) that is draped in the usual sterile fashion. After prepping the arm from the hand to the elbow, we place the entire arm in a sterile stockingette (Figure 5.2), which helps to maintain sterility. This step is by no means mandatory, and many operators just place an aperture drape over the operative area once it has been prepped. The arm is then extended with the hand supinated and the wrist hyperextended on a rolled sterile towel (Figure 5.2). If the stockingette is used, the operative area is exposed by cutting an opening over the radial artery. Once access is achieved and the sheath inserted, an aperture drape is placed, and the sheath is secured with a Tegaderm® adhesive or a suture. After the sheath is inserted and secured, the arm can be returned to the side so that the ergonomics are no different from those for transfemoral access as the wrist at the patient's side is at the same level as the femoral artery.

I find it useful to employ an ambidextrous technique (see Figure 5.4) for access, as the artery may be felt much better by the operator's left hand standing laterally to the patient or by the right hand when the operator is standing between the patient's arm and chest, depending on the anatomy and the position of the radial artery relative to the radius (see Figures 5.4a and 5.4b). There are 2 standard ways of accessing the artery—one using the micropuncture technique and the second using the Seldinger technique with angiocath (catheter over the needle). With either technique, the artery may be best accessed proximal to the wrist crease. This is usually approximately 2 to 3 finger-breadths proximal to the tip of the styloid process of the radius. The radial artery is larger and straighter in this area than it is as it courses more distally and superficially (see Chapter 3). Even though it may be easier to feel the artery more distally because it is superficial, it is usually more difficult to access because of the smaller size and tortuosity of the vessel in this area. Furthermore, because the vessel is smaller distally, it is more prone to closure as a result of the access. Ninety percent of the time, I stand lateral to the patient and

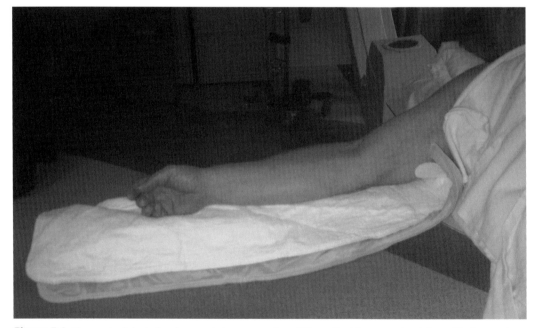

Figure 5.1 The arm is abducted and supported on an arm board. The patient is prepped and draped in the usual fashion. The arm is then prepped from the hand to the elbow and placed in a sterile stockingette. A sterile drape is then placed on the arm board and the arm supported. (See Figures 5.2 and 5.3.) Once access is achieved, the arm is adducted and placed back in a sterilely draped arm holder next to the body. The arm board is then removed except in the situation of a very obese patient, when the arm board can be rotated and placed under the body to help support the arm.

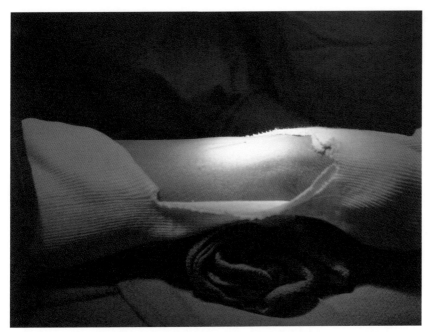

Figure 5.2
Preparation of the patient. To help maintain sterility and still be able to visualize as well as feel the bony landmarks, the arm is placed in a sterile stockingette. The arm is supinated and the wrist hyperextended on 2 rolled sterile towels.

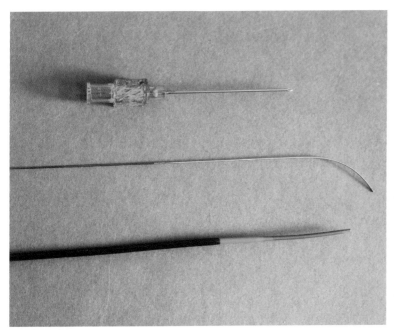

Figure 5.3 Micropuncture needle (21 gauge), nitinol wire, and micropuncture sheath. Note that this hydrophilic sheath is coated with silocone and should be wiped with a wet sponge prior to insertion. If this is not done, the excess silocone on the sheath may be deposited in the subcutaneous tissue and result in a sterile abscess 1–2 weeks following the procedure. This is easily avoided by wiping the sheath with a wet sponge. This occurs only with the Cook sheath but does not occur with other micropuncture sheaths. Note also the 2-stage taper of the dilator that allows for smooth transition into the radial artery.

feel the pulse with the left hand lining up the artery beneath the tips of my first and second fingers (see radial artery access video—❿ Video 5.1). The skin is anesthetized with 1 cc of 1.0% lidocaine given subcutaneously through a 25-gauge needle. More than this amount is definitely not necessary and only makes it more difficult to feel the pulse for

access. In addition, I give 100 µg of nitroglycerine that helps to dilate the artery locally. The needle is then withdrawn, and subcutaneous nitroglycerine and lidocaine are massaged into the tissues.

Now you are ready for access. Using the micropuncture technique (see Figure 5.3 and radial artery access video—Video 5.1), the

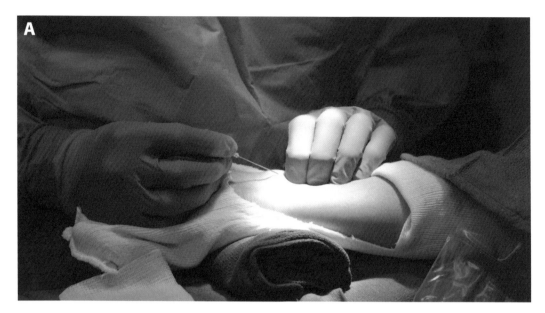

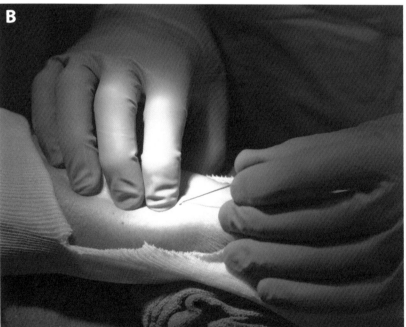

Figure 5.4 Ambidextrous technique. Depending on the location of the artery and the surrounding tissues, the artery may be better palpated by the left hand while standing lateral to the patient or by the right hand while standing between the patient's body and the extended arm. I have found it advantageous, therefore, to be able to access with either hand depending on how easy it is to palpate the artery. (**A**) Standing laterally to the patient with right arm extended on an arm board. The artery is palpated by the fingertips of the left hand, and the micropuncture needle is advanced with the right hand. Notice the shallow angle of approach. (**B**) Standing between the patient and the right arm extended on an arm board, the artery is palpated by the fingertips of the right hand, and the needle is advanced with the left hand. Again, notice the shallow angle of approach.

radial artery is stabilized by the first and second fingers of the left hand. The micro-puncture needle is inserted at a shallow angle, bevel up, toward the pulse; then the needle is released by the right hand, and the "bounce" of the needle is assessed. The shallow angle is important because the vessel is small, and the shallow angle allows for more room to enter the artery with an anterior wall puncture only without engaging the posterior wall. The operator should attempt to access the artery directly above the vessel and not from the side. If the approach is correct, the needle will bounce up and down and not sideways. If the needle is bouncing from side to side or not bouncing at all, the needle can be withdrawn and readvanced until the appropriate bounce is obtained. I attempt to do only an anterior wall puncture, and the needle is advanced only 1–2 mm at a time and then released to follow the bounce (see radial artery access video—Video 5.1). If the bounce increases, it lets you know that you are getting closer to the artery, and if the bounce decreases, it lets you know that you have passed the artery or are going in the wrong direction. You can usually feel when the tip of the needle engages the anterior wall of the artery. Then advancing ever-so-slowly and with gentle pressure, the artery is entered. This process takes only about 15–20 seconds but allows for confidence in your approach. It is not uncommon that the artery is not well felt but very well seen by the bounce, and you are assured that you are going in the right direction. This technique is a "poor man's Doppler" for locating the artery. At times, the patient (usually an obese patient) will have a normal Doppler signal but a pulse that is very difficult to feel. In this setting, the pulse can be identified with a Doppler and marked with an indelible pen. This then allows for reliable transradial access despite the inability to feel the pulse. When the needle is inserted over the pulse marked by the Doppler, you will be able to see the needle bounce without actually feeling the artery. This technique allows for arterial access despite the inability to feel a good pulse. Alternatively, ultrasound can be used to visualize the artery in an effort to obtain access.

Visualization with ultrasound may be helpful to the novice, but for the experienced operator it is rarely necessary. Once there is free flow of arterial blood, an 0.018 slightly angled-tip nitinol guidewire is advanced into the artery. This should go absolutely smoothly and without resistance or any pain felt by the patient. On occasion, it may be necessary to torque the guidewire until it advances easily and fully into the artery (see radial artery access video—Video 5.1). Depending on the sheath type used, a small incision may be necessary with a #11 blade either before or after the needle is withdrawn. The operator should be careful to keep the blade "flat to the skin" with a side-to-side incision to avoid penetrating the artery. The sheath can then be placed safely over the guidewire.

If there is pain, with the initial insertion of the wire it is undoubtedly subintimal, and the wire and needle should be withdrawn and the process started over again. Advancement of the guidewire should be completely painless. If there is resistance once the artery has been entered without difficulty, the wire tip is probably in a small side branch (see radial artery access video—Video 5.1). The wire can be withdrawn slightly and rotated to avoid the side branch. If the wire cannot be fully inserted, it is wise in this circumstance to advance a short 4-Fr micropuncture catheter and perform an angiogram (digital subtraction with road map if possible) through this catheter. This will allow for visualization of the artery with safe navigation with a 0.035 hydrophilic, steerable, angled-tip wire, mirco J-tipped wire or 0.014 coronary guidewire.

The artery may also be entered via the Seldinger technique. Again, the artery is stabilized with the first and second finger of the left hand, and the catheter over the needle assembly is advanced at a shallow angle with the right hand with the bevel up. The assembly will pass through the anterior and posterior wall of the artery at a shallow angle. The needle is then withdrawn, and the catheter is retracted slowly until there is a free, pulsatile flow of blood. A 0.25 hydrophilic guidewire is then inserted in the same fashion as noted above with the micropuncture technique, and the dilator and sheath can then be inserted in the standard fashion. Some hydrophilic sheaths are coated with a thin film of silicone. If the silicone comes off the catheter when it is removed, it can cause a sterile abscess. In an effort to avoid this, wiping the sheath with a wet sponge will remove the excess silicone and avoid the problem of a sterile abscess. A hydrophilic sheath is very useful because it is easy to remove even if there is some degree of spasm. Because it is slippery, it must be well secured when it is inserted with either a sterile adhesive or a suture; otherwise, it may inadvertently come out during catheter exchanges.

■ PREVENTING SPASM AND HYPOTENSION

The radial artery is very susceptible to spasm. Once spasm occurs, it may be difficult to reverse. It is, therefore, imperative to treat the patient with medication to prevent spasm because it is much easier to prevent spasm than it is to reverse it. To begin with, it is helpful to adequately sedate the patient, as anxiety and certainly pain will make spasm more likely to occur. Accordingly, treating the patient expectantly with sedation is helpful. You must be careful not to make the patient hypotensive because the radial artery will be more difficult to palpate in this circumstance. In addition, a spasmolytic cocktail may be given through the sheath once access is obtained in an effort to prevent spasm. Every operator has his or her favorite combination of intra-arterial drugs that usually contains 100 µg of nitroglycerine plus a calcium channel blocker (verapamil, diltiazem, or nicardipine). In addition, we slowly give 90–100 µg of intra-arterial lidocaine, diluting it constantly with blood as it gives the patient a sensation of extreme heat locally. This is well tolerated as long as the patient is averted to the sensation and the drug is diluted as it is administered. The purpose of the intra-arterial lidocaine is to anesthetize the artery, which it does very successfully. Once the artery is anesthetized with intra-arterial lidocaine, intra-arterial heparin may be administered without any sensation by the patient. Alternatively, the heparin may be given intravenously, typically 2,500–5,000 units

depending on the size of the patient. The use of heparin has been shown to decrease radial artery occlusion postprocedure (see Chapter 6 on patent hemostasis).

Finally, it should be noted that the use of intra-arterial nitroglycerine and a calcium channel blocker may predispose the patient to hypotension, particularly if the patient is volume depleted as may occur with patients who have been fasting and who are treated late in the day. This hypotension is easily treated with volume administration. If there is evidence of a vasovagal reaction, this is treated in the standard fashion with volume and intravenous atropine.

■ ACCESSING THE CENTRAL AORTA FROM THE RIGHT RADIAL

Several different types of guidewire may be used for accessing the central aorta. We generally use a 0.035 small, J-tipped Glidewire®. The wire generally passes easily into the brachial artery with the J-tip avoiding small side branches. If an angled Glidewire is used, it is important to fluoroscopically visualize the wire traversing the forearm and the upper arm, as well as the subclavian artery, in an effort to avoid small side-branch access and resultant perforation that can occur easily. If there is any resistance in advancing a guidewire or catheter, an angiogram of the radial artery with diluted contrast (50% contrast and 50% saline) is exceedingly helpful in delineating the problem encountered (see brachial loop videos—▶ Videos 5.2 and 5.3—and radial tortuosity video—▶ Video 5.4). Some operators routinely perform an angiogram prior to advancing a catheter. Although this may not be necessary in every case, the threshold to perform an angiogram should be low. Once in the subclavian artery, it is obviously important to avoid the carotid and vertebral arteries. On occasion, the guidewire will enter the descending rather than the ascending aorta. In this instance, it is helpful to have the patient take a deep breath (see videos from descending aorta to ascending aorta—▶ Videos 5.5, 5.6, and 5.7). This will elongate the ascending aorta and make it much easier to obtain central aortic access. At times, it may be necessary to advance a catheter to the aorta and ask the patient to take a deep breath as the guidewire is then directed toward the ascending aorta with the tip of the catheter (see Videos 5.5, 5.6, and 5.7). When the takeoff of the right subclavian artery arises from the left side of the aorta and courses behind the esophagus (arteria lusoria), it can be difficult to access the central aorta, with the guidewire preferentially selecting the descending aorta. In this circumstance, a Vitek® or Simmons® catheter can be placed in the descending aorta, with the tip pointed cephalad. An 0.035 hydrophilic angled Glidewire can then be directed cephalad and toward the ascending aorta coming from below. Once the wire is in the ascending aorta, the catheter can be advanced over the guidewire, with a gentle "pull-push" technique (push on the catheter and pull on the guidewire) until it is in the ascending aorta. An exchange-length guidewire can then be placed in the ascending aorta for the delivery of subsequent catheters. Severe tortuosity and radial loops can present technical challenges (see dilated and tortuous subclavian and aorta videos—▶ Videos 5.8 and 5.9—and videos of severe tortuosity straightened out by guidewire—▶ Videos 5.10 and 5.11). A radial loop can usually be overcome with a soft guidewire, and frequently a coronary guidewire is useful (see radial tortuosity video—Video 5.4). Once the loop is straightened out, a soft catheter is placed, and a stiffer guidewire is then introduced, but manipulation of the catheter is usually not a problem (see brachial loop videos—Videos 5.2 and 5.3). Smaller catheters (and hydrophilic catheters, if available) are usually preferable in this situation. Severe tortuosity and/or marked dilatation of the subclavian artery can also present a challenge. This generally can be overcome using a stiffer guidewire to help straighten out the curves (see videos of dilated and tortuous subclavian and aorta—Videos 5.8 and 5.9). At times, it is necessary to place a long sheath in the subclavian artery to overcome the tortuosity. (Please see the excellent and comprehensive "tips and tricks" recommended by Patel, Shah, and Pancholy in Chapter 15.

■ ACCESSING THE ASCENDING AORTA FROM THE LEFT RADIAL

As from the right radial, a J-tipped Glidewire may be inserted and advanced without difficulty. If an angled Glidewire is used, it should be visualized in the forearm, the upper arm, and the subclavian artery. Entering the ascending aorta from the left subclavian artery is generally very easy. Some operators prefer the left radial approach because, once in the subclavian artery, the remainder of the access of the ascending aorta and the coronary arteries is similar to the femoral approach. Once access is achieved, the left arm and wrist can be positioned across the body toward the right groin. This allows the procedure to progress as if one were working from the right radial or right femoral access.

Please see the chapter on diagnostic and guide catheter manipulation to engage the coronary arteries.

■ SUMMARY

Transradial access is technically more difficult than transfemoral access because of the size of the artery, the increased incidence of severe spasm, and anatomic variation such as loops and tortuosity. Nevertheless, the technique can be easily learned and mastered if the operator is committed.

■ VIDEO LEGENDS

Radial Artery Access Video

Video 5.1 Note the low angle of insertion and the bounce of the needle as it advances slowly toward the artery using gentle palpation of the artery with the tips of the first two fingers of the left hand. The needle should be bouncing up and down and not side to side. As you get closer to the artery, the bounce increases. If you press too hard with your left hand, you may obliterate the bounce. Apply just enough pressure to trap the needle between your fingertips and the artery. The flow may be pulsatile, but in many cases the flow may be slow. The bright red color of the blood will assure you that the artery has been entered. The wire should advance easily and without any pain. If there is any pain, it is likely that the wire is subintimal and should be withdrawn with the flow rechecked. If there is resistance to advancement of the wire, it is either subintimal or in a side branch. In this case, you can see that the wire can be torqued and advanced but then meets resistance. Finally, the wire should pass the side branch and advance easily. The needle is withdrawn, and a small nick in the skin is made with a #11 blade. (Some catheter and dilators do not require a dermatotomy with a #11 blade.) Once the sheath has been inserted, medications can be administered prophylactically to prevent spasm.

Brachial Loop

Video 5.2   The loop in the brachial artery above the elbow is overcome with an angled Glidewire gradually advanced through the loop. It is advisable to overcome the loop with a soft-tipped angled or J-tipped guidewire followed by a catheter in order not to dissect the artery or cause spasm.

Video 5.3   Note that the loop is now straightened by the guidewire and is now safe to traverse with a catheter. All subsequent catheter exchanges should be made over an exchange-length guidewire.

Severe Tortuosity of the Radial Artery

Video 5.4   Note the severe tortuosity of the radial artery with the angled-tipped Glidewire entering a small branch at the top of the curve (recurrent radial artery). You can see how advancing a catheter into this vessel at the very least would cause severe spasm and at worst could cause perforation. This is why any resistance of a guidewire or a catheter should be interrogated with an angiogram through the sheath. The severe loop shown in this example may be overcome with a J-tipped guidewire (which will probably not enter the small branch) or, if this is unsuccessful, a transition-less 0.014 soft coronary guidewire can overcome the bend. Once the severe curve is overcome, a Glide Catheter can be passed over the guidewire and the coronary guidewire then exchanged for an 0.035 J-tipped Glidewire.

From Descending Aorta to Ascending Aorta

Video 5.5   Note tortuosity of the subclavian artery with the tip of the angled Glidewire appearing to be in the ascending aorta.

Video 5.6   Note how the guidewire and the following Judkins Left 3.5 diagnostic catheter have straightened out the tortuosity, but the tip of the guidewire is now in the descending aorta.

Video 5.7   With the tip of the diagnostic catheter at the aortic knob and the guidewire in the descending aorta, the patient is asked to take a deep breath, and the catheter is torqued toward the ascending aorta as the guidewire is retracted and then readvanced when the catheter is pointing toward the ascending aorta. Once the position in the ascending aorta is achieved, any catheter exchange should be made over a long guidewire to maintain position in the ascending aorta and to obviate the need of renegotiating the severe tortuosity.

Dilated and Tortuous Subclavian and Aorta

Video 5.8   Note extreme tortuosity of subclavian artery. This may be negotiated with a J-tipped guidewire advancing a catheter over the curves and ultimately into the ascending aorta.

Video 5.9   The left main coronary artery (LMCA) is engaged with a 110-cm-long multipurpose catheter with the guidewire in place in order to overcome the extreme tortuosity. The guidewire is carefully withdrawn once the LMCA is approached in the left coronary cusp with the adjustment of advancing or withdrawing the catheter until the LMCA is selectively engaged.

Severe Tortuosity Straightened Out by Guidewire

Video 5.10   Note the severe tortuosity of the subclavian artery that is negotiated with an angled Glidewire. A J-tipped Glidewire may be equally effective in negotiating the tortuosity. The advantage of the J-tipped Glidewire is that it may be helpful in avoiding side branches because it usually selects the large main branch and stays out of smaller side branches that can be perforated by the angled Glidewire. The disadvantage of the J-tipped Glidewire is that it has no steerability. The angled Glidewire can be "steered away" from unwanted branches.

Video 5.11   The tortuosity is overcome by the angled Glidewire that is now in the ascending aorta.

chapter 6

Closure and Hemostasis after Transradial Access

Samir B. Pancholy, MD
Tejas Patel, MD, DM
Sanjay C. Shah, MD, DM

■ HEMOSTASIS

Hemostasis after transradial access (TRA) is probably the most important reason for popularity of TRA. It is effective, well tolerated, and cheap. The anatomy of the distal forearm allows for liberal compression of the radial artery against a flat base of the radius bone. This combined with the absence of any major nerves or other structures in the vicinity makes it a very well-tolerated procedure.

Traditionally, hemostasis after TRA is obtained using multiple techniques, varying from manual compression to the use of dedicated compression devices. The common denominator, among all these techniques, is continuous compression at the site of arterial puncture. Available hemostatic compression devices range from plastic bands to inflatable devices.

Although hemostatic compression is effective in achieving its primary goal, which is arterial hemostasis, it frequently leads to interruption of flow in the radial artery lumen and, not infrequently, causes radial artery occlusion. Hemostasis is probably the only modifiable procedural component of the transradial procedure, which can affect radial artery occlusion.

■ RADIAL ARTERY OCCLUSION

Radial artery occlusion is the most common complication of transradial access, which leads to permanent obliteration of radial artery lumen and limits future transradial access. Its incidence varies from 2% to 10% and is dependent on the attributes of the population studied. In the majority of cases, it

Transradial Access: Techniques for Diagnostic Angiography and Percutaneous Intervention
©2013 Howard A. Cohen (Editor). Cardiotext Publishing, ISBN 978-1-935395-41-6.

is completely asymptomatic and well tolerated from an ischemia standpoint. From the outset, it has been realized that prevention of radial artery occlusion is of paramount importance, as the majority of patients with coronary artery disease require repeat procedures, and hence maintenance of radial artery patency will provide the benefits of TRA for future procedures. Patients with smaller-caliber radial arteries and those with diabetes mellitus, as well as women and those with end-stage renal disease, have a higher incidence of radial artery occlusion.

The pathophysiology of radial artery occlusion appears to be a thrombotic process, initiated by local injury due to introduction of the introducer sheath in the radial artery lumen, which forms a nidus for local thrombus formation. This is then supported by stasis created by a combination of radial artery spasm and the profile of the equipment dwelling in the radial artery lumen decreasing the radial flow during the procedure, usually to a standstill. Once the procedure is completed, this thrombus, formed at the site of entry, usually progresses to a transmural occlusive thrombus, in the presence of flow cessation, created by hemostatic compression. The creation of this occluded segment of the radial artery at the site of catheter entry leads to excellent hemostasis and also creates acute radial artery occlusion. A large subset of these patients will then recanalize this occluded segment, with the establishment of radial artery patency. A small portion, though, fails to recanalize, and rapid organization with eventual fibrotic obliteration of the lumen results.

Prevention of radial artery occlusion starts at the beginning of the transradial procedure, with special emphasis on minimizing trauma to the radial artery. Smaller-caliber introducers, as well as catheters, have been associated with a lower incidence of radial artery occlusion. Systemic anticoagulation using heparin has also been shown to significantly reduce the incidence of radial artery occlusion. Other systemic anticoagulants, such as bivalirudin and enoxaparin, have shown similar efficacy. The protective effect of heparin appears to be systemic, as there is no difference noted with intra-arterial or intravenous administration. The effect also appears to be dose dependent, as lower doses have been associated with a higher rate of radial artery occlusion (RAO).

Postprocedural care has probably the largest effect on occurrence of RAO. A strong relationship exists between the interruption of radial artery flow and occurrence of RAO. Maintenance of radial artery patency during hemostatic compression, described as "patent hemostasis technique," has been shown to have an incremental effect in lowering the incidence of radial artery occlusion. Duration of hemostatic compression has also been shown to have an effect, with longer duration of compression associated with a higher incidence of radial artery occlusion. In a systemically anticoagulated patient, a 2-hour duration of hemostatic compression appears to be an optimal duration for achieving hemostasis, as well as providing the lowest incidence of radial artery occlusion.

■ PATENT HEMOSTASIS TECHNIQUE

As the name implies, this technique revolves around using the lowest necessary pressure for hemostatic compression with establishment of hemostasis, as well as maintenance of radial artery patency. These 2 goals are simultaneously achievable in 60% to 75% of patients. The description of the technique is as follows.

Step 1: Purge the static contents of the radial artery, proximal to the introducer sheath, by opening the side arm stopcock bleeding and removing 3 to 5 mL of blood.

Step 2: Apply the hemostatic compression device, 2 to 3 mm proximal to the skin entry site (Figure 6.1), and tighten or inflate it (Figure 6.2), then remove the introducer sheath (Figure 6.3).

Step 3: Decrease the pressure of the hemostatic compression device, to the point of mild pulsatile bleeding, at the skin entry site. After 2 to 3 cycles of bleeding, retighten the hemostatic compression device to eliminate this pulsatile bleeding. At this point, you have applied the least necessary pressure to maintain hemostasis.

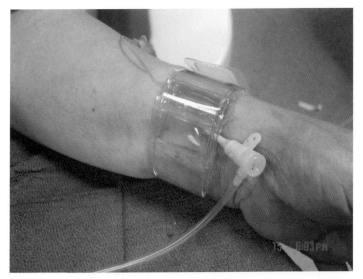

Figure 6.1 Application of compression band at the puncture site.

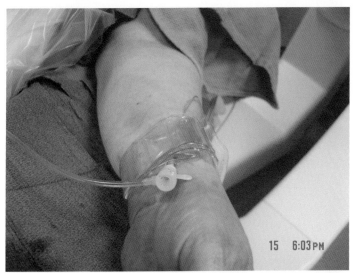

Figure 6.2 Inflate/tighten the compression band.

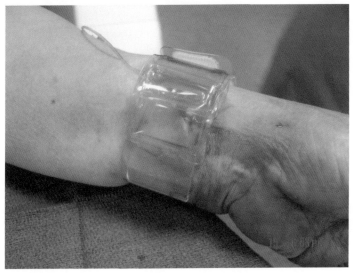

Figure 6.3 Remove introducer sheath.

Step 4: Documentation of radial artery patency status is performed by using the reverse Barbeau's test. A plethysmographic sensor is placed on the index finger of the involved upper extremity, with the observation of pulsatile waveforms. The ulnar artery is then compressed at the level of the wrist, and the behavior of the waveform is observed. Absence of plethysmographic waveform is indicative of interruption of radial artery flow (Figure 6.4). At this point, the hemostatic compression pressure is promptly lowered (Figure 6.5), to the point where plethysmographic waveform returns, confirming the establishment of radial artery flow (Figure 6.6). If bleeding occurs before the return of plethysmographic waveform, hemostatic compression pressure is increased to eliminate bleeding, as this is the primary goal of the process of hemostasis. In 25% to 35% of patients, the radial artery patency cannot be maintained while achieving hemostasis. These patients are especially at a high risk for developing radial artery occlusion.

Step 5: Periodic evaluation of radial artery patency is necessary to prevent subsequent flow cessation causing radial artery occlusion. Our protocol presently requires evaluation of radial artery patency by monitoring staff every 15 minutes throughout the duration of compression by using the reverse Barbeau's test. If plethysmographic evidence of absence of radial flow is noted, hemostatic pressure is further decreased, as long as hemostasis is maintained.

Step 6: After 2 hours of hemostatic compression, gradually decrease the pressure of compression, weaning the pressure to zero. Carefully remove the hemostatic pressure device without tenting the skin, as this may dislodge the hemostatic plug and restart bleeding.

■ PREDISCHARGE CARE

After removal of the hemostatic compression device, it is especially important to not apply encircling dressings with compression bandages. Covering the entry site with a bandage, without application of any pressure, is not only sufficient but also necessary to prevent subsequent interruption of radial artery flow.

Key Points

- Use the lowest French size required for successfully completing the procedure.

- Use at least 50 U/Kg unfractionated heparin administered intra-arterially or intravenously at the beginning of the procedure after obtaining radial artery access, or at the latest after entering ascending aorta. Bivalirudin may be substituted for heparin for percutaneous coronary intervention.

- Never leave the introducer sheath in place after completion of the procedure. Reaccess, if needed, for a following procedure, even if it is anticipated on the same day.

- Patent hemostasis technique is a must.

- Wean the hemostatic pressure to zero before removal of the band.

- Never apply hemostatic compression longer than 2 hours, except when subsequent bleeding occurs.

■ SUMMARY

Hemostasis after radial artery access is a simple, highly successful, cheap, and extremely effective portion of the transradial procedure. Its effect on subsequent radial artery occlusion is frequently unrecognized and needs to be underscored, with special attention paid to maintenance of radial artery flow throughout hemostatic compression in order to prevent radial artery occlusion. Radial artery occlusion, although asymptomatic from an ischemia standpoint, eliminates the use of that radial artery in the future. Radial artery occlusion deprives the patient of a low-risk vascular access site for future percutaneous coronary intervention. Patent hemostasis is an extremely successful technique that preserves the radial artery as an access site.

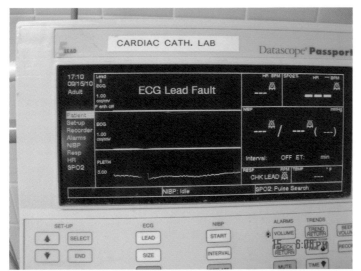

Figure 6.4 Plethysmographic evaluation of radial artery patency by performing reverse Barbeau's test (absence of patency evident in this instance).

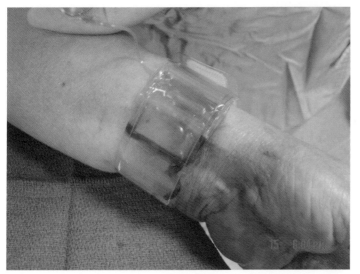

Figure 6.5 Deflate/loosen the band to decrease compression pressure, maintaining hemostasis.

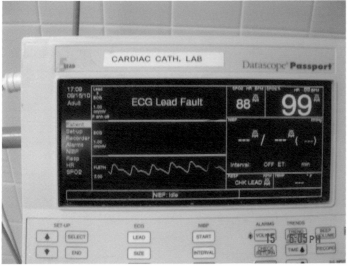

Figure 6.6 Reevaluate radial artery patency (patency evident by presence of plethysmographic signal).

◼ REFERENCES

1. Pancholy SB. Transradial access in an occluded radial artery: new technique. *J Invasive Cardiol*. Dec 2007;19(12):541–544.

2. Sanmartin M, Gomez M, Rumoroso JR, Sadaba M, Martinez M, Baz JA, Iniguez A. Interruption of blood flow during compression and radial artery occlusion after transradial catheterization. *Catheter Cardiovasc Interv*. 2007 Aug 1;70(2):185–189.

3. Saito S, Ikei H, Hosokawa G, Tanaka S Influence of the ratio between radial artery inner diameter and sheath outer diameter on radial artery flow after transradial coronary intervention. *Catheter Cardiovasc Interv*. 1999:46(2):173–178.

4. Spaulding C, Lefevre T, Funck F, Thebault B, Chauveau M, Ben Hamda K, Chalet Y, Monsegu, J, Tsocanakis O, Py A, Guillard N, Weber S. Left radial approach for coronary angiography: results of a prospective study. *Cathet Cardiovasc Diagn*. 1996;39:365–370.

5. Plante S, Cantor WJ, Goldman L, Miner S, Quesnelle A, Ganapathy A, Popel A, Bertrand OF. Comparison of bivalirudin versus heparin on radial artery occlusion after transradial catheterization. *Catheter Cardiovasc Interv*. Nov 1 2010;76(5): 654–658.

6. Feray H, Izgi C, Citiner D, et al. Effectiveness of enoxaparin for prevention of radial artery occlusion after transradial cardiac catheterization. *J Thromb Thrombolysis*. 2010;29:322–325.

7. Pancholy S, Coppola J, Patel T, Roke-Thomas M. Prevention of radial artery occlusion-patent hemostasis evaluation trial (PROPHET study): a randomized comparison of traditional versus patency documented hemostasis after transradial catheterization. *Catheter Cardiovasc Interv*. 2008;72(3): 335–340.

8. Pancholy SB, Patel TM. Effect of duration of hemostatic compression on radial artery occlusion after transradial access. *Catheter Cardiovasc Interv*. Jan 1 2012;79(1):78–81.

chapter 7

Basic Catheter Techniques for Diagnostic Angiography and PCI

Tift Mann, MD

■ INTRODUCTION

The cannulation of coronary arteries using radial artery access requires a different set of skills than access from the femoral artery. It should be emphasized that the skills are different but not difficult. Indeed, once learned, selective cannulation of the coronary ostia can expeditiously be performed from either arm. Fluoroscopy times among experienced operators are similar between radial and femoral approaches.[1,2] Furthermore, several recent studies have demonstrated no difference in door-to-balloon times in patients with ST-elevation myocardial infarction (STEMI) undergoing emergency procedures.[3–8] The purpose of the present chapter is to review the techniques and catheters required for a successful transradial procedure.

■ PATIENT SELECTION

Although discussed in more detail elsewhere, patient demographics and the operator's previous experience with the technique should be considered before proceeding with transradial procedures. For example, it is prudent to begin one's radial experience with middle-aged males who have large radial arteries and straightforward aortic arches. Similarly, Type A and B1 lesions in the left anterior descending (LAD) and right coronary arteries should be undertaken initially before moving to more complex interventions. Patients with bypass grafts, short stature, older age, previous radial procedures, and dilated aortic roots should be approached only after acquiring radial experience. It also should be emphasized that patients who have contraindications to

Transradial Access: Techniques for Diagnostic Angiography and Percutaneous Intervention
©2013 Howard A. Cohen (Editor). Cardiotext Publishing, ISBN 978-1-935395-41-6.

femoral access are often the most difficult to approach transradially, and the use of radial access should not be limited to these patients.

■ RIGHT VERSUS LEFT RADIAL ACCESS

The cannulation of coronary arteries from left radial access is similar to that from femoral access. Furthermore, the subclavian artery, the aortic arch, and the ascending aorta anatomies are favorable for the use of standard Judkins catheters. Thus, many institutions initially teach fellows using left radial access. In the TALENT trial, fluoroscopy times for fellows were significantly lower when left radial access was utilized as opposed to right radial access.[9] In this same study, left radial access was associated with a significantly lower fluoroscopy time when compared to right radial access in patients over 70 years of age. Advanced age is associated with straightening and unwinding of the aorta, creating subclavian tortuosity that makes catheter manipulation from the right radial approach challenging. Obtaining access from the right side of the table, however, may be difficult due to the awkward position of the left wrist. Thus, some centers obtain access from the left side of the table, then redrape and perform the procedure from the right side. Some operators who work routinely from the left

radial will work from the left side and reverse the monitors and the the radiation shielding.

■ GENERAL CATHETER TECHNIQUES

Generally speaking, more catheter manipulation is required for coronary ostial cannulation from the radial approach as compared to the femoral. An important technique is the use of the J-wire to improve catheter torquability and control. Coronaries may be engaged with the J-wire still within the catheter by passing the J-wire through the Tuohy Borst, which allows contrast injection during catheter engagement (Figure 7.1).

A more advanced technique is the use of the stiff end of the J-wire to make subtle changes in the catheter curve to improve coaxial engagement of the proximal coronary. Of course, care is taken to ensure the guidewire remains within the catheter. For example, the universal TIG catheter (Terumo Corporation, Somerset, NJ) often selectively engages the proximally arising conus branch of the right coronary because of its superior angle. Straightening the secondary curve with the stiff end of the J-wire converts this catheter to a Judkins Right-like curve, thus avoiding the conus branch (Figure 7.2). Maneuvers such as these can avoid time-consuming and spasm-inducing catheter exchanges.

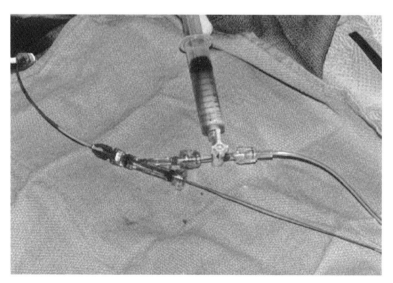

Figure 7.1 The J-wire inserted through a Tuohy Borst improves catheter control while allowing contrast injection.

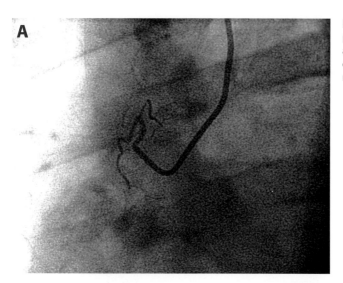

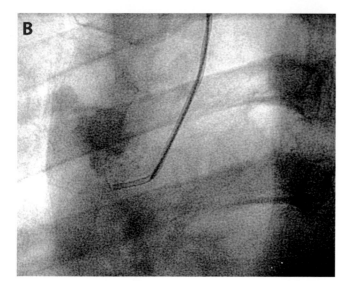

Figure 7.2 The TIG catheter is particularly prone to select the conus artery branch of the proximal right coronary (**A**), but a J-wire can usually redirect the tip into the primary lumen (**B**).

■ DIAGNOSTIC CORONARY ANGIOGRAPHY

The indications for transradial *diagnostic* angiography are less clear than for transradial coronary *intervention* because bleeding complications from transfemoral diagnostic angiography performed without anticoagulation are rare. Thus, as a general rule, the radial artery should be preserved for interventional procedures. However, patient preference and the need for transradial training may necessitate performing diagnostic procedures. Furthermore, ad hoc interventional procedures

are increasingly common. (In fact, in some centers the majority of patients are booked as "left heart cath-possible PCI [percutaneous coronary intervention].")

When diagnostic procedures are performed, it is imperative that techniques to avoid postprocedural radial occlusion be compulsively used. The smallest catheter size possible is a requirement because the incidence of radial occlusion is directly related to catheter size.[10] Diagnostic procedures should be performed with at most a 5-Fr system, and some catheterization laboratories use 4-Fr catheters. A variable-rate power injection system may improve angiographic images.[11] Furthermore, the use of a 5-Fr *guide* catheter as opposed to a *diagnostic* catheter for angiography may provide better opacification in high-flow states.

It should be emphasized that adequate sedation and intra-arterial verapamil to reduce spasm, heparinization (50 units/kg), and minimization of catheter exchanges will all reduce postprocedural radial occlusion after diagnostic procedures. Hemostasis devices must be applied using patent hemostasis and removed as rapidly as possible after angiographic procedures.[12–15] Transradial angiography is often criticized for subselective injections with poor opacification, but excellent angiography can always be attained using proper technique. The debate of "transfemoral versus transradial" is very reminiscent of the "Sones versus Judkins" debate in the early days of coronary angiography. The differences are clearly a reflection of the experience of the operators with either technique.

Left Radial Approach

Catheters utilized from the left radial approach are essentially the same as from femoral access. Standard Judkins curves work well although a variety of femoral catheters including Amplatz curves may also be used in special situations. Positioning the left wrist near the left femoral area either before or after access allows the procedure to be performed from the right side of the table with minimal back strain. Left subclavian tortuosity is usually not an issue, and catheter manipulation is similar to the femoral approach.

Right Radial Approach

The most common diagnostic catheters used from the right radial approach worldwide are standard Judkins curves.[16] Cannulating the left coronary ostium involves torquing the catheter 180 degrees into the left coronary cusp followed by advancement or withdrawal into the coronary ostium. This maneuver is distinctly different from the femoral approach and may be challenging, particularly when right subclavian tortuosity is present or the ascending aorta is short. As previously

mentioned, keeping the J-wire within the catheter during this maneuver may be necessary. A Judkins 3.5 curve rather than the standard femoral 4.0 curve is preferred from the right radial approach.

Cannulation of the right coronary is usually easily accomplished with the standard Judkins R4 catheter. Occasionally, a Judkins R5 or an Amplatz R2 is required, particularly when the takeoff of the coronary is inferior. An Amplatz R2 or an Amplatz L1 is used for anterior takeoff of the right coronary (Figure 7.3).

Universal Curves

Many experienced radialists prefer to use universal curves for angiography of both coronary arteries, thus avoiding catheter exchanges. Most catheter manufacturers currently have a 5-Fr diagnostic universal curve. These curves are essentially variations of the Kimny curve originally designed by Dr. Ferdinand Kiemeneij (Figure 7.4).

Cannulation of the left coronary with these curves involves torquing the catheter into the left cusp and then advancing forward into the left coronary ostium (▶ Video 7.1). Alternatively, the catheter is positioned above the left coronary cusp, the *U* is opened with a J-wire, and the left coronary ostium is engaged from above (▶ Video 7.2). As previously noted, the J-wire, is actively used with these universal curves for support and to straighten the curve through subclavian tortuosity, thus improving tortuosity, and to make subtle changes in the curve itself to actively engage the coronary ostium.

The right coronary cusp is lower than the left in most patients. Thus, to engage the right coronary ostium, the catheter must be advanced forward in addition to being torqued clockwise (▶ Video 7.3). It is recommended that new operators practice this maneuver initially with a 6-Fr Kimny catheter using the J-wire through the Tuohy to allow visualization.

An important criticism of universal catheters is their lack of coaxial alignment within the proximal segment of the coronary arteries. These curves tend to point superiorly in both coronaries, potentially causing subintimal dissection. The initial contrast injection in the

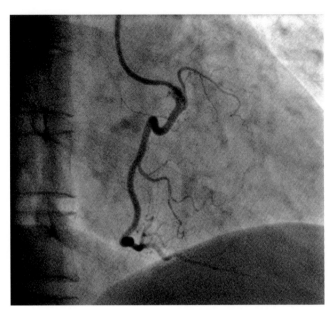

Figure 7.3 Anterior takeoff of the right coronary artery cannulated with Amplatz L1.

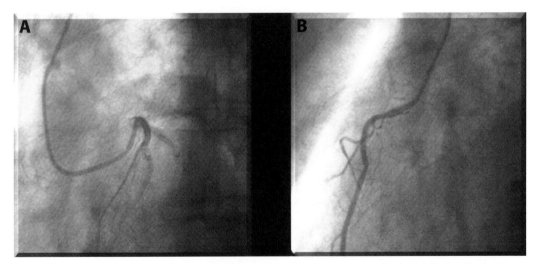

Figure 7.4 Kimny guide catheter (Boston Scientific, Watertown, MA) can be utilized for both left (**A**) and right (**B**) coronary interventions. It is uniquely applicable for patients with STEMI.

vessel must be done carefully, and compulsive attention must be paid to damping of the arterial pressure. The TIG catheter (Terumo Corporation, Somerset, NJ) is particularly prone to select the conus artery branch of the proximal right coronary, but active use of the J-wire can usually redirect the tip into the primary lumen (see Figure 7.2). The operator should have a low threshold to exchange catheters to attain coaxial alignment and

optimum angiography. The Jacky (Terumo Corporation, Somerset, NJ) catheter may cannulate coronaries with better coaxial alignment (Figure 7.5).

A minority of operators, particularly those with experience using the Sones technique, may use a multipurpose catheter as a universal curve to select both coronaries. In most centers, this technique is a lost art, but skilled operators may obtain excellent

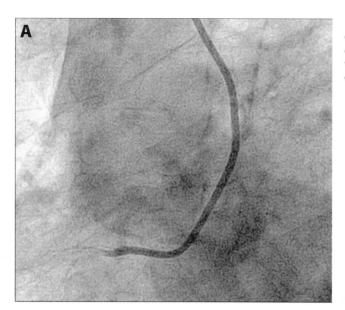

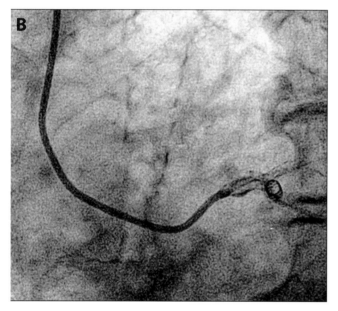

Figure 7.5 The Jacky catheter (Terumo Corporation, Somerset, NJ) allows cannulation of both coronary arteries with excellent coaxial alignment. (**A**) Right coronary and (**B**) left coronary.

arteriograms relatively quickly using this technique.

Arteria lusoria is a congenital condition in which a retroesophageal right subclavian joins the arch on the left side, creating an extremely acute angle to access the ascending aorta. This anatomical challenge can usually be overcome with either a JL 3.5 or universal curve with a 0.035 unit angled Glidewire, having the patient take very deep breaths. However, cannulation of the coronary is extremely difficult, and it is

usually preferable to use an alternative access such as left radial when encountered.

Diagnostic angiography in patients with previous bypass surgery may be challenging. Cannulating the left internal mammary graft or left coronary saphenous vein bypass grafts from the right radial approach is challenging and may involve specialized techniques.[17] It is generally best to perform diagnostic angiography from the femoral approach in these patients and subsequently stage interventional procedures. In the presence of a compelling indication for ad hoc intervention, diagnostic angiography should be performed from the left radial approach.

■ CATHETERS USED FOR PCI

Early concerns about transradial guide catheters providing sufficient backup for interventional procedures have largely proven baseless. Most transradial curves provide support from the contralateral wall, and backup becomes an issue only in complex procedures. In fact, with continued miniaturization and improvement of devices, the majority of interventions can now be performed through 5-Fr guide catheters. Furthermore, the smaller guiding catheters used from the radial approach allow for safe "deep seating" of the guide to obtain superior backup in some cases and obviate the need for a GuideLiner type of approach.

Catheter Size

The first consideration in selecting a guide for an interventional procedure is catheter size. Although transradial coronary interventions have traditionally been performed through a 6-Fr guide catheter, significant intimal and medial damage to the radial artery may occur with the introduction of a 6-Fr sheath.[18] There has recently been an increased focus on radial artery preservation because postprocedure

radial occlusion can often be prevented (see Chapter 6). Using the smallest catheter possible for a given lesion complexity is essential. Most straightforward interventions today can easily be performed using 5-Fr guides. This is particularly important in women with smaller radial arteries.

Sheathless Guides

The external diameter of a sheath must be sufficiently large to provide an internal diameter that will allow passage of the same French guide catheter. Thus, the external diameter of a 6-Fr guide catheter is actually smaller than that of a 5-Fr sheath. This concept has led to the use of "sheathless" insertion of catheters. The Asahi Eaucath (INPECC Company, Aichi, Japan) is a designated sheathless guide that comes with an inner dilator for ease of insertion.[19] Sheathless guide catheters from other manufacturers are also available, but as of the date of publication, these catheters are not available in the United States.

The insertion of standard guide catheters using a sheathless technique has been described.[20] With this technique, a telescoped "pseudodilator" is used as an introducer to improve the transition between the guidewire and the tip of the guide catheter. A 4-Fr 125-cm Glide catheter (Terumo, Somerset, NJ) is used as the "pseudodilator" for sheathless 5-Fr guide catheters, and a 5-Fr 125-cm

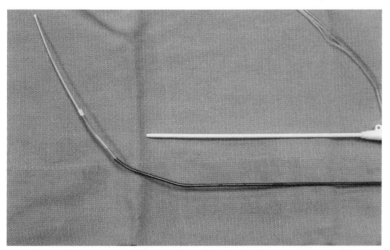

Figure 7.6 Sheathless technique. A telescoped 4-Fr 125-cm Glide catheter (Terumo, Somerset, NJ) is used as the "pseudodilator" for a sheathless 5-Fr standard guide. A 125-cm 5-Fr diagnostic catheter is used as the "pseudodilator" for 6-Fr guides. Note that the external diameter of the 6-Fr guide is smaller than a 5-Fr sheath.

JR4 is used for 6- and 7-Fr guide catheters (Figure 7.6).

These sheathless guides are inserted over a 0.035-in J-wire positioned in the ascending aorta. The issue of transitioning from a 0.018-in guidewire utilized for radial access to this J-wire is overcome by using 1 of 2 techniques. The first is simply to obtain access with a standard 4- or 5-Fr sheath through which the J-wire is inserted. The second technique is to use a Cook Silhouette double dilator. With this system, an inner 0.018-in compatible dilator is removed, leaving a 0.036-in compatible introducer for deployment of the J-wire.

The transition between the "pseudodilator" and the standard guide catheter, whether it is 5 or 6 Fr, is not smooth as a designated introducer. Thus, care must be taken in introducing the guide catheter to avoid damage at the arteriotomy site. Although this technique has theoretical advantages due to the smaller external diameter of the guide catheter, a definitive study demonstrating actual reduced radial occlusion is not available.

Catheter Selection for PCI

Once catheter size has been determined, consideration should be given to the shape of the guide catheter curve. Although experienced operators can utilize universal curves for interventions in both coronary arteries, most operators will vary catheter shape selection depending on the artery involved. This is particularly true for more complex interventional procedures. In a recent survey, standard femoral curves were most commonly used for transradial interventions; however, specific transradial curves may improve backup in certain situations.[16]

LAD Interventions

The most commonly utilized guide catheters for radial LAD interventions in the Bertrand survey were EBU 3.5 (28%), Judkins Left 3.5 (22%), and XB 3.5 (18%). Downsizing to the JL 3.5 has been shown to increase backup support in in vitro studies.[21,22] The Kimny guide (Boston Scientific Corporation, Watertown, MA) tends to be coaxial with the LAD and provides excellent support from the contralateral aortic wall. This catheter is also currently available in 5 Fr. The RBLBT (Cordis Corporation, Bridgewater, NJ) and MRADIAL (Medtronic, Minneapolis, MN) are also excellent 5-Fr guides. The Ikari guide (Terumo, Somerset, NJ) was specifically designed to provide excellent backup from the right radial approach. The size of the curve corresponds to Judkins sizes. The Cordis Fajadet L4 is an excellent guide for the LAD and circumflex, particularly if there is a long left main coronary artery.

Right Coronary Interventions

The most frequently used guide catheter for right coronary interventions is a Judkins curve, either JR4 or JR5, with an Amplatz Right being a distant second.[16] However, neither of these catheters provides excellent support from the contralateral wall that is attained using universal curves. Thus, a Kimny or other universal curve is useful in this situation. Other catheters that provide better backup are an Amplatz Left 0.75 or 1 or an Ikari Right. The Cordis Hockey Stick also is an excellent guide catheter for the majority of right coronary artery (RCA) interventions. This catheter can be "deep seated" safely, by experienced operators, and provides excellent support. All RCA guides need to be "coaxial" and not merely engaged in the ostium of the RCA. This is best seen in the right anterior oblique (RAO) projection and can be achieved by a gentle clockwise rotation of the guide when it appears to be not coaxial.

Left Circumflex Interventions

Interventions involving the left circumflex are often the most difficult encountered by the interventionalist. Therefore, careful guide catheter selection is imperative. In the Bertrand survey, EBU 3.5 (26%), XB 3.5 (21%), and Judkins Left (12%) were the most commonly utilized.[16] A Voda 3.5 is also an option. Generally speaking, Judkins curves are avoided in LCX interventions because they tend to point superiorly into the LAD. For 5-Fr circumflex interventions, the EBU 3.5 or 3.75 or MRADIAL (Medtronic, Minneapolis,

MN) provides satisfactory backup and opacification. The Cordis Fajadet L4 is similar in shape to the Voda catheter and is quite good for the circumflex. Clearly, these choices are personal, just as they are when working from femoral access.

Bypass Graft Interventions

Left internal mammary artery (IMA) graft interventions are performed from the left radial artery.[23] A standard IMA guide catheter or a Mann IM (Boston Scientific, Watertown, MA) is utilized (Figure 7.7). The latter catheter provides excellent support and is 90 cm in length, thus allowing balloons and stents

to reach even distal lesions in the LAD. Right IMA interventions are performed from right radial access.

Right saphenous vein bypass graft interventions can be performed from the right radial artery using an Amplatz R2, multipurpose, or Amplatz Left catheter. An Amplatz L1 curve is used in 59% of right saphenous vein graft interventions in Japan. With a dilated aortic root, an AL2 catheter may be helpful (Figure 7.8).

Left saphenous vein bypass graft interventions are best performed from the left radial approach. These interventions, particularly high-takeoff left circumflex vein grafts, are difficult and should not be performed until

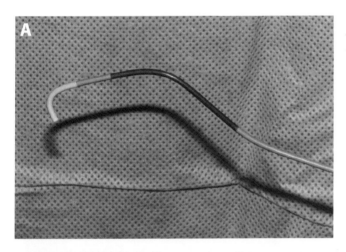

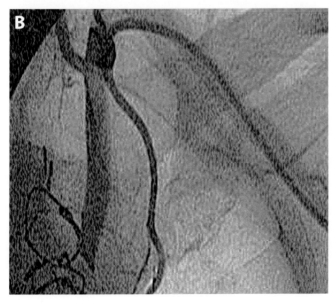

Figure 7.7 Mann IM catheter in left IMA graft using left radial approach. (**A**) 6-Fr Mann IM. (**B**) LIMA cannulated via left radial artery using Mann IM.

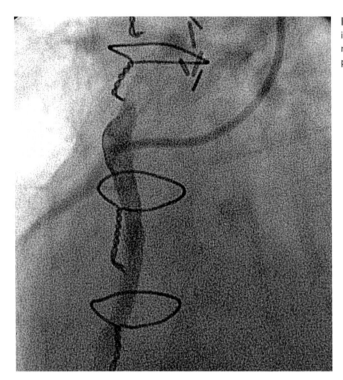

Figure 7.8 Right saphenous vein graft interventions can be performed from the right radial approach. An AL1 or AL2 guide provides excellent support.

well into the learning curve. Amplatz Left and left bypass graft curves are most commonly used. However, the Kimny catheter provides excellent support from the left radial artery and is also an excellent option (Figure 7.9). A buddy wire is commonly used for stability, particularly during deployment of embolic protection devices. A GuideLiner will provide additional support and is commonly used for these interventions.

■ TIPS TO IMPROVE TRANSRADIAL PCI SUCCESS

Buddy wires positioned either in the target vessel or in an adjacent vessel are very useful to improve guide catheter coaxiality and support (Figure 7.10). Operators should have a low threshold to insert a second wire if difficulties are encountered with either predilatation or stent deployment. They can be utilized with any size or shape catheter but are particularly useful with 5-Fr guides.

Deep seating of 5-Fr guide catheters is a technique that has been long associated with transradial access. This technique is utilized

much less frequently now with the continued improvements in the deliverability of balloons and stents. However, when additional support is necessary, a mother-daughter extension catheter (GuideLiner, Vascular Solutions, Minneapolis, MN) may be useful. When used transradially, the proximal port of the GuideLiner may be located in an angulated segment in the shoulder and may entrap the stent (Figure 7.11). Thus, stents should be passed into the GuideLiner in a straight segment, and then both should be passed together into the target vessel.

Rotational atherectomy may be a necessary pretreatment in heavily calcified vessels and lesions. Burr sizes up to 1.75 mm can be used for standard 6-Fr guide catheters. A 1.25-mm Burr can be passed through a 0.058-in 5-Fr guide catheter such as the Launcher MRADIAL (Medtronic, Minneapolis, MN) (Figure 7.12). Although standard-shape curves are generally utilized, Q curves provide good support and allow smooth passage of the Burr into the target vessel.

In patients with STEMI, most operators utilize catheters with which they are most familiar. Experienced radialists will perform

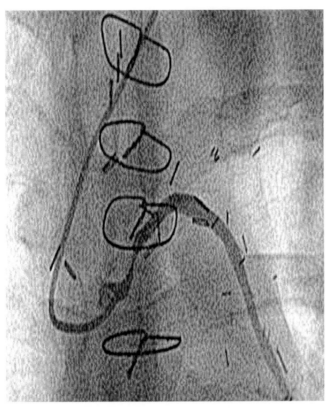

Figure 7.9 Kimny guide in left coronary saphenous vein bypass graft. The left radial approach is utilized for left coronary saphenous vein bypass graft interventions, and the Kimny catheter provides excellent support. An AL1 with or without a GuideLiner catheter is also commonly used.

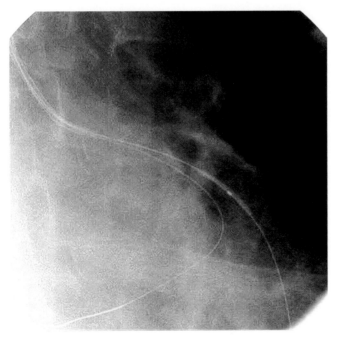

Figure 7.10 Buddy wire. A buddy wire in the target vessel or an adjacent vessel provides additional support.

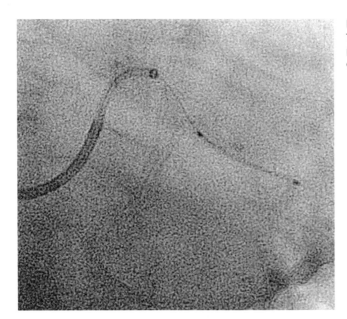

Figure 7.11 GuideLiner in 6-Fr guide. This system is commonly utilized to provide additional support for stenting complex lesions.

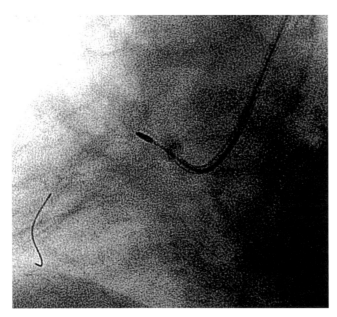

Figure 7.12 Rotational atherectomy with a 1.25-mm Burr performed through a 5-Fr 0.58-in ID Launcher MRADIAL catheter (Medtronic, Minneapolis, MN).

the entire procedure with a universal guide catheter to eliminate time-consuming catheter exchanges. This benefit is obviously negated if the coronaries cannot be expeditiously cannulated, and previous experience with these curves in elective procedures is mandatory. In these emergency procedures, catheter exchanges should be made over an exchange-length guidewire or a standard guidewire anchored in the right coronary cusp to avoid renegotiating subclavian tortuosity. STEMI is one clinical situation where 6-Fr guides are preferred because insertion of a thrombectomy catheter may be necessary.

If Burrs larger than 1.75 mm are required, a 7-Fr guide catheter should be inserted using the sheathless technique; it should be pointed out that the external diameter from a 7-Fr guide catheter is actually smaller than that of a 6-Fr sheath. Thrombectomy catheters including the AngioJet system are all compatible with 6-Fr guide catheters.

Guide catheter use in women requires special mention. In general, the radial artery is a small artery and more prone to spasm. Thus, smaller guide catheters are required, and operators should have a low threshold to repeat doses of spasmolytic agents if arm pain is encountered; intra-arterial verapamil is utilized in 3-mg increments. Straightforward interventions should be performed with 5-Fr guide catheters, which can be utilized in most women. If a 6-Fr guide is thought to be necessary, consideration of insertion using a sheathless technique is appropriate. For the smallest arteries, a 5-Fr guide catheter can be inserted sheathless using the 4-Fr Terumo glide catheter as an introducer.

In conclusion, patient selection, appropriate use of the right as opposed to left radial access, and thoughtful catheter selection are crucial to easing the transition to the radial approach. The benefits of transradial access are well documented but are fully experienced only with its routine use. A commitment to transradial access is essential.

■ SUMMARY

This chapter recognizes that patient selection, appropriate use of right as opposed to left radial access, and thoughtful catheter selection are crucial to easing the transition to the radial approach. The benefits of transradial access are well documented but are fully experienced only with its routine use. A commitment to transradial access is essential.

■ REFERENCES

1. Geijer H, Persliden J. Radiation exposure and patient experience during percutaneous coronary intervention using radial and femoral artery access. *Eur Radiol*. 2004;14:1674–1680.
2. Neill J, Douglas H, Richardson G, et al. Comparison of radiation dose and the effect of operator experience in femoral and radial arterial access for coronary procedures. *Am J Cardiol*. 2010;106:936–940.
3. Louvard Y, Ludwig J, Lefevre T, et al. Transradial approach for coronary angioplasty in the setting of acute myocardial infarction: a dual-center registry. *Catheter Cardiovasc Interv*. 2002;55:206–211.
4. Philippe F, Larrazet F, Meziane T, et al. Comparison of transradial vs. transfemoral approach in the treatment of acute myocardial infarction with primary angioplasty and abciximab. *Catheter Cardiovasc Interv*. 2004;61:67–73.
5. Saito S, Tanaka S, Hiroe Y, et al. Comparative study on transradial approach vs. transfemoral approach in primary stent implantation for patients with acute myocardial infarction: results of the test for myocardial infarction by prospective unicenter randomization for access sites (TEMPURA) trial. *Catheter Cardiovasc Interv*. 2003;59:26–33.
6. Hetherington SL, Adam Z, Morley R. Primary percutaneous coronary intervention for acute ST-segment elevation myocardial infarction: changing patterns of vascular access, radial versus femoral artery. *Heart*. 2009;95:1612–1618.
7. Pancholy S, Patel T, Sanghvi K, Thomas M, Patel T. Comparison of door-to-balloon times for primary PCI using transradial versus transfemoral approach. *Catheter Cardiovasc Interv*. 2010;75:991–995.
8. Weaver AN, Henderson RA, Gilchrist IC, Ettinger SM. Arterial access and door-to-balloon times for primary percutaneous coronary intervention in patients presenting with acute ST-elevation myocardial infarction. 2010;75:695–699.
9. Sciahbasi A, Romagnoli E, Burzotta F, et al. Transradial approach (left vs. right) and procedural times during percutaneous coronary procedures: TALENT study. *Am Heart J*. 2011;161(1):172–179.
10. Saito S, Ikei H, Hosokawa G, Tanaka S. Influence of the ratio between radial artery inner diameter and sheath outer diameter on radial artery flow after transradial coronary intervention. *Catheter Cardiovasc Interv*. 1999;46:173–178.
11. Hou I, Wei YD, Song J, et al. Comparative study of 4 French catheters using the ACIST variable rate injector system versus 6 French catheters using hand manifold in diagnostic coronary angiography via transradial approach. *Chin Med J*(Engl). 2010;123:1373–1376.
12. Pancholy S, Coppola J, Patel T, Roke-Thomas M. Prevention of radial artery occlusion - patent hemostasis evaluation trial (PROPHET study): a randomized comparison of traditional versus patency documented hemostasis after transradial catheterization. *Catheter Cardiovasc Interv*. 2008;72: 335–340.
13. Sanmartin M, Gomez M, Rumoroso, J, et al. Interruption of blood flow during compression and radial artery occlusion after transradial catheterization. *Catheter and Cardiovasc Interv*. 2007;70: 185–189.
14. Cubero J, Lombardo J, Pedrosa C, et al. Radial compression guided by mean artery pressure versus standard compression with a pneumatic device (RACOMAP). *Catheter and Cardiovasc Interv*. 2009;73:467–472.
15. Gilchrist I. Laissez-faire hemostasis and transradial injuries. *Catheter Cardiovasc Interv*. 2009;73:473.
16. Mamas MA, Fath-Ordoubadi F, Fraser DG. Atraumatic complex transradial intervention using large bore sheathless guide catheter. *Catheter Cardiovasc Interv*. 2008;72:357–364.

17. From A, Gulati R, Prasad A, Rihal CS. Sheathless transradial intervention using standard guide catheters. *Catheter Cardiovasc Interv.* 2010;76:911–916.

18. Ikari Y, Nagaoka M, Kim JY, Morino Y, Tanabe T. The physics of guiding catheters for the left coronary artery in transfemoral and transradial interventions. *J Invasive Cardiol.* 2005;17:636–641.

19. Ikari Y, Masuda N, Matsukage T, et al. Backup force of guiding catheters for the right coronary artery in transfemoral and transradial interventions. *J Invasive Cardiol.* 2009;21(11):570–574.

20. Bertrand O, Rao SV, Pancholy S, et al. Transradial approach for coronary angiography and interventions: results of the first international transradial practice survey. *J Am Coll Cardiol Intv.* 2010;3:1022–1031.

21. Mann T, Cubeddu G, Schneider J, and Arrowood M. Left internal mammary artery intervention: the left radial approach with a new guide catheter. *J Invasive Cardiol.* June 2000;12(6):298–302.

22. Burzotta F, Trani C, Hamon M, et al. Transradial approach for coronary angiography and interventions in patients with coronary bypass grafts: tips and tricks. *Catheter Cardiovasc Interv.* 2008;72: 263–272.

■ VIDEO LEGENDS

Video 7.1   Left coronary cannulation technique using universal catheter. A 5-Fr RBLBT (Cordis, Bridgewater, NJ) is positioned in the left coronary cusp and advanced to engage the left coronary.

Video 7.2   Cannulation of the left coronary with a universal catheter using the superior approach with a 5-Fr RBLBT (Cordis, Bridgewater, NJ). The curve is opened from above using a J-wire, and the catheter is advanced into the left coronary.

Video 7.3   Right coronary cannulation technique using universal catheter. The right coronary cusp is usually inferior to the left coronary cusp. Thus, engagement of the right coronary involves counterclockwise rotation and forward advancement into the right coronary artery.

chapter 8

Sheathless Transradial Intervention

Rajiv Gulati, MD, PhD

Aaron M. From, MD

Charanjit S. Rihal, MD

■ INTRODUCTION

Although it is becoming the standard in many catheterization laboratories, a limitation of transradial intervention has historically been the inability to perform 7- or 8-Fr interventions due to the inability of most radial arteries to accommodate large-caliber introducer sheaths. The outer diameter of introducer sheaths is approximately 2 Fr sizes larger than the outer diameter of the corresponding guide catheters (Figure 8.1). Using a guiding catheter alone (without an introducer sheath) allows for a larger internal lumen without a corresponding increase in outer diameter (Figure 8.1). An 8-Fr sheathless guide, with the same outer diameter as a 6-Fr sheath, will thus enable complex transradial intervention to be undertaken in most radial arteries. A similar strategy allows for 5- and 6-Fr sheathless interventions, equivalent to

the use of 3- and 4-Fr sheaths, in patients with small radial arteries or in those whom maintenance of radial patency is paramount.

■ DEVICES AND TECHNIQUES

Central to success with such an approach is to minimize trauma on insertion of the sheathless guiding catheter into the radial artery. In this regard, the Eaucath (Asahi Inc, Japan) is a custom-made commercial sheathless guiding catheter whose tapered central dilator provides a seamless transition between wire, dilator, and guiding catheter for atraumatic entry into the radial artery. More so, the guide has a hydrophilic coating along its entire length to aid with forward advancement and to minimize friction and risk of spasm with catheter torquing. The guiding catheters are available with 6.5- and 7.5-Fr inner working lumens and

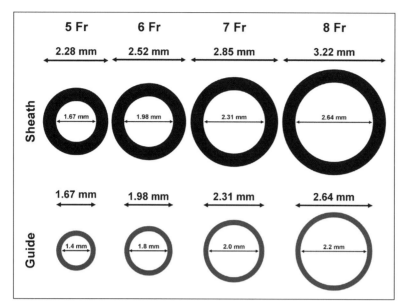

Figure 8.1 Example of a sheath to guide catheter comparison. In this example, the outer diameter of a 7-Fr guiding catheter is similar to that of a 5-Fr sheath but allows for a larger internal diameter. *Source:* From AM, Gulati R, Prasad, A, Rihal CS. Sheathless transradial intervention using standard guide catheters. *Cath Cardiovasc Interv.* 2010;76(7):911–916. Used with permission from Wiley.

carry the outer footprints equivalent to 5- and 6-Fr introducer sheaths. Although a number of series have shown feasibility and safety of these guides,[1,2] it should be noted that their cost is significantly greater than the cost of standard guides and that they are not available in all countries, including the United States.

It is also possible to use standard equipment available in all cath labs to fashion an inner dilator for use with standard guiding catheters.[3,4] Although we have not found spasm to be a limitation, the lack of a hydrophilic coating on standard guiding catheters makes this theoretically more likely to be an issue compared with the custom-made devices. Likewise, we have not yet encountered problems at the radial entry point, but the lack of a protective sheath raises the probability of hematoma formation or ongoing oozing during the procedure, particularly if significant guide torquing is required. Our approaches are as follows.

Larger-Caliber Guides

First, obtain access to the radial artery with a 5- or 6-Fr sheath in a standard manner. The entry site arteriotomy created by the sheath will facilitate subsequent guide advancement. Next, advance any diagnostic catheter into the aortic root and use this to switch for an exchange-length 0.035-in stiff guidewire. A regular wire will also work, but the stiff wire will serve as a stronger rail over which the guide/dilator can be advanced into the radial artery. To create a taper for standard 7- and 8-Fr guides of any configuration, insert a 125-cm 5- or 6-Fr multipurpose diagnostic catheter (Figure 8.2) or a 125-cm 6.5-Fr Shuttle Select hydrophilic catheter through the guide. The Shuttle catheter has a gentle taper on its tip and is therefore easier to pass through the skin than multipurpose diagnostic catheters and creates a smoother transition from diagnostic catheter to guide. After removing the sheath, advance the guide/dilator over the 0.035-in wire into the radial artery (Figure 8.3). It is helpful for the assistant to apply traction on the wire, actually physically pulling it back slowly, as this provides a taut rail that facilitates guide entry. A quick moderately forceful push may be required to enter the radial because the transition between wire, dilator, and catheter is not perfect. Remember to keep forward pressure on the dilator at the same time. Once the guide is in the radial artery, it can be advanced with its dilator and then used to cannulate the coronary in the usual manner. On occasion, there may be minor ooze at the skin entry site, but this will settle with a minute of gentle compression.

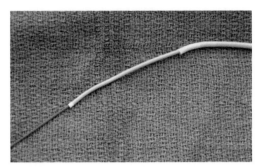

Figure 8.2 A 5-Fr diagnostic catheter inserted into and through a 7-Fr guiding catheter and over a 0.035-in standard J-tip wire for easier percutaneous insertion of the guiding catheter into the radial artery. *Source:* From AM, Gulati R, Prasad A, Rihal CS. Sheathless transradial intervention using standard guide catheters. *Cath Cardiovasc Interv.* 2010;76(7):911–916. Used with permission from Wiley.

Smaller-Caliber Guides

For 5- and 6-Fr sheathless guide insertion, first access the radial with a micropuncture kit and advance an exchange-length 0.035-in wire to the aortic root. The dilator that is associated with the greatest ease of guide catheter insertion is a 110-cm Cook 4-Fr sheath dilator through a 5-Fr guiding catheter (Figure 8.4). For a 6-Fr guide, a 5-Fr × 125-cm Shuttle Select diagnostic catheter also provides a reasonable transition. Alternatives include a 4-Fr 125-cm multipurpose diagnostic catheter or a 5-in-6 GuideLiner, but these require more forward push for successful guide entry to the radial artery.

■ CASE EXAMPLE

An 84-year-old female with a body mass index (BMI) of 18, history of mild chronic renal insufficiency, and chronic anemia presented with chest pain at rest, ST-segment depression in V2-V5, and a positive troponin-T. Despite immediate commencement of antiplatelet and anticoagulant therapy, she experienced recurrent chest pain with dynamic electrocardiogram (ECG) changes on the day of admission, prompting urgent angiography. A right radial approach was selected. After adequate intravenous sedation, a 6-Fr short hydrophilic sheath (Terumo) was placed uneventfully. A standard intra-arterial vasodilator cocktail and an activated clotting time (ACT)-guided

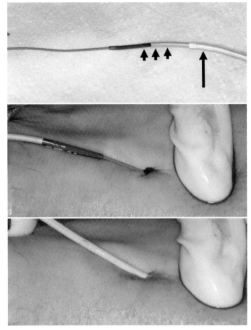

Figure 8.3 Tapering of a standard guide catheter for sheathless insertion in the radial artery using a telescoping shuttle select diagnostic catheter. *Source:* From AM, Bell MR, Rihal CS, Gulati R. Minimally invasive transradial intervention using sheathless standard guiding catheters. *Catheter Cardiovasc Interv.* 15 Nov 2011;78(6):866–871. Used with permission from Wiley.

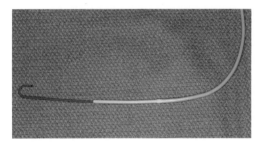

Figure 8.4 Tapering of a standard 6-Fr guide catheter for sheathless insertion into the radial artery by insertion of a 5-in-6 GuideLiner catheter (Vascular Solutions Inc, Minneapolis, MN) over a 0.035-in wire. *Source:* From AM, Bell MR, Rihal CS, Gulati R. Minimally invasive transradial intervention using sheathless standard guiding catheters. *Catheter Cardiovasc Interv.* 15 Nov 2011;78(6):866–871. With permission from Wiley.

intravenous heparin bolus were administered. Angiography with 5-Fr Judkins Left 3.5 and Judkins Right 4 diagnostic catheters indicated critical bifurcation disease in mid-left anterior descending (LAD) and second diagonal branch (Medina classification 0,1,1) with additional distal LAD disease (Figure 8.5a).

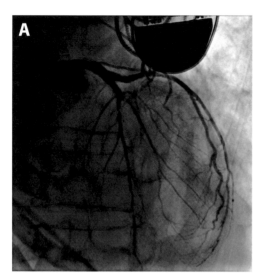
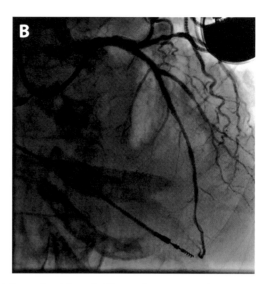

Figure 8.5 (**A**) Transradial left coronary angiography in the left anterior oblique (LAO) cranial projection indicating a critical LAD bifurcation stenosis. (**B**) Excellent final result after sheathless transradial intervention using an 8-Fr XB 3.5 guiding catheter. A simultaneous *V* stent approach was employed at the bifurcation with an additional distal LAD stent.

The decision was made to proceed with intervention using an 8-Fr sheathless guide, which carries approximately the same outer diameter as the in situ 6-Fr sheath. A 260-cm 0.035-in Amplatz extra-stiff wire was advanced to the aortic root. Following removal of the diagnostic catheter and sheath, an 8-Fr XB 3.5 Vista Brite Tip® guiding catheter (Cordis Corporation, Miami, FL) was advanced into the radial artery with a 6.5-Fr 125-cm Shuttle Select diagnostic catheter as the inner taper. To facilitate entry into the radial artery, the second operator applied back traction on the wire while maintaining forward pressure on the tapering Shuttle catheter within the guide. The guide and taper were advanced into the aortic root, and the taper was removed. Guide fit was good, and subsequent intervention was performed unremarkably. After predilation, the mid-LAD and second diagonal bifurcation were treated using simultaneously deployed stents in a V configuration. A distal LAD stent was then deployed with an excellent final result (Figure 8.5b). The guiding catheter was then removed over a standard 0.035-in wire, and a hemostasis band was applied in the usual manner. There were no issues with access site spasm or bleeding, and the radial artery was confirmed to be patent the following day.

■ SUMMARY

Sheathless guides are currently available outside the United States but not yet approved in the United States. This chapter explains how the sheathless technique can be utilized with currently available technology. As the guide's outer diameter is 2-Fr sizes smaller than the sheath, a 7-Fr guide used without a sheath can be exchanged, for example, for a 5-Fr sheath over a long guidewire without upsizing the access site. The advantages and disadvantages of this approach are discussed.

■ REFERENCES

1. Mamas MA, Fath-Ordoubadi F, Fraser DG. Atraumatic complex transradial intervention using large bore sheathless guide catheter. *Catheter Cardiovasc Interv*. 2008;72:357–364.
2. Mamas M, D'Souza S, Hendry C, Ali R, Iles-Smith H, Palmer K, El-Omar M, Fath-Ordoubadi F, Neyses L, Fraser DG. Use of the sheathless guide catheter during routine transradial percutaneous coronary intervention: a feasibility study. *Catheter Cardiovasc Interv*. 2010;75:596–602.
3. From AM, Gulati R, Prasad A, Rihal CS. Sheathless transradial intervention using standard guide cathe- ters. *Catheter Cardiovasc Interv*. 2010;76(7):911–916.
4. From AM, Bell M, Gulati R, Rihal CS. Minimally invasive transradial intervention using sheathless standard guiding catheters. *Catheter Cardiovasc Inter*. 15 Nov 2011;78(6):866–871.

chapter 9

Transradial Access and Outpatient PCI: State-of-the-Art and Persisting Challenges

Eltigani Abdelaal, MD
Olivier F. Bertrand, MD, PhD

■ INTRODUCTION

Percutaneous coronary intervention (PCI) is an integral part of tackling the global burden of coronary artery disease (CAD). Since its introduction more than 30 years ago, continuous refinement of PCI, coupled with constant evolution of adjunctive pharmaco-therapy, has dramatically increased its safety and success and resulted in a wider application of this technique.[1–3] Although the number of patients with stable angina undergoing PCI has relatively plateaued, the increased activity worldwide has been primarily due to an increased number of patients with acute coronary syndrome (ACS) referred for coronary intervention. This is supported by a large body of evidence showing improved outcomes with fast-track PCI compared with conservative medical therapy as shown in several multicenter, international trials.[4]

The growing number of PCI procedures worldwide, coupled with rising health care costs, has led to significant logistic constraints on hospitals. Therefore, strategies that drive down the cost of PCI, such as outpatient PCI practice, are contemplated, because they may facilitate treatment of more patients without significant increments in actual budget. Over the last 15 years or so, there has been a mounting body of compelling evidence from observational studies and a few randomized trials that outpatient PCI in selected groups of patients is perfectly feasible and safe.

Transradial Access: Techniques for Diagnostic Angiography and Percutaneous Intervention
©2013 Howard A. Cohen (Editor). Cardiotext Publishing, ISBN 978-1-935395-41-6.

Contemporary practice is moving increasingly toward outpatient practice in an unremitting endeavor to limit health care costs.

Historically, 2 main reasons were associated with hospitalization after PCI procedures, even when these were performed electively. The most commonly quoted reasons for overnight stay are fear of abrupt target vessel closure and acute stent thrombosis, with their associated morbidity and mortality, and the need for scrutiny of access site complications (for the transfemoral access). Besides, there are potentially other reasons as to why a traditional overnight hospitalization approach is often adopted, and these include legal, financial, psychosocial, and cultural reasons.

In this chapter, we attempt to systematically address all these facets and narrate in a chronological manner the mounting body of evidence, which has strongly built the case for outpatient PCI practice, not only from the transradial approach (TRA) but also with more conventional transfemoral access.

■ ISCHEMIC RISK IS NEGLIGIBLE IN CONTEMPORARY PCI PRACTICE

In the early days of percutaneous transluminal coronary angioplasty (PTCA), abrupt target vessel closure occurred in 5%–8% of patients treated with plain old balloon angioplasty (POBA), usually within the first 24 hours.[5] It usually follows vessel dissection, acute thrombus formation, or both, with important clinical consequences, including myocardial infarction, emergency coronary surgery, or death. Such an adverse event is usually evident in the first 6 hours post PTCA, with the incidence sharply falling thereafter,[6,7] and even more precipitously after 48 hours.[8] Furthermore, the advent of coronary stents has been associated with dramatic reduction in the incidence of abrupt target vessel closure. In the early days, this ischemic risk (of abrupt vessel closure or stent thrombosis) was closely linked not only to the clinical presentation but also to the angiographic appearance prior to balloon dilatation.

The rare but catastrophic event of stent thrombosis occurs in < 1% in the current era of PCI but remains associated with serious

clinical consequences.[9–11] Nonetheless, this usually occurs in the first 3 to 5 days post PCI and would therefore not be related directly to the chosen discharge strategy.[12]

■ TRANSRADIAL ACCESS: CONSISTENTLY LOWER RISK OF BLEEDING AND VASCULAR COMPLICATIONS

Traditionally, coronary angiography (CA) and PCI have been performed through femoral puncture, but in the late 1980s, a French Canadian physician, Dr. L. Campeau, introduced the radial approach. By 1992, Dr. Ferdinand Kiemeneij, the pioneer of transradial intervention, had already begun to experiment with techniques to perform coronary intervention via the TRA and demonstrated the safety and efficacy of TRA procedures.[13] Access site complications associated with the transfemoral approach (TFA) to PCI range from 3% to 5% and include bleeding, superficial or retroperitoneal hematomas, pseudoaneurysms, and arteriovenous fistulae. These have a detrimental effect on patient outcomes and inevitably delay ambulation, prolong hospitalization, and thereby increase the procedural cost. The TRA potentially eliminates or substantially reduces most of these complications, resulting in faster mobilization and quicker discharge.

There is currently a large body of evidence that transradial PCI is safer and potentially more cost-effective than transfemoral PCI.[14] Several randomized trials have demonstrated fewer access site complications after transradial compared with transfemoral PCI, even when femoral artery closure devices were used.[12,15] A more recent meta-analysis showed that the risk of bleeding and vascular complications was consistently lower for the TRA compared to the TFA.[16]

Over the past 15 years, the TRA for coronary procedures has continued to grow in popularity among the interventional community, although its penetration in clinical practice remains scattered. Whereas parts of Europe and Asia perform as high as 30%–40% of coronary interventions through the TRA, the uptake in the United States remains as low as 5%–10%. Parallel to the expected increase in the use of TRA in the United States, it can be anticipated that current reform in the US health care system will promote same-day-discharge programs as well. At this time, several reasons play a part in the limited utilization of the TRA in the United States; the most important is that only a relatively small percentage of interventional cardiologists in the United States are trained in this technique, although this is changing rapidly. Other reasons for this low penetration may include lack of financial incentive due to the reimbursement structure in US health care institutions and relative lack of patient knowledge that this alternative access exists. In addition, the relatively steep learning curve for transradial access probably plays a role as well. Most operators in the United States are "low-volume operators" performing fewer than 200 cases per year, making it difficult for them to learn and to feel comfortable with the technique. On the other hand, the high-volume operator may feel "too busy" to learn and apply transradial access to routine angiography and PCI.

■ SAME-DAY-DISCHARGE PCI: BUILDING THE EVIDENCE IN EARLY DAYS

The concept of outpatient PCI is not new. Over the past 2 decades, a series of registries and a number of randomized trials with same-day discharge after transradial PCI have been reported (Table 9.1). These studies utilized well-defined clinical criteria for carefully selecting patients who would be eligible for same-day discharge, and those who had predictors of adverse outcome were naturally excluded.

The upsurge in PTCA activity urged Laarman et al in the early 1990s to assess the practicality and safety of same-day discharge after uncomplicated transbrachial PTCA.[17] They tested the hypothesis that by carefully selecting a group of patients (stable angina) who are at low risk of postprocedural complications identified using pre- and post-PTCA criteria, these patients may

be discharged on the same day of procedure. Limited-risk PTCA was performed through the brachial artery using 6-Fr catheters in 61 patients (70 lesions); 2 were excluded due to failed access. Following this, patients with angiographic evidence of dissection and/or thrombosis and complications were assigned to an inpatient group, and those with good angiographic result were assigned to an outpatient group. Following successful PTCA, 50 patients (82%) with 57 lesions (81%) were considered eligible for discharge but remained hospitalized overnight without monitoring. No ischemic complications occurred in this group. Eleven patients (18%) in whom 13 lesions (19%) were attempted were assigned to the inpatient group. Three of these sustained abrupt vessel closure (2 within 1 hour of observation, and 1 just 20 minutes post PTCA). Out of all 61 patients, only 5 had vascular complications (despite using the brachial access and 6-Fr catheters), and 2 of those required local surgical repair. This pilot study highlighted the importance of defining patients at ischemic risk following PTCA and demonstrated the potential feasibility of discharging low-risk patients after a short observation period post PTCA.

Out of 1,911 elective PTCA patients, Knopf et al[18] stratified 262 (14%) as low-risk candidates for same-day discharge, and out of these, 90 patients (34%) were prospectively randomized to either an inpatient ($n = 47$) or an outpatient ($n = 43$) strategy. Similar procedural and clinical outcomes were observed in the 2 groups, with 33 out of 43 outpatients (77%) discharged on the same day of the procedure. Crucially, no late complications (between 1 and 7 days postprocedure) were observed in the outpatient group. A satisfaction survey of all patients and their families showed an overwhelming preference for same-day discharge. Similarly, Koch et al evaluated the safety of short-term observation (4 hr) after elective PTCA in a prospective study of 1,900 patients.[19] One of 1,680 patients triaged to discharge after 4 hours developed acute recurrent ischemia, and 7 patients (0.4%) required repeat PTCA during the observation period. Of the 187 patients assigned for overnight hospitalization, mainly due to suboptimal angiographic

Table 9.1 Published Studies of PCI with Same-Day Discharge.

Reference	Type of study	Number eligible/ number discharged	Access site	Anticoagulant	Time to discharge (hr)	Major complications in the first 24 hours	Comments
Kiemeneij et al.	SC, NR, P	188/100	Radial	Heparin, Coumadin	6	None	Palmaz-Schatz stent used; on Coumadin INR > 2.5
Koch et al.	SC, NR, R	1,015/922	Femoral	Heparin	~8		Many patients "discharged" back to referring hospital for care overnight; mostly balloon angioplasty; 20% received stents; manual compression
Carere et al.	SC, R, P	50/41	Femoral	Heparin	Mean 11.2	None	Suture closure of site and same-day discharge versus manual compression and discharge the following day; no difference in events
Slagboom et al.	SC, NR, P	159/106	Radial	Heparin	4–6	None	Balloon angioplasty alone in some patients; exclusions from early discharge defined
Gilchrist et al.	SC, NR, R	–/26	Radial	Heparin	Mean 6.5	None	Only stents used; 6-hr infusion of eptifibatide after bolus
Ormiston et al.	SC, NR, P	100/26	Femoral	Bivalirudin	Mean ~7	None	Restrictions to early discharge, but safe
Dalby et al.	SC, NR, P	70/51	Femoral	Heparin	~4	None	Angio-Seal closure used
Banning et al.	SC, NR, P	487/409	Femoral	Heparin	6–12	None	Manual compression, high patient satisfaction
Ziakas et al.	SC, NR, R	2,072/943	Radial	Heparin	~4	No serious complications	Outcome data self-reported by questionnaire sent to patients
Porto et al.	SC, NR, P	196/233	Femoral	Heparin	6–10	None	70% of PCIs were excluded, manual compression used, 5 patients discharged had an elevated troponin
Slagboom et al.	SC, NR, P	644/375	Radial/ Femoral	Heparin	4–6	1	Randomized radial versus femoral, exclusions from early discharge defined, 1 stent thrombosis with nonfatal MI after early discharge
Lasevich et al.	SC, NR, P	100/51	Femoral	Heparin	8–12	None	46 patients sent to "minimal care area" after PCI
Kumar et al.	SC, NR, P	150/120	Radial	Heparin	Unknown	1	Cases selected, incomplete abciximab infusions, 1 stent thrombosis with nonfatal MI
Bertrand et al.	SC, NR, P	504/444	Radial	Heparin + abciximab	4–6	None	Randomized to radial, bolus-only abciximab, and early discharge (n = 504) versus femoral, bolus, and infusion abciximab and overnight stay (n = 501)
Wiper et al.	SC, NR, R	442/378	Radial	Heparin	Mean 9.75	None	Abciximab used in some, mostly bolus-only
Heyde et al.	SC, R, P	403/326	Femoral	Heparin	~4	None	Randomized (n = 800) to early discharge versus overnight stay
Jabara et al.	SC, NR, R	450/12	Radial	Heparin	Unknown	None	No adverse events occurred between 6 and 24 hr with no discharge delays in this interval

MI, myocardial infarction; NR, not randomized; P, prospective data collection; PCI, percutaneous coronary intervention; R, retrospective data collection; SC, single center. *Source:* Modified from Blankenship JC. Here today, gone today: time for same-day discharge after PCI. *Catheter Cardiovasc Inter.* 2008;72:626-628. Reprinted with permission.

result, 66 developed complications. It could, therefore, be concluded that a short observation period after uncomplicated PTCA is safe, and a large proportion of patients could be safely discharged home the same day, with a trivial risk of recurrent ischemia (abrupt vessel closure) after this period. Similarly, based on the angiographic postprocedural result, patients could be triaged for overnight hospitalization as appropriate.

■ OUTPATIENT PCI IN THE ERA OF CORONARY STENTS

After the Laarman et al PTCA pilot study in 1994,[17] Kiemeneij and Laarman et al were keen to explore the feasibility of coronary Palmaz-Schatz stent implantation on an outpatient basis.[20] A total of 188 patients who underwent stent implantation through the radial artery were recruited between May 1994 and July 1995 for this prospective study. In the initial phase, patients received anticoagulation with Coumadin, and stenting performed at an international normalized ratio (INR) of > 2.5, but from December 1994 onward, patients were treated with aspirin and ticlopidine, and heparin was administered during the procedure. Suitability for same-day discharge was determined on the basis of pre-, post-, and periprocedural criteria. Of the 188 patients included, 88 were assigned for overnight hospitalization for various reasons. In the 100 outpatients, 110 lesions were covered with 125 stents, 92 patients were discharged home the same day, and 8 returned to their referring center. In the outpatient group, no cardiac or bleeding complications were encountered in the first 24 hours. At 2 weeks' follow-up, only 1 patient was readmitted (Day 4) due to a bleeding abdominal aortic aneurysm, which was treated surgically. The authors concluded that after an optimal-result Palmaz-Schatz coronary stent performed transradially, patients could safely be discharged home the same day.

Following their initial report of the safety of short-term observation of patients for 4 hours post PTCA, Koch et al[21] reported an update of their experience between January 1995 and May 1997. To evaluate the triage of patients

for short-term observation, and to study the predictors of failure of same-day discharge after elective PTCA, 1,015 consecutive patients were prospectively included for short-term observation, and patients with unstable angina Braunwald Class 3 were excluded. In all, 922 (90.8%) patients were selected for short-term observation and had an uncomplicated course for the next 72 hours. Observation was prolonged in 87 patients (8.6%), and 40 patients developed complications. Two patients died, including 1 of 6 patients who required emergency bypass surgery. Several independent predictors of procedural complications emerged from this study, including acute target vessel closure, side branch occlusion, ostial lesions, lack of angiographic success, and female sex. It is imperative to note that, despite its growing use during the study period, the rate of stenting was still very low at < 30%. Once again, this study showed the safety of a short 4-hour observation period after PTCA. Furthermore, it also emphasized the strength of procedural and periprocedural variables as predictors of complications, and that immediate procedural results can safely permit triage for short observation.

As PCI techniques evolved, the outpatient approach was also introduced with the transfemoral access. Wilentz et al[22] reported the use of vascular sealing devices, in conjunction with small transfemoral guiding catheters to decrease time to mobilization and achieve early discharge. They recruited both stable and unstable patients (unstable angina or positive ETT following a recent MI) into their study. Of the 50 patients originally recruited, 49 underwent vascular sealing, and 45 were safely discharged home the same day without ischemic or bleeding adverse events. One patient developed a femoral pseudoaneurysm requiring surgical repair.

In a retrospective study of 539 patients who underwent PCI in the province of Quebec between January 1997 and December 1999, via either femoral or radial approach, Clement-Major and Lemire[23] demonstrated that 383 patients (71%) were discharged home the same day, and 156 patients were hospitalized overnight after suboptimal PCI results. Although the use of stents was heterogeneous during the study period, ranging from < 25%

in the first 6 months to 75% in last 6 months, this analysis showed the feasibility and the potential safety of outpatient angioplasty.

Ziakas et al[24] described the first western Canadian experience on same-day discharge after transradial PCI. Between April 1998 and March 2001, a total of 943 had same-day-discharge radial PCI and represented patients with stable and unstable angina, single or multilesion PCI, and all types of lesion characteristics. Out of 943 patients who were discharged the same day of PCI, 811 responded to a mailed questionnaire, 38 patients had died, and 94 refused to participate. Within 24 hours post discharge, 27 patients (3.3%) visited their doctor and/or the hospital for access site–related complications, and 38 (4.6%) visited within 1 month. Notably, however, none of these patients had a major entry site complication or required hospital admission. Only 1 patient (0.1%) underwent a repeat coronary angiogram in the first 24 hours because of chest pain but did not require repeat intervention. During the first month, 11 patients (1.4%) needed a repeat coronary angiogram, out of which 4 had subacute vessel closure. Overall, 718 patients (89%) affirmed their satisfaction with same-day discharge.

As time evolved in the last decade, outpatient PCI was described in different scenarios, using both radial and femoral access, PTCA with or without stenting, and with or without glycoprotein IIb/IIIa inhibitors.

Carere et al[25] sought to determine whether immediate suture closure of 8-Fr femoral puncture site could facilitate same-day discharge after PCI. They randomly assigned 100 patients to immediate femoral arterial sheath removal and suture-based device closure versus delayed sheath removal with the application of a C-clamp. Following pertinent bed rest and subsequent mobilization, same-day discharge was possible in 41 patients (84%) assigned to a closure device, with economic analysis indicating potential hospital cost savings. Overall, patients preferred the suture closure method when they answered a simple questionnaire.

In 2001, Slagboom et al[6] reported the results of the OUTCLAS pilot study that tested the feasibility and safety of outpatient PCI in 159 patients treated with PTCA or coronary stent implantation exclusively performed through the radial artery using 6-Fr guiding catheters. This was intended to substantiate the significance of their sets of 7 clinical and 5 angiographic criteria barring same-day discharge. One hundred and six patients (66%) were selected for same-day discharge in the absence of any adverse predictors of acute/subacute vessel closure or unfavorable clinical outcome in the first 24 hours post successful PTCA. Despite the low use of stents, only 40% in total, there were no cardiac or vascular complications during the observation phase or up to 24 hours post PTCA in the outpatient group. One hospitalized patient had acute in-lab vessel occlusion, and 3 others required repeat PTCA during the observation period.

Following this, and utilizing these predefined clinical and angiographic predictors of adverse outcomes, Slagboom et al[7] went on to conduct a randomized trial in which 644 patients were randomly assigned to either transradial or transfemoral PTCA (322 in each group) using 6-Fr guiding catheters and same-day discharge. After successful PCI (62% were stented in both groups), 177 patients (55%) in the femoral group and 198 patients (61%) in the radial group were selected for same-day discharge based on the predefined set of predictors of an adverse outcome. Outpatient management appeared to be safe, with only 1 major adverse outcome (stent thrombosis) in 375 patients (0.3%) and 5 bleeding events (1.3%) in the first 24 hours after successful PCI. Predictably, more ischemic and bleeding events were observed in the higher-risk group staying in the hospital overnight, as 19 (7%) of the 269 patients sustained an adverse event.

■ TRADE-OFF BETWEEN ISCHEMIC AND BLEEDING RISK AND OUTPATIENT PCI

With the higher rate of stenting and inclusion of higher-risk patients, several registries and randomized studies have demonstrated the feasibility and safety of same-day discharge after successful PCI (through either the TRA or the TFA once hemostasis is achieved). Using a combination of clinical and angiographic criteria, patients identified to be at high risk remained hospitalized overnight.

As vascular complications and access site–related bleeding remained a substantial concern, however, the use of platelet glyco-protein IIb/IIIa inhibitors was still considered to be an exclusion criterion and prohibited same-day discharge.

Using a curtailed course of the intravenous antiplatelet agent eptifibatide, Gilchrist et al[26] explored the feasibility of same-day outpatient coronary stent implantation in 26 patients with both stable and unstable angina. Intervention was performed via the TRA using 5- or 6-Fr guiding catheters, and patients received a 6-hour infusion of eptifiba-tide. All patients were successfully discharged home the same day after a mean observation period of 6.5 hours, and neither vascular site complication nor readmission occurred.

In the RADICAL study, Kumar et al[27] reported their initial experience with a consecutive group of 150 patients referred for elective PCI for noncomplex coronary lesions. Following successful PCI, same-day discharge was possible in 80% of patients.

Using abciximab as a bolus-only, Wiper et al[28] reported a higher incidence of same-day discharge following transradial PCI compared to both OUTCLAS[6] and RADICAL[27] studies. They reviewed their experience of 442 consec-utive patients undergoing elective PCI over a 4-year period (between 2001 and 2005). Patients were selected for day-case tran-sradial PCI based on clinical (CCS 1-3) and angiographic criteria including Type A, B, and C lesions (as per NHLBI criteria), chronic total occlusion (CTO), and localized lesions in degenerate vein grafts. Bifurcation lesions were treated using 7-Fr guiding catheters. Patients requiring unprotected LMS inter-vention and those with ACS were excluded. Abciximab as a bolus-only was administered in 216 cases, used at operators' discretion, both electively and in "bailout" circumstances. PCI was successful in 95% of the cases, and 367 patients (83%) were discharged home the same day after minimum 4-hour observation period. There were no major or minor bleeding complications. Stent thrombosis occurred in 3 patients, leading to STEMI in 2 patients within 48 hours post PCI and 1 cardiac death

at 72 hours, confirmed on autopsy to be secondary to stent thrombosis.

Overall, these aforementioned studies demonstrated the feasibility and safety of same-day discharge after PCI, even when intravenous antiplatelet agents were used as a bolus-only or in an abbreviated protocol, in conjunction with the transradial approach. An important question remained unanswered: Was abciximab bolus-only, or an abbreviated treatment with eptifibatide equivalent to standard recommended protocols? To expand the utilization of outpatient PCI into a higher-risk group, a randomized trial to answer this question was required.

■ EVIDENCE FROM RANDOMIZED TRIAL—THE EASY STUDY: THE BUILDING BLOCK FOR A STRUCTURED OUTPATIENT CLINICAL PROGRAM

Published in 1994, the EPIC study (Evaluation of c7E3 for the Prevention of Ischemic Complications) long established the impor-tance of platelet aggregation in the occurrence of acute ischemic events in patients under-going PTCA.[1] It was shown that the adminis-tration of the monoclonal antibody c7E3 Fab directed against the platelet glycoprotein IIb/IIIa receptor as bolus, and infusion resulted in a 35% reduction in the composite-event rate compared to placebo, mainly in the rate of nonfatal MI and need for emergency PTCA or coronary artery bypass graft (CABG). The bolus-only approach resulted in only a 10% reduction compared to placebo. It was therefore recommended to prolong platelet inhibition by a 12-hour infusion of abciximab following a bolus. However, this was at the cost of an increase in bleeding complications. On close analysis, the worse outcomes in the EPIC bolus-only group were driven entirely by rates of urgent repeat revascularization at 30 days (3.6% bolus group vs. 0.8% bolus and infusion group, $P < 0.001$), a complication probably related to the lack of stent use at that time (< 1%).

This led to the conception in 2001 of the EASY trial (Early Discharge After Transradial Stenting of Coronary Arteries) by our group.[29] The investigators hypothesized that with coronary stent implantation and use of the transradial approach to PCI, abciximab as a bolus-only would be as effective as bolus and 12-hour infusion, and that a wider spectrum of low-, moderate-, and high-risk patients treated with bolus-only abciximab during PCI could be discharged home the same day. The study was conducted at Institut Universitaire de Cardiologie et de Pneumologie de Québec (IUCPQ) (formerly Laval Hospital, Quebec) between October 2003 and April 2005; this center began its transradial program in 1994 and to date has treated more than 70,000 patients through the radial access, making it one of the world's largest centers using this approach. Patients referred for cardiac catheterization with the view to proceeding to ad hoc PCI were eligible if they were > 18 years old and underwent successful transradial PCI. For clinical reasons, patients with any of the following were excluded: recent (< 72 hours) STEMI; history of EF < 30%; transient vessel closure or hemodynamic collapse during PCI; allergy or intolerance to aspirin or thienopyridine; INR > 2.0; or contraindication to abciximab.

During the study period, a total of 4,621 PCIs were performed. Of these, 3,277 clinically eligible patients were approached, but 1,929 were excluded for various reasons. Of the 1,348 remaining patients, all of whom received a standard bolus of abciximab with an uncomplicated ad hoc PCI with stent, 1,005 patients (75%) were randomized to either overnight hospitalization or early discharge after 4–6 hours of observation. All patients received aspirin, clopidogrel, and a bolus dose of abciximab prior to balloon dilation. In addition, only those assigned to overnight stay received a 12-hour infusion of abciximab. The remaining 343 patients (25%) who had unsuccessful PCI were entered into a registry and received a standard 12-hour infusion of abciximab overnight. Unsuccessful PCI was defined by persistent Type B or greater dissection, TIMI flow < 3, compromised side branch ≥ 1 mm, or thrombus.

The primary composite endpoint included any of the following 7 events at 30 days: death from any cause, Q- and non-Q-wave MI,

any unplanned revascularization (including PCI or CABG) for ischemia, major bleeding according to REPLACE-2 criteria (Randomized Evaluation in PCI Linking Angiomax to Reduced Clinical Events), rehospitalization for any cause related to index procedure, severe thrombocytopenia (platelets < 50,000), and access site complications. The overall population of this study was at moderate to high risk, as two-thirds of patients presented with unstable angina and 25% presented with ACS and positive troponins.

The primary composite endpoint, including ischemic and bleeding events, was equivalent in the 2 randomized groups. As expected, the registry patients with unsuccessful stenting had more events when compared with both randomized groups (34.1% with troponin T-based definition of MI, and 21% with CK-MB-based definition, $P < 0.0001$ for both). No death occurred during the 30-day follow-up period.

Indeed, the study also reported a very low overall rate of bleeding of 0.5% (1.4% when registry is included). This contrasts favorably with the contemporary benchmark for current incidence of bleeding complications, which exists in the control arm of the REPLACE-2 trial.[30] In this, the femoral approach was utilized, and major bleeding occurred in 4.1% of control patients receiving heparin and glycoprotein IIb/IIIa inhibitor, and in 2.4% after bivalirudin and provisional glycoprotein IIb/IIIa inhibitors.

The EASY study provided further resolute assurance to operators and referring physicians, and further consolidated the existing body of evidence in the literature stressing safety of the transradial approach. Decisively, however, it provided the building block for the development of a structured, clinical outpatient program for PCI.

In 2008, Jabara et al reported the results of the STRIDE study (Same-day TransRadial Intervention and Discharge Evaluation).[31] In this large observational study, conducted in a tertiary US center setting, 450 patients undergoing TR-PCI between 2004 and 2007 were included. The intention was to describe, in a US setting, the safety and cost-effectiveness of same-day discharge after TR-PCI. The primary endpoint was in-hospital adverse clinical outcomes between 6 and 24 hours postprocedure. Indications for intervention included stable angina (49%), unstable angina (31%), non-ST-elevation MI (NSTEMI, 17%), and STEMI (3%), with primary PCI performed in 11 cases. Fourteen percent of patients received GpIIb/IIIa inhibitors, and bivalirudin was used in 41%. In 450 patients, a total of 630 lesions were treated, and 540 stents were implanted. Of the lesions treated, 20% were complex, including chronic total occlusion (CTO), calcified lesions, and bifurcations (treated using 7-Fr catheters). The right transradial access was used in 99% of cases, and left radial and ulnar composed the remainder. Procedural success was 96%. In total, in-hospital adverse clinical events occurred in 24 patients (5.3%). Based on the timing of these events, they were divided into 3 groups: those that occurred between 0 and 6 hours, between 6 and 24 hours, and beyond 24 hours. Twenty postprocedural complications (4.4%) were observed during the first 6 hours, and 4 (0.9%) occurred after 24 hours. Crucially, no complications occurred between 6 and 24 hours (ie, the assessed time interval between same-day and following-day discharge). Minor access site–related bleeding complications were observed in 2.4% of patients in the first 6 hours and resolved with manual compression. Postprocedural MI occurred in 8 patients (1.8%), all within the first 6 hours post PCI. Four underwent repeat revascularization. Likewise, 4 patients (0.9%) suffered acute stent thrombosis in the first 6 hours, and all underwent successful revascularization without in-hospital mortality. Not surprisingly, all 4 patients were high risk, with initial indication for PCI being STEMI in 2 patients and NSTEMI in 2 patients. All had complex lesions.

In the third group (> 24 hours post PCI), procedural complications occurred in 4 cases: One patient suffered a cerebrovascular accident (CVA), and a second developed paroxysmal atrial fibrillation (PAF), 28 and 30 hours post PCI, respectively. A third patient was referred for CABG 2 days after unsuccessful PCI of a CTO, and the fourth (0.2%) patient died 3 days post complicated attempt at PCI

of a CTO. Fifty-seven patients (13%) had prolonged hospitalization, but only in 3.8% was the reason for this procedure related.

In this observational study, Jabara et al demonstrated that no ischemic or bleeding adverse events occurred between 6 and 24 hours, and no discharge delays occurred, further emphasizing the importance of a short observation period but also demonstrating the safety of this approach in selected patient groups. This was a key observation. Importantly, any adverse events occurring in the first 6 hours post PCI would have disqualified the patient from early discharge, and complications after 24 hours would not have been influenced by overnight hospitalization.

More recently, Rao et al[32] reported the prevalence and outcomes of same-day discharge after elective PCI among older patients in the United States. In this multicenter cohort study, data from 107,018 patients 65 years or older undergoing elective PCI procedures at 903 sites participating in the CathPCI Registry between November 2004 and December 2008 were included and divided into 2 groups based on their length of stay post PCI: same-day discharge or overnight stay. The primary endpoints for this study were death or rehospitalization for any cause occurring within 2 days of discharge and at 30 days. The 2 days' time was selected to reveal an early outcome that might be influenced by overnight observation. Other endpoints included procedural success, bleeding, and vascular complications.

Of the total 107,018 patients included, only 1,339 (1.25%) were discharged home on the same day after their elective PCI. Procedural characteristics varied between the 2 groups. Patients who were discharged home the same day underwent shorter, less complex procedures and received a lower contrast volume. Overall, the transfemoral approach was utilized in the majority of patients (97.7%), with transradial in 1.55% and brachial in the remainder. A slightly higher proportion of same-day-discharge patients underwent transradial interventions (3.14%) compared to the overnight group (1.55%). Adjuvant pharmacotherapy differed significantly between the groups, with fewer same-day-discharge patients receiving glycoprotein IIb/IIIa inhibitors or bivalirudin compared with overnight-stay patients.

The majority of hospitals discharged less than 3% of patients on the same day as their PCI, and the practice of same-day discharge varied significantly across PCI facilities in the United States. There was no significant difference between the groups in the incidence of primary endpoints of 2-day mortality or rehospitalization or 30-day rehospitalization, and extremely low rates of bleeding and vascular complications (< 1%).

■ CURRENT GUIDELINES FOR OUTPATIENT PCI PRACTICE

According to a published SCAI (Society for Cardiovascular Angiography and Interventions) statement[33] endorsed by the American College of Cardiology (ACC), same-day discharge can be considered in patients undergoing successful PCI stratified as low risk based on clinical criteria but without prolonged IV antithrombotic treatment and, especially in the elderly, those who have adequate social support. Major inclusion criteria include:

1. Stable angina on presentation without elevated cardiac biomarker preprocedure;

2. Asymptomatic, with an abnormal stress test;

3. Absence of significant comorbidities (including congestive heart failure [CHF], significant or symptomatic chronic obstructive pulmonary disease [COPD], symptomatic peripheral vascular disease [PVD], known bleeding diathesis or coagulopathy, significant other organ system disease, or history of contrast allergy);

4. Normal renal function (estimated glomerular filtration rate [e-GFR] ≥ 60 mL/min);

5. Normal or near-normal left ventricular ejection fraction (LVEF) in the absence of valvular regurgitation;

6. Fully loaded with a thienopyridine and no glycoprotein IIb/IIIa inhibitor used (the guidelines state that "the abbreviated bolus-only administration of glycoprotein IIb/IIIa inhibitors as has been used by some has not been adequately studied either in terms of safety or efficacy");

7. Single-vessel PCI with a < 28-mm stent, no balloon angioplasty alone or other interventional devices used;

8. Successful uncomplicated procedure without the occurrence of "no reflow," acute closure during the procedure, vessel dissection, or compromised side-branch flow; immediate postprocedure access site stabilization with the successful deployment of a closure device or secure manual compression, or PCI performed via radial artery access or brachial artery cutdown; and

9. A patient and family willing to consider early discharge, appropriate at-home support structure, and rapid access to a health care facility and advanced emergency services, should unexpected complications develop.

These recommendations appear extremely conservative, as numerous centers have developed same-day-discharge programs with higher-risk clinical scenarios and much more complex lesions. In the United States, Gilchrist et al[34] reviewed their own same-day-discharge experience according to the SCAI/ACC criteria. In their series of > 100 patients successfully discharged the same day of the procedure, < 15% would have qualified for same-day discharge if the SCAI/ACC criteria were strictly applied.

■ SETTING UP OUTPATIENT PCI PROGRAM

Outpatient PCI is both feasible and safe in selected patients as highlighted above, but the key to success is judicious selection of patients who would be eligible for this approach, based on both clinical and angiographic criteria. Prudence and adjudication is still required in the higher-risk patients receiving ASA, clopidogrel, and abciximab bolus.

Although outpatient PCI can be simply implemented, home discharge requires the allocation of suitable resources to develop a structured program. There are essential requirements for establishing a successful and safe outpatient PCI program:

1. Transradial approach is preferred to femoral approach ± vascular closure devices;

2. Triage criteria for suitable patients;

3. Dedicated and trained nursing and cath lab staff;

4. Optimal patient information (risk factors and medications) and education before and after PCI and before discharge;

5. Early (next-day) follow-up phone call to provide reassurance and early guidance and serve as a safety net; and

6. (Optional) Dedicated infrastructure (lounge).

Quality Assurance: "The Safety Net" and Beyond

Although the outpatient approach to PCI has lately been described also utilizing the transfemoral approach, there are many advantages on top of this of using the TRA as demonstrated in several randomized trials and meta-analyses, which show that the risk of access site bleeding and vascular complications is consistently lower with TRA. Other advantages of TRA include increased patient comfort and preference. It allows immediate mobilization of patients following PCI, reducing dependency on nursing staff and logistically creating more beds for sicker patients. It is clearly more cost-effective, leads to increased turnover and shorter waiting lists for PCI, and facilitates speedy return to work for the patient. Furthermore, TRA is particularly useful and safer for several patient groups, including the obese, the elderly, and restless patients, as well as those with severe peripheral vascular disease or with musculoskeletal disorders. The advantage of TRA is also abundantly clear in patients with ACS requiring heavy antiplatelet and antithrombotic therapy, as it is associated with less bleeding risk.

Judicious application of triage criteria for patients who would be eligible for same-day discharge after PCI could not be more emphasized. The major inclusion criteria for potentially suitable patients are outlined in the SCAI guidelines above, as based on several registries and 3 randomized trials of same-day discharge after PCI. The exclusion criteria for early discharge according to randomized trials of early discharge after PCI are summarized in Table 9.2.

Any outpatient program of PCI needs to be supported by adequately trained personnel to provide a "safety net" that is best suited for the particular local practice. An example would be a liaison nurse whose first role after completion of PCI would be to verify with the operator and referring physician whether the patient could be safely discharged. The liaison nurse would then meet with the patient and his or her family to organize discharge and address any logistic concerns. During the observation period of potential same-day-discharge patients, a liaison hospital pharmacist would check with the referring physician/hospital as to the exact list of medications that patient is already on, and with the operator as to the desired list of therapies the patient should remain on until the next follow-up appointment. Of particular relevance is the length of dual antiplatelet therapy, especially in the context of drug-eluting stents (DES), and patient education.

Prior to discharge, the liaison nurse verifies the absence of any procedural complications, schedules a telephone contact for the following day, and provides the patient with a procedural summary and leaflet detailing aspects of the procedure undertaken and the expected timeframe for recovery and return to work.

Of paramount importance are post-PCI patient rehabilitation and risk factor modification. The obvious risk, besides safety concern, of high-turnover PCI procedure is that aspects related to secondary prevention may be overlooked. However, a built-in quality control with dedicated personnel ensures that these important aspects are all appropriately addressed and emphasized. Beyond a safety

Table 9.2 Exclusion Criteria for Early Discharge in Randomized Reports of Early Discharge Following PCI.

Study	Carere et al.	Bertrand et al.	Heyde et al.
Clinical	Operator did not believe early discharge appropriate Clinical evidence of peripheral artery disease Preexisting femoral artery hematoma Serum creatine > 150 mmol/l BP > 180/100 mm Hg	Recent (< 72 hr) STEMI LVEF ≤ 30% Allergy or intolerance to aspirin or thienopyridines INR > 2.0 Contraindication to abciximab	Hospitalized patient Acute coronary syndrome Ad hoc PCI Need for long-term oral anticoagulation
Procedural		In-lab transient vessel closure during PCI Hemodynamic collapse during PCI Access other than radial artery PCI without stent placement Stented length > 25 mm in one vessel Compromised or suboccluded branch with diameter > 1 mm Residual dissection of ≥ B of NHLBI classification Persisting chest pain after PCI TIMI flow < 3 after stenting Entry site complication Thrombus after PCI Resuscitation before PCI	Catheters > 6 Fr GP IIb/IIIa inhibitors used Severe dissection with failed or suboptimal stent Occluded side branch Angiographic thrombus/no reflow Suspected guidewire perforation Suspected CVA
Social	Unspecified other factors		Lives > 60 min from PCI center Difficult follow-up Care person not available at home No transportation available

CVA, cerebrovascular accident; GP, glycoprotein; INR, international normalized ratio; LVEF, left ventricular ejection fraction; NHLBI, National Heart, Lung, and Blood Institute; STEMI, ST-segment elevation myocardial infarction; TIMI, thrombolysis in myocardial infarction; PCI, percutaneous coronary intervention.

net to ensure short- as well as long-term safety of such patients, a built-in feedback and follow-up program to ensure patient and family satisfaction is also vital.

Radial Lounge

A dedicated "Radial Lounge" for patients' recovery following transradial procedures can significantly enhance the patients' experience, save money, and reduce workload on hospital staff. Inspired by an idea from a KLM airport lounge, Dr. Ferdinand Kiemeneij, Department of Interventional Cardiology, Onze Lieve Vrouwe Gasthuis, Amsterdam, The Netherlands, created the first "elite-class," airport-like lounge, dedicated radial access recovery room in Europe (see Figure 9.1). His idea was to create a café-like atmosphere, with reclining chairs (instead of beds) and Internet access, where independently ambulant radial PCI patients will be able to surf the net and be less anxious about having an invasive procedure.

Following their successful experience, more and more health institutions in Europe, Asia, and North America have adopted this patient-friendly and cost-effective approach of a dedicated minimalistic recovery lounge, moving away from the sterile look of traditional hospitals to a warm, inviting, and friendly atmosphere, which immediately makes patients feel more comfortable and in control (see Figure 9.2).

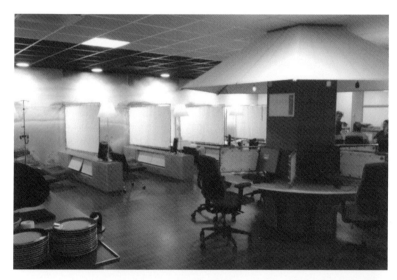

Figure 9.1 The first warm and inviting, airport-like radial lounge in Europe created for the Department of Interventional Cardiology, Onze Lieve Vrouwe Gasthuis, Amsterdam (The Netherlands). Photo courtesy of Dr. Ferdinand Kiemeneij.

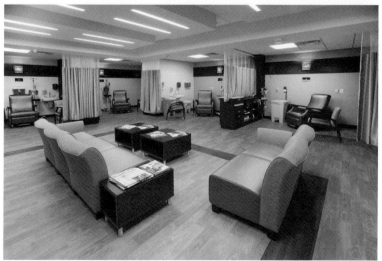

Figure 9.2 Lounge design by Dr. Jack Chen. Photo courtesy of St. Joseph's Hospital in Atlanta, GA.

Brewster et al reported their first-year experience after the introduction of such a lounge in a tertiary center in London, UK (*European Heart Journal* [2011] 32 [Abstract Supplement, 399]). During the 1-year study period, 1,548 patients were managed in the radial lounge. Of these, 1,109 patients underwent coronary angiography, 114 of whom also underwent PW study or intravascular ultrasound (IVUS), and 439 had PCI. The latter was performed radially in 81.8%, allowing same-day discharge in 84.7%. No postprocedural complication was observed in the radial lounge during the observation period prior to discharge. In Pilsen Hospital (Czech Republic), elective patients are offered to transit only through a dedicated radial lounge. Every day, 4 patients are treated in this more relaxed environment. This further emphasizes the fact that a dedicated radial lounge free of cardiac monitors is a safe environment in which the majority of patients undergoing elective PCI procedures could be managed.

■ SUMMARY

In summary, same-day-discharge practice after uncomplicated PCI is both safe and extremely effective in selected patients. In this regard, the transradial approach offers a tremendous advantage over the conventional femoral approach as hemostasis can be obtained while the patient is already ambulatory. As hemostasis is usually completed within 2 hours of radial access, it remains prudent to have an observation period of 4 to 6 hours to detect any severe complications prior to hospital discharge. Because a recent survey revealed that less than 50% of radial operators in the world discharge patients the same day of the procedure,[35] several nonmedical issues and obstacles remain to be resolved in order to promote outpatient practice.

■ REFERENCES

1. Use of a monoclonal antibody directed against the platelet glycoprotein IIb/IIIa receptor in high-risk coronary angioplasty: the EPIC Investigation. *N Engl J Med*. 1994;330:956–961.

2. Platelet glycoprotein IIb/IIIa receptor blockade and low-dose heparin during percutaneous coronary revascularization: the EPILOG Investigators. *N Engl J Med*. 1997;336:1689–1696.

3. Umans VA, Kloeg PH, Bronzwaer J. The CAPTURE trial. *Lancet*. 1997;350:445.

4. Braunwald E, Antman EM, Beasley JW, et al. ACC/AHA guideline update for the management of patients with unstable angina and non-ST-segment elevation myocardial infarction—2002: summary article: a report of the American College of Cardiology/American Heart Association Task Force on Practice Guidelines (Committee on the Management of Patients With Unstable Angina). *Circulation*. 2002;106:1893–1900.

5. Lincoff AM, Popma JJ, Ellis SG, et al. Abrupt vessel closure complicating coronary angioplasty: clinical, angiographic and therapeutic profile. *J Am Coll Cardiol*. 1992;19:926–935.

6. Slagboom T, Kiemeneij F, Laarman GJ, et al. Actual outpatient PTCA: results of the OUTCLAS pilot study. *Catheter Cardiovasc Interv*. 2001;53:204–208.

7. Slagboom T, Kiemeneij F, Laarman GJ, van der Wieken R. Outpatient coronary angioplasty: feasible and safe. *Catheter Cardiovasc Interv*. 2005;64:421–427.

8. Rodes J, Tanguay JF, Bertrand OF, et al. Late (> 48 hr) myocardial infarction after PTCA: clinical and angiographic characteristics of infarction related or not to the angioplasty site. *Catheter Cardiovasc Interv*. 2001;53:155–162.

9. Cutlip DE, Baim DS, Ho KK, et al. Stent thrombosis in the modern era: a pooled analysis of multicenter coronary stent clinical trials. *Circulation*. 2001;103:1967–1971.

10. Urban P, Gershlick AH, Guagliumi G, et al. Safety of coronary sirolimus-eluting stents in daily clinical practice: one-year follow-up of the e-Cypher registry. *Circulation*. 2006;113:1434–1441.

11. Iakovou I, Schmidt T, Bonizzoni E, et al. Incidence, predictors, and outcome of thrombosis after successful implantation of drug-eluting stents. *JAMA*. 2005;293:2126–2130.

12. Mann T, Cowper PA, Peterson ED, et al. Transradial coronary stenting: comparison with femoral access closed with an arterial suture device. *Catheter Cardiovasc Interv*. 2000;49:150–156.

13. Kiemeneij F, Laarman GJ. Percutaneous transradial artery approach for coronary stent implantation. *Cathet Cardiovasc Diagn*. 1993;30:173–178.

14. Cooper CJ, El-Shiekh RA, Cohen DJ, et al. Effect of transradial access on quality of life and cost of cardiac catheterization: a randomized comparison. *Am Heart J*. 1999;138:430–436.

15. Choussat R, Black A, Bossi I, et al. Vascular complications and clinical outcome after coronary angioplasty with platelet IIb/IIIa receptor blockade: comparison of transradial vs. transfemoral arterial access. *Eur Heart J*. 2000;21:662–667.

16. Agostoni P, Biondi-Zoccai GG, de Benedictis ML, et al. Radial versus femoral approach for

percutaneous coronary diagnostic and interventional procedures: systematic overview and meta-analysis of randomized trials. *J Am Coll Cardiol.* 2004;44:349–356.

17. Laarman GJ, Kiemeneij F, van der Wieken LR, et al. A pilot study of coronary angioplasty in outpatients. *Br Heart J.* 1994;72:12–15.

18. Knopf WD, Cohen-Bernstein C, Ryan J, et al. Outpatient PTCA with same day discharge is safe and produces high patient satisfaction level. *J Inv Cardiol.* 1999;11:290–295.

19. Koch KT, Piek JJ, de Winter RJ, et al. Short-term (4 hours) observation after elective coronary angioplasty. *Am J Cardiol.* 1997;80:1591–1594.

20. Kiemeneij F, Laarman GJ, Slagboom T, van der Wieken R. Outpatient coronary stent implantation. *J Am Coll Cardiol.* 1997;29:323–327.

21. Koch KT, Piek JJ, Prins MH, et al. Triage of patients for short term observation after elective coronary angioplasty. *Heart.* 2000;83:557–563.

22. Wilentz JR, Mishkel G, McDermott D, et al. Outpatient coronary stenting using the femoral approach with vascular sealing. *J Inv Cardiol.* 1999;11:709–717.

23. Clement-Major S, Lemire F. Is outpatient coronary angioplasty and stenting feasible and safe? Results of a retrospective analysis. *Can J Cardiol.* 2003;19:47–50.

24. Ziakas AA, Klinke BP, Mildenberger CR, et al. Safety of same-day-discharge radial percutaneous coronary intervention: a retrospective study. *Am Heart J.* 2003;146:699–704.

25. Carere RG, Webb JG, Buller CE, et al. Suture closure of femoral arterial puncture sites after coronary angioplasty followed by same-day discharge. *Am Heart J.* 2000;139:52–58.

26. Gilchrist IC, Nickolaus MJ, Momplaisir T. Same-day transradial outpatient stenting with a 6-hr course of glycoprotein IIb/IIIa receptor blockade: a feasibility study. *Catheter Cardiovasc Interv.* 2002;56:10–13.

27. Kumar S, Anantharaman R, Das P, et al. Radial approach to day case intervention in coronary artery lesions (RADICAL): a single centre safety and feasibility study. *Heart.* 2004;90:1340–1341.

28. Wiper A, Kumar S, MacDonald J, Roberts DH. Day case transradial coronary angioplasty: a four-year single-center experience. *Catheter Cardiovasc Interv.* 2006;68:549–553.

29. Bertrand OF, De Larochelliere R, Rodes-Cabau J, et al. A randomized study comparing same-day home discharge and abciximab bolus only to overnight hospitalization and abciximab bolus and infusion after transradial coronary stent implantation. *Circulation.* 2006;114:2636–2643.

30. Lincoff AM, Bittl JA, Harrington RA, et al. Bivalirudin and provisional glycoprotein IIb/IIIa blockade compared with heparin and planned glycoprotein IIb/IIIa blockade during percutaneous coronary intervention: REPLACE-2 randomized trial. *JAMA.* 2003;289:853–863.

31. Jabara R, Gadesam R, Pendyala L, et al. Ambulatory discharge after transradial coronary intervention: preliminary US single-center experience (Same-day TransRadial Intervention and Discharge Evaluation, the STRIDE Study). *Am Heart J.* 2008;156:1141–1146.

32. Rao SV, Kaltenbach LA, Weintraub WS, et al. Prevalence and outcomes of same-day discharge after elective percutaneous coronary intervention among older patients. *JAMA.* 2011;306: 1461–1467.

33. Chambers CE, Dehmer GJ, Cox DA, et al. Defining the length of stay following percutaneous coronary intervention: an expert consensus document from the Society for Cardiovascular Angiography and Interventions. Endorsed by the American College of Cardiology Foundation. *Catheter Cardiovasc Interv.* 2009;73:847–858.

34. Gilchrist IC, Rhodes DA, Zimmerman HE. A single center experience with same-day transradial-PCI patients: a contrast with published guidelines. *Catheter Cardiovasc Interv.* 2011.

35. Bertrand OF, Rao SV, Pancholy S, et al. Transradial approach for coronary angiography and interventions: results of the first international transradial practice survey. *JACC Cardiovasc Interv.* 2010;3:1022–1031.

chapter 10

Transradial Access for PCI in Acute Myocardial Infarction

Sameer J. Khandhar, MD

Oscar C. Marroquin, MD

Suresh R. Mulukutla, MD

◼ INTRODUCTION

Acute coronary syndromes (ACS) consist of both ST-segment elevation myocardial infarctions (STEMI) and unstable angina/non-ST-segment elevation myocardial infarction (NSTEMI). Although the optimal strategy has not yet been fully defined for ACS, an invasive approach, primarily driven by percutaneous coronary intervention (PCI), has become the cornerstone of therapy. The most recent American College of Cardiology (ACC) and American Heart Association (AHA) practice guidelines recommend initiation of anticoagulation to inhibit platelet aggregation and thrombin formation combined with revascularization when warranted. Rapid revascularization in less than 90 minutes from presentation is strived for in STEMI patients,[1] and an early invasive strategy is preferred for moderate- to high-risk NSTEMI patients.[2] These evolving strategies of revascularization and anticoagulation have significantly decreased the morbidity and mortality associated with ACS.

Years ago, ischemic complications dominated outcomes after intervention for ACS. Therefore, bleeding at either access site or elsewhere was largely ignored or thought to be an unavoidable necessity to reduce events such as myocardial infarction (MI) and stent thrombosis. These ischemic events have become less common as treatment regimens have advanced, and more attention is now given to bleeding as we acknowledge its association with adverse events. Additionally, the Centers for Medicare & Medicaid Services (CMS) have included bleeding postcardiac catheterization as an indicator of quality, and it may ultimately be linked with reimbursement for procedures (see Chapter 14).

Transfemoral access historically has been the preferred method of access for PCI in the United States over the past 30 years. Despite comfort with femoral access, it remains one of the most common sites of bleeding.[3-11] The relationship between bleeding complications and poor outcomes has now made prevention a priority. A major strategy to reduce bleeding is radial arterial access because it is a superficial artery that is easily compressible. Performing PCI by means of radial access can be challenging initially and require training and experience in the nonacute setting to gain proficiency. However, ACS patients have a higher risk of bleeding, and therefore, despite the technical challenges, performing PCI by means of the radial artery may improve outcomes. Given the potential benefit of radial access in ACS, considerable research has been done to answer concerns of whether the radial approach can be performed safely and effectively. Specifically, these studies address whether equal rates of success can be achieved while effectively reducing major adverse cardiac events (MACE) without a delay in door-to-balloon times or need for crossover to femoral access.

This chapter is dedicated to reviewing (1) the procedural component of performing radial catheterizations in the ACS setting, (2) the harmful effects of bleeding, and (3) the role of radial access in acute coronary syndromes.

■ TRENDS IN ACS MANAGEMENT

It is currently estimated that there are about 1.1 million hospitalizations a year in the United States for ACS, and between 29% and 48% of these are for STEMI.[12] This is despite a decline in the overall number of MIs in the past decade due to advancements in medical therapy.

More than 90% of patients presenting with ACS now receive the combination of aspirin and at least 1 anticoagulant, and more than 80% receive thienopyridine-based therapy.[14-15] In addition, revascularization rates have increased to 70%–80% of STEMI and 50%–55% of NSTEMI patients. Thrombolytic use has significantly decreased over time, and even STEMI patients initially treated with those thrombolytics are more often referred for cardiac catheterization. Increasing revascularization and more aggressive utilization of antiplatelet and antithrombotic agents over the past decade have led to an important reduction in cardiogenic shock, recurrent ischemia, and 30-day mortality rates from 10.5% to 7.8% ($P < 0.001$), after ACS.[13-15] We have clearly witnessed the benefits of modern-day therapy; however, strategies to identify patients at risk of bleeding and to reduce their risk are critical.

Transradial Access in ACS

As revascularization rates have grown, the majority of cases worldwide (80%) and in the United States (98%) continue to be performed via femoral access.[16-17] There is great variability in radial access use between countries and regions, with Japan and France performing the highest percentage at 60% and 55%, respectively.[17] The use of radial access has grown recently, albeit slowly, especially in the United States. It is also important to note that these numbers are for all coronary interventions, and reports show lower usage rates in ACS patients despite potentially having a greater benefit in this group. The reason for slow adaptation to radial access revolves around the fact that most interventionalists and laboratory personnel are trained and comfortable with femoral access. Only lately has there been a focus in fellowship training to teach radial artery access, and most recently even simulation-based learning has been developed specifically for this purpose.

■ PROCEDURAL ASPECTS

In this section, we will review techniques and recommendations for use of transradial access (TRA) in coronary interventions for ACS. Detailed descriptions of the technique are described in earlier chapters, and from a procedural standpoint, many aspects of performing PCI by means of radial access for ACS are similar to the elective setting. Conversely, performing PCI in this setting can be more challenging and carry greater risk than in an elective case. Rapid and successful revascularization is essential, and therefore it is prudent to be comfortable and proficient with TRA prior to attempting its use for ACS. Studies have shown that there is a learning curve with TRA, and we recommend that operators be proficient with TRA in the elective setting prior to attempting TRA in ACS patients and particularly in STEMI patients. There is no formal training requirement, but based on studies, at least 50 cases are required for proficiency. For most operators, performing 50–100 cases appears to significantly increase success rates to 98% while decreasing procedure times, contrast use, and radiation exposure.[18–21] (See Chapter 13 on the learning curve for TRA.) ACS patients stand to benefit the most, but these are also the patients at highest risk. Operators should feel totally comfortable with all aspects of the technique prior to utilizing in this high-risk cohort.

In the ACS setting, it is imperative that the operator and the staff are comfortable with radial access as the RIVAL trial demonstrated that centers with the highest radial volumes achieved the best outcomes.[22] Just as it is important for the operator to be well trained, it is crucial that the staff be trained with radial access cases prior to use in ACS.

Medication and Anticoagulation

Regional practices for anticoagulation vary greatly when treating ACS. We recommend that once a patient is identified as having ACS, aspirin, a thienopyridine, and an antithrombotic be administered in conjunction with ACC/AHA guidelines.[1–2] Forms of antithrombotics supported by the ACC/AHA include unfractionated heparin, low-molecular-weight heparin, and bivalirudin. Bivalirudin in the ACUITY[23–24] and HORIZONS-AMI[25] trials was associated with a decrease in bleeding and improvement in outcomes. The concept of combing radial access with bivalirudin is very appealing to prevent both access site and non-access site bleeding, though further data are needed to define the potential benefit and cost-effectiveness of this strategy.

Please refer to Chapter 5 for the combination of medications to prevent spasm and radial artery thrombosis. Intra-arterial nitroglycerin and calcium channel blockers should be used cautiously in patients with low blood pressures or in cardiogenic shock due to their ACS as this can worsen hypotension. At the conclusion of the case, the sheath should be removed, and a hemostasis device of choice should be placed.

Technique

When the patient arrives emergently for PCI in the ACS setting, we quickly obtain consent and transfer the patient to the catheterization table. Usually preparing the arm for a radial approach can be done simultaneously as the patient, the equipment, and the catheterization lab are being readied. Radial arterial access can be obtained once the patient's arm is sterilized, even before the drapes over the rest of the body are placed. We do recommend also sterilizing and preparing the femoral region in the event that need for crossover or additional mechanical assistance is required.

Choice of right or left radial artery is based on the discretion of the performing physician and patient preference as both have similar success rates and procedural times.[26] Once access is obtained, we usually reposition the arm next to the patient's body and begin the procedure. Most PCI equipment including aspiration catheters, balloons, and stents will fit through a 6-Fr system; therefore, we recommend placing a 6-Fr radial sheath as the initial sheath in acute MI patients. This avoids complications related to sheath exchange especially given that less than 10% of PCIs worldwide are performed with a 5-Fr system.[27] It is operator choice whether to start with diagnostic catheters or to start with a guiding catheter appropriate for the suspected infarct artery.

In a worldwide survey, the Judkins Right guiding catheter was preferred for right coronary artery (RCA) interventions, and extra backup guiding catheters such as the EBU 3.5 (Medtronic, Minneapolis, MN) or XB 3.5 (Cordis, Bridgewater, NJ) were preferred for the left coronary system.[27] The Ikari guides (Terumo, Somerset, NJ) are also gaining popularity and offer additional backup support compared to the Judkins catheters. Once proper guide position is obtained, the remainder of the procedure is similar compared to the femoral route. It is important when performing PCI through radial access to be flexible in choice of guiding catheters and to adapt to allow for the best fit and support. Familiarity with various guiding catheters allows the operator to select the best guide for a particular clinical scenario. Gaining experience with various guides during non-ACS cases when time to reperfusion is not as critical allows one to gain comfort prior to attempting radial access in ACS.

We advocate for also sterilizing and preparing the groin for femoral arterial access up front in the event crossover or additional access is necessary. Especially as operators are gaining experience with TRA, having the femoral artery accessible allows for quick conversion if necessary. Up to 10% of early cases may require crossover, and if the femoral site is already prepared and draped, additional time is not wasted. Also, in the event of hemodynamic instability, having the femoral artery site easily accessible can allow for prompt insertion of additional support such as intra-aortic balloon pump, Impella (Abiomed, Danvers, MA), TandemHeart (CardiacAssist, Pittsburgh, PA), or extra-corporeal membrane oxygenation (ECMO).[28] Use of femoral arteries for mechanical support in conjunction with radial access for PCI also has several benefits in the setting of cardiogenic shock. First, in the event of acute collapse, guide catheter and wire position does not have to be sacrificed for arterial access to insert additional support. And second, the most common complications with mechanical support are access site related and from poor distal extremity perfusion. When mechanical support and PCI are performed by the femoral route, both lower extremities are at jeopardy for complications related to poor perfusion, whereas utilizing the radial artery for the PCI component only puts 1 lower extremity at risk for hypoperfusion and allows the operator to choose the leg with better perfusion.

Radial access should not be dismissed in ACS, as its benefit may be larger in this population that is at higher risk for bleeding. However, prior to attempting radial access for PCI in the ACS setting, it is important that operators and staff be comfortable and proficient with this means of access.

■ BLEEDING IN ACS

The principal benefits of TRA revolve around reducing bleeding, so it is important to understand the consequences of bleeding when it occurs in this setting. In this section, we will review bleeding specifically in the ACS setting, whereas other chapters discuss in detail bleeding complications during and after PCI. Historically, the cardiology community has focused its efforts on strategies to reduce mortality associated with ACS by lowering ischemic events, and until recently, little attention was paid to bleeding and its potential negative role in outcomes.

The notion that bleeding or need for blood transfusion after PCI was associated with poor outcomes including death was starting to be accepted based on registry and retrospective data; however, OASIS-5 was the first randomized study to support this.[29] This brought scientific and public attention to the detrimental effects of bleeding and began the search for bleeding avoidance strategies.

Contemporary studies have now clearly shown that bleeding and transfusions after PCI for ACS are associated with an increase in mortality and other MACE such as repeat ischemic events, stent thrombosis, and stroke.[30-31] The effect of bleeding and anemia on outcomes is complex and multifactorial. Despite advances in our understanding of the harm associated with bleeding, further research is still warranted on the true incidence of bleeding, the significance of the site of bleeding, and mechanistically how bleeding leads to adverse outcomes.

Comparing bleeding events between trials is difficult because important variables differ significantly. These include clinical presentation for PCI (stable coronary artery disease, NSTEMI, or STEMI), choice of arterial access site, anticoagulation strategy (antiplatelet and antithrombotic) being utilized, and perhaps most importantly the definition of bleeding. Despite attempts to control for these variables, comparing results between trials is difficult and may lead to error.

Periprocedural bleeding is in large part related to access site and the anticoagulation regimen utilized during the procedure. Of bleeding events, 30%–70% are related to femoral access site,[3–11] although bleeding does occur at other sites such as the gastrointestinal tract, genitourinary system, and intracranial. Causality of femoral access site bleeding and death has not been firmly established. However, bleeding does lead to patient dissatisfaction and morbidity, and may affect mortality. Patients certainly find radial access more comfortable and prefer this method of access.[22] Ultimately, if we can identify which

patients are most susceptible to bleeding and associated harmful consequences, a bleeding avoidance strategy such as TRA can be implemented to improve clinical outcomes.

Definitions of Bleeding

Table 10.1 summarizes the definition of bleeding from various trials, and demonstrates how some are based on clinical events while others are based on lab values. Again, these differences make the comparison of definitions difficult. Combining data from various trials and implementing a single definition further support that all levels of bleeding are associated with mortality,[30,32] and consistent across studies is that the more severe the bleeding, the greater the risk of death as seen in Figure 10.1. However, there

Table 10.1 Bleeding Definitions from Major Trials.

ACUITY DEFINITION[24]	
Major	ICH, intraocular, access site bleed requiring intervention, hematoma > 5 cm, Hgb drop > 4 g/dL without source, or > 3g/dL with source
CRUSADE[35]	
Any transfusion	
GRACE DEFINITION[11]	
Major	ICH, life threatening, transfusion > 2 units, hematocrit drop > 10%, death
GUSTO DEFINITION[10]	
Mild	Bleeding that does not meet criteria for moderate-severe
Moderate	Requires blood transfusion but no hemodynamic compromise
Severe	ICH, causes hemodynamic compromise, or requiring intervention
OASIS-5 DEFINTION[29]	
Minor	Clinically significant but does not meet definition of major, and leads to interruption of study drug for > 24 hours, surgical intervention, or transfusion of 1 unit of PRBC
Major	Fatal, symptomatic ICH, RP, intraocular leading to vision loss, decrease in Hgb > 3 g/dL adjusted for transfusion, or requiring transfusion of >2 units
TIMI DEFINITION[85]	
Minimal	Any sign of bleeding but decrease in Hgb of < 3 g/dL
Minor	Observed bleeding with decrease in Hgb 3–5 g/dL, unobserved bleeding but decrease in Hgb > 4 g/dL, hematuria, or hematemesis
Major	Decrease in Hgb > 5 g/dL or any ICH
NCDR[16]	Hematoma > 10 cm, RP, GI, GU, transfusion, prolonged hospital stay due to bleed or Hgb drop > 3 g/dL
RIVAL-major[22]	Fatal bleed, transfusion > 2 units, hypotension requiring inotropes, surgical intervention, disabling sequelae, ICH, intraocular

ICH: intracranial bleed, Hgb: hemoglobin g/dL, RP: retroperitoneal bleed, GI: gastrointestinal bleed, GU: genitourinary bleed.

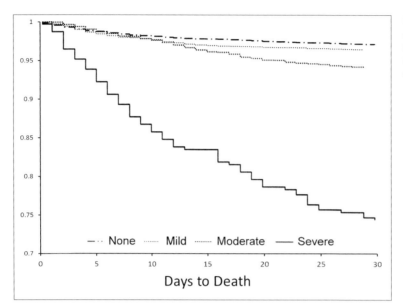

Figure 10.1 Kaplan-Meier estimates of 30-day survival by GUSTO definition of bleeding.[32] *Source*: Courtesy of Elsevier.

remains to be a consensus among trials for the optimal definition of bleeding that is most predictive and representative of outcomes.

Fortunately, the Academic Research Consortium created a committee with the task to develop a standard bleeding scale to be utilized in future trials. This committee, named the Bleeding Academic Research Consortium (BARC), has created a scale with 5 levels of bleeding, which are listed in Table 10.2. The final definitions of bleeding will be published once the scale is validated and will soon provide a universal definition of bleeding, making comparison of trials more meaningful.

Incidences of Bleeding in ACS

Relying on trials and registries to estimate the true incidence of bleeding in ACS is difficult given the influence of multiple confounders. Key confounders include definition of bleeding, trial design, and anticoagulation strategy being studied. Because of these issues, the true incidence of bleeding after PCI for ACS ranges between 1% and 10%.[3,24–25,33–37]

Table 10.2 Bleeding Definition from the Bleeding Academic Research Consortium (BARC).

Type 0	No bleeding
Type 1	Bleeding that does not require action and requires no further testing or treatment
Type 2	Any overt sign of bleeding (but not Type 3–5) that requires evaluation (visit to health care professional or diagnostic testing), requires intervention to stop bleeding (surgical treatment, medical treatment, altering of medications), or leads to change in routine care (require hospitalization, prolong hospital stay, or increase level of care)
Type 3	
Type 3a	Overt bleeding with Hgb drop between 3 and 5 g/dL, tamponade, bleeding requiring surgical or percutaneous intervention
Type 3b	Need for transfusion or overt bleeding with drop in hemoglobin of > 5 g/dL, tamponade, or bleeding requiring surgical/percutaneous intervention or inotropes
Type 3c	Intracranial bleed, intraocular bleed
Type 4	CABG-related bleeding
Type 5	Fatal bleeding (bleeding primary cause of death)

CABG: coronary artery bypass grafting, Hgb: hemoglobin g/dL.

The definition of major bleeding can significantly change the incidence of bleeding. For example, patients from the PURSUIT and PARAGON trials were reexamined using both the TIMI and GUSTO definitions. The incidence of major bleeding ranged from 1.2% by GUSTO criteria to 8.2% for TIMI criteria, and when these definitions were compared in the same patient population, only the GUSTO definition correlated with outcomes.[34]

Because most randomized trials had strict inclusion criteria, registries have attempted to provide a real-world look at bleeding. The 3 largest registries are the Global Registry of Acute Coronary Events (GRACE), Can Rapid Risk Stratification of Unstable Angina Patients Suppress Adverse Outcomes with Early Implementation of the ACC/AHA Guidelines (CRUSADE), and the National Cardiovascular Data Registry (NCDR).

GRACE recently published data on more than 50,000 patients from 2000 to 2007 and found that 2.3% of all ACS patients had a major bleeding event, with STEMI patients at an even higher risk. Additionally, major bleeding decreased over the study period from 2.6% in 2000 to 1.8% by 2007 ($P = 0.0001$), showing that more modern practice patterns are associated with better outcomes.[33] CRUSADE found the incidence of bleeding to be 10.4% in ACS patients when bleeding is defined merely as need for blood transfusion. This definition is likely not ideal because criteria for transfusion vary greatly between centers.[35,37] The rate of bleeding in the subgroup of patients from the NCDR registry with ACS ranged from 2.07% for NSTEMI to 3.07% for STEMI patients.[16]

Bleeding appears to have a bimodal peak and occurs either at the time of the procedure or several days after PCI. Early bleeding appears to be related to access site and anticoagulation use during PCI, and bleeding that occurs later is likely related to dual antiplatelet therapy and tends not to be related to access site choice.[36] It is easy to see now why truly estimating the incidence of bleeding based on these trials and registries is so difficult. As we move into the future, most trials will follow a more standardized definition based on the BARC criteria and allow us to better compare trials and appreciate the real risk of bleeding in ACS.

Consequences of Bleeding

Although the optimal definition of bleeding is still being debated, it is clear from studies that patients who experience periprocedural and in-hospital bleeding during treatment for ACS are at higher risk of death and adverse events.

Bleeding is predictive of adverse events including death, nonfatal MI, stroke, and stent thrombosis in both the short and the long term. OASIS-5 was the first randomized clinical trial that showed that bleeding was associated with long-term morbidity and mortality. This trial of 20,000 patients with ACS randomized to either fondaparinux or low-molecular-weight heparin (LMWH) found that fondaparinux reduced bleeding events from 9.0% to 7.3% (hazard ratio 0.81, $P < 0.001$), and this was the driving force of lower mortality at 30 and 180 days.[29]

Others have pooled data from several large trials or registries and have shown that bleeding is associated with adverse events, and the more severe the bleeding, the greater the adjusted hazard ratio for death. Combining data from GUSTO IIb, PURSUIT, and PARAGON A and B trials revealed an adjusted hazard ratio of death of 10.6 (90% CI 8.3–13.6) with severe bleeding using the GUSTO definition at 30 days and 7.5 (CI 6.1–9.3) at 180 days.[32]

In addition, bleeding leads to additional procedures and increased length of stay, and can delay patient recovery. Major bleeding adverse events can directly increase hospital costs by more than $8,000 per event.[38,39] This, however, does not take into account the effects and costs of pain, time off from work, and associated morbidity, making the true cost of bleeding likely to be many times higher.

Mechanism

The exact mechanism by which bleeding is linked to MACE is not clear, but is likely due to multiple factors. There currently is a strong association between bleeding and MACE, but causality has not been established, and it remains possible that bleeding may just be a marker of more severe comorbidities.

Short-Term Effects of Bleeding. The most obvious mechanism by which bleeding leads to death is related to the actual blood loss. Acute blood loss can lead to hypotension and shock, and worsen coronary ischemia. In addition, acute blood loss will activate the adrenergic system, therefore increase oxygen demand, and further worsen myocardial ischemia.[40] When bleeding occurs in areas that cannot accommodate this large volume, such as intracranial, the mass effect can directly lead to death.

Patients who experience bleeding or present with anemia are more likely to have proven beneficial therapies withheld. Trials show that 13%–23% of patients presenting with ACS have baseline anemia, and these patients are treated less aggressively. They have lower rates of aspirin, clopidogrel, and heparin use combined with higher rates of blood transfusion, all of which are associated with higher rates of short-term mortality.[37,41,42] Even medical therapies such as beta-blocker and angiotensin-renin-aldosterone inhibitors that do not cause bleeding are more likely to be withheld. These agents blunt the negative effects of the adrenergic and neurohormonal systems that are activated during ACS, and withholding can accelerate negative left ventricular remodeling.

Long-Term Effects of Bleeding. Bleeding and anemia may activate clotting factors and platelet aggregation, and promote erythropoietin release. These adaptive mechanisms were meant to prevent further blood loss and be protective. However, in the ACS setting, this creates a relative hypercoagulable state that can worsen ischemia and lead to future myocardial infarctions. These effects likely last beyond the acute phase, and may explain why patients are at increased risk for MACE up to a year after the index event.

Predicting Bleeding

Identifying patients prior to PCI at increased risk of bleeding is crucial so that bleeding reduction strategies can be implanted. Clinical risk scores assigning point values have been developed from 2 large registries and validated to predict bleeding in the ACS setting.

The CRUSADE bleeding score was created from a registry of 71,000 real-world patients and validated in nearly 18,000 patients with NSTEMI. Bleeding was defined as intracranial

bleed, retroperitoneal bleed, hematocrit drop > 12%, and any red blood cell transfusion when baseline hematocrit was either > 28% or < 28% with a witnessed bleed. The algorithm developed is based on 8 clinical factors (baseline hematocrit, creatinine clearance, heart rate, sex, signs of congestive heart failure [CHF], prior vascular disease, diabetes, and systolic blood pressure), and the scoring system can be found at www.crusadebleedingscore.org. The sum of these points predicts major in-hospital bleeding as defined above, and scores are graded from very low risk to very high risk[43] as seen in Figure 10.2.

The NCDR developed another risk score from its database of 300,000 PCI procedures performed at more than 400 US hospitals. Bleeding was defined as femoral hematoma of > 10 cm, retroperitoneal bleed, gastrointestinal bleed, genitourinary bleed, blood transfusion, prolonged hospital stay, or drop in hemoglobin > 3 g/dL. Although this risk score wasn't created in ACS patients, calibration plots testing the bleeding risk score in ACS patients were performed and showed that the model was in fact predictive in this setting. This scoring system assigns a point value for 9 clinical variables (ACS type, angina, shock, sex, previous heart failure, previous PCI, New York Heart Association Class IV heart failure, peripheral vascular disease, and estimated glomerular filtration rate) and generates a risk score based on the sum of these[44] as seen in Figure 10.3.

Both of these scoring systems are easy to use and allow for quick and accurate risk assessment for bleeding. Therefore, routine use of these bleeding calculators prior to PCI may allow for better planning and implementation of bleeding reduction strategies.

Bleeding Avoidance Strategies

As the negative effects of bleeding are better recognized, ways to improve outcomes have been sought. The evolution of medical therapy over the past decade has led to a reduction in unfractionated heparin and glycoprotein IIb/IIIa use, with an increase in LMWH, bivalirudin, and thienopyridine use.[13–14,33] Despite the potential benefits of new anticoagulation strategies, use remains low even in groups

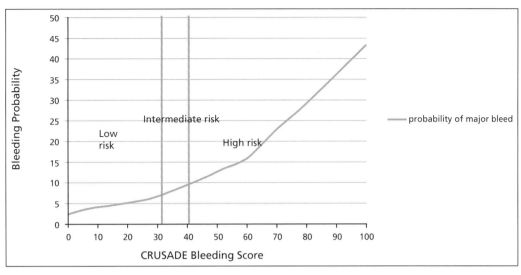

Figure 10.2 Probability of major bleeding based on CRUSADE bleeding risk calculator.[43]

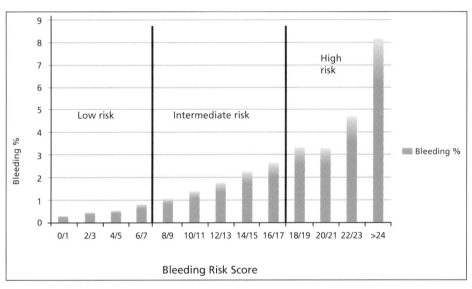

Figure 10.3 Probability of major bleeding based on NCDR bleeding risk calculator.[44]

identified to be at higher risk of bleeding and adverse events.[14] Recently, newer strategies including transradial access, bivalirudin, and vascular closure devices have been studied.

Transradial Access in ACS. With our better understanding of the real risk associated with bleeding and in particular access site bleeding, the use of radial artery access has been growing. In the United States, despite increased awareness of radial access, its actual usage remains low at only about 2% of cases[16] and is limited to select

interventionalists and hospitals. Globally, radial artery use varies tremendously between countries with select countries such as Sweden now performing nearly half of their ACS interventions by the radial artery. However, the majority of radial access use appears to be in low-risk cases, not in the ACS setting. Even high-volume operators seem to use radial access in only about 30% of PCI cases.[27] Further detail and trials assessing TRA use for ACS will be discussed later in this chapter.

Bivalirudin and ACS. Most recently, bivalirudin, a direct thrombin inhibitor, has gained popularity as studies showed its use led to lower rates of bleeding in both NSTEMI and STEMI settings. The ACUITY trial, which enrolled NSTEMI patients, found that bivalirudin alone was noninferior in rates of composite ischemic endpoints, but had statistically lower rates of bleeding (3.0% vs. 5.7%, $P < 0.001$) compared to heparin and glycoprotein IIb/IIIa inhibitors.[25]

Of the 13,819 patients enrolled in the ACUITY trial, only 6.2% underwent PCI by TRA, and this was based on physician and patient preference. In a retrospective review of this population, there was no difference in ischemic outcomes between radial and femoral access at 30 days (8.1% vs. 7.5%, $P = 0.18$) or at 1 year, although the radial access group had fewer major bleeding events (3.0% vs. 4.8%, $P = 0.03$). This is likely because bivalirudin lowered access site bleeding in the femoral group and non–access site bleeding in both groups.[23]

The HORIZONS-AMI trial showed bivalirudin lowered 30-day adverse event rates (death, reinfarction, target-vessel revascularization, stroke, and major bleeding) from 12.1% to 9.2% in STEMI patients compared to heparin plus glycoprotein IIb/IIIa inhibitors. This was driven primarily by a significant reduction in bleeding from 9.6% to 5.9% when defined by TIMI criteria and from 5.6% to 3.5% by the GUSTO definition.[25] This study further supported the notion that bleeding was associated with poor outcomes.

Bivalirudin is clearly beneficial at lowering bleeding events in the ACS setting and is now a Class I recommendation for use in patients at increased risk of bleeding.[1,2] Further studies and randomized trials are needed to assess if radial access and bivalirudin together are superior to either alone for reducing bleeding events.

Vascular Closure Devices for Femoral Access in ACS. Vascular closure devices (VCDs) have gained tremendous popularity with both physicians and patients given their ease in placing and greater patient comfort. However, their safety and role in reducing bleeding have not been clear and previously have even been thought to be harmful.[45,46]

The NCDR found that both bivalirudin and VCD were associated with lower rates of bleeding, and the combination of the 2 was even more beneficial. This was especially true in the group with a predicted risk of bleeding greater than 3% based on the NCDR calculator, where the number needed to treat was only 33 patients to prevent 1 episode of major bleeding. However, this higher-risk group was found to be the least likely to receive a VCD, providing more reason to identify and target strategies toward this higher-risk group.[44]

Similarly, the authors from the ACUITY trial found VCD reduced both access site bleeding (ASB) (2.5% vs. 3.3%, $P = 0.01$) and ACUITY major non-CABG (coronary artery bypass graft) bleeding (3.9% vs. 5.3%, $P = 0.0003$). The combination of a VCD and bivalirudin was associated with the least amount of bleeding (0.7%).[47]

Again, there is limited head-to-head data on TRA versus femoral access with bivalirudin, VCD, or both. All are acceptable strategies to lower risk of bleeding, and further studies are warranted to determine the most beneficial combination. Perhaps the most important message from these trials is that patients at the highest risk of bleeding are not receiving these strategies and need to be identified and targeted.

■ STUDIES COMPARING RADIAL WITH FEMORAL ACCESS

Current treatment for ACS involves intensive anticoagulation often combined with an early invasive strategy. This approach has clearly lowered adverse ischemic events, however, at the expense of bleeding and its associated poor outcomes. Radial access nearly eliminates access site bleeding and therefore has been felt to be of greatest benefit in ACS patients who are at higher risk for bleeding. The radial artery is a superficial artery that can be easily compressed, nearly eliminating large hemodynamically significant bleeds. The concern with radial access has been whether it can be performed with equal efficacy in the ACS setting as femoral access. Specifically, can TRA be successfully utilized without an increase in procedure/door-to-balloon times and need for crossover to femoral access, all while reducing MACE and bleeding events?

Retrospective, observational studies, and now large multicenter international randomized trials, have attempted to answer these questions. The number of studies and the amount of coverage this topic has received in recent years point to how important an issue this has become. In this section, we will review key trials and the data on transradial success, door-to-balloon times, and outcomes with radial access.

Transradial Procedural Success

Multiple observational studies have compared the feasibility of TRA in the setting of ACS with femoral access. Prompt revascularization in this setting is of the utmost importance and requires a high rate of success. Early observational studies suggested that TRA was feasible in the ACS setting as summarized in Table 10.3. Most of these series were small and nonrandomized, were conducted at single centers, and only involved experienced operators, allowing selection bias and other confounders to potentially affect outcomes. Despite limitations, these trials demonstrated that 88% success rates with acceptable low levels of crossover to femoral access could be achieved.

Several randomized trials provide further insight into the role and benefits of radial access in ACS and are summarized below and in Table 10.4.[48] The first and only multicenter international trial to date on this issue was recently published and will therefore be discussed separately.[22]

Shortly after Kiemeneij et al first described radial artery use for PCI, the first randomized clinical trial (RCT) in ACS was conducted. In this single-center trial, 142 consecutive patients were randomized to femoral or radial access, and only 2 experienced operators performed the radial cases. Although this was an ACS trial, more than 50% of patients had unstable angina, and only 14% were truly STEMI patients. Also, 20% of patients received thrombolytics and therefore underwent rescue PCI. Success rates were high (96%) with 12% of patients crossing over to femoral access (8% due to negative Allen's test and 4% due to access failure).[49]

Several years later, the TEMPURA trial randomized 157 patients with STEMI to radial or femoral access in Japan. This trial was powered to prove equivalence for in-hospital MACE between TRA and TFA. The average age was 67 years, 82% were male, and thrombolytics and IIb/IIIa inhibitors were not used in this trial. Successful reperfusion of the infarct-related artery was achieved in > 95% of patients in both groups ($P = 0.94$), and no patients in the TRA group required crossover to femoral access. Surprisingly, the TRA group was even associated with a shorter procedural time by 6 minutes ($P = 0.033$).[50]

In the FARMI trial, 114 patients with STEMI were randomized to either femoral access or radial access with 5-Fr interventional equipment being utilized. Greater than 90% of patients in both groups had successful reperfusion ($P = 0.43$); however, 12% of patients in the TRA group required crossover to femoral access due to technical difficulties compared with 1.8% of femoral patients requiring crossover to radial access ($P = 0.03$).[51]

In a single-center study from Poland, 100 patients with STEMI were randomized to femoral or radial access. In the radial group, 8% of patients were unable to have PCI performed via the radial approach (1 due to excessive tortuosity and 3 due to abnormal Allen's test), and procedural success defined as TIMI III Flow at the completion of the procedure was similar between groups (88% vs. 92%, $P > 0.05$).[52]

The results of the above-mentioned trials support radial access as feasible and perhaps even superior to femoral access for ACS patients; however, a large randomized international trial had been lacking. In response to this, the RIVAL trial was designed to help compare outcomes based on access site.

RIVAL Study. The trial was designed to compare femoral and radial access in the ACS setting, began as a substudy of the CURRENT-OASIS 7 study,[68] and continued as an independent trial after its completion. Patients were eligible for enrollment if their presenting diagnosis was either STEMI or NSTEMI and if they underwent an invasive strategy. Patients had to be suitable candidates for either access route, meaning they had to have palpable radial pulse with normal

Table 10.3 Summary of Observational Studies.

Study	# Patients radial	# Patients femoral	Age years	Male %	IIb/IIIa use %	Antithrombotic regimen	Bleeding definition used	Radial success %	Femoral success %	Radial bleeding events %	Femoral major bleeding events %	Femoral crossover need %
Kim[53]	30	26	57	100	–	–	–	90	96	0	–	–
Mulukutla[54]	29	–	58	69	86	Aspirin + clopidogrel/ticlopidine	–	100	–	0	–	0
Louvard—Site A[55]	180	889	60	80	6.1		Hgb drop > 3g	98	97	0	2	1
Louvard—Site B[55]	87	58	59	79	79.3		Hgb drop > 3 g	96	98	0	7	3.5
Valsecchi[56]	163	563	61.5	77	–	Aspirin/clopidogrel/abciximab		96.9	95.5	0	1.2	1.2
Philippe[57]	64	55	59.1	75	100					0	5.5	0
Diaz de la Llera[58]	103	59	55	90	68		Transfusion, hematoma prolonging stay, surgical repair	96.1	94.9	0	8.5	4.6
Kim[59]	132	220	62	67	–		Hgb drop 3.2 g/dL, transfusion, surgical repair, prolong stay	88	89	1	5	4.1
Hetherington[60]	571	480	62	75	92	Aspirin + heparin and clopidogrel after procedure	Transfusion, delaying discharge, pseudoaneurysm	92	90	2.3	3.1	7.7
De Carlo[61]	130	531	66	68.5	83.8	Aspirin + heparin/LMWH and abciximab encouraged	TIMI criteria	91.0	93.1	1.9	13.1	–
Siudak[62]	169	917	63	76	0	Aspirin/clopidogrel + heparin/LMWH	Hematoma, transfusion, intracranial bleed	–	–	2.4	11.6	1.8
PRESTO-ACS[63]	307	863	65	73	39	Aspirin/thienopyridine, heparin/LMWH, +/– IIb/IIIa	TIMI	–	–	0.7	2.7	–
Pancholy[64]	109	204	66.4	61	98	Heparin	Transfusion, hematoma, pseudoaneurysm, retroperitoneal bleed	89	91	0.9	9.8	–
Weaver[65]	124	116	60	82	–		TIMI major	98.3	97.4	5.7	13.8	4.8
Larsen[26]	135	–	69.7	73	83.7	Heparin (97%) or bivalirudin (3%)		98.5	–	1.5	–	0.7

IIb/IIIa: glycoprotein IIb/IIIa inhibitor, Hgb: hemoglobin g/dL, CABG: coronary artery bypass grafting, LMWH: low-molecular-weight heparin, TIMI: thrombolysis in myocardial infarction.

Table 10.4 Summary of Randomized Clinical Trials.

Study	# patients radial	# patients femoral	Age in years	% male	Antithrombotic regimen	IIb/IIIa use %	Bleeding definition used	Radial success (TIMI III) %	Femoral success (TIMI III) %	Radial bleeding events %	Femoral bleeding events %	Femoral crossover need %	MACE radial %	MACE femoral %
Mann[48]	65	77	62	64	Aspirin, heparin, +/– IIb/IIIa	13	–	96	96	0	4	5	0	0
TEMPURA[50]	77	72	61	81	–	0	Transfusion, surgical repair, ICH	96	97	0	3.0	1.5	5.2	8.3
RADIAL-AMI[66]	25	25	55	88	Aspirin/clopidogrel, heparin, IIb/IIIa	94	ICH, RP, Hgb drop > 5 g/dL, transfusion	87	88	0	0	4	0	2
FARMI[51]	57	57	59	84	Aspirin, heparin/ LMWH, IIb/IIIa	100	TIMI	91	97	5.3	5.3	12.3	5.3	5.3
Li[67]	184	186	56	67	ASA/clopidogrel and heparin	0	Hematoma, A-V fistula, pseudoaneurysm, spasm	95	94	1.1	3.8	1.6	–	–
RADIAMI[52]	50	50	60	68	Heparin +/– IIb/IIIa inhibitor	43	Fatal, transfusion, operation, ICH, Hgb drop > 3 g/dL	88	92	6	14	8	2	4
RIVAL[22]	3,507	3,514	62	74	Discretion of physician	25	ACUITY	95	95	1.9	4.5*	7	3.7	4

*statistically significant at $P < 0.05$

IIb/IIIa: glycoprotein IIb/IIIa receptor inhibitor, TR: transradial, TF: transfemoral, LMWH: low-molecular-weight heparin, MACE: major adverse cardiac events, ICH: intracranial hemorrhage, RP: retroperitoneal bleed, Hgb: hemoglobin, A-V: anterior-venous, TIMI: Thrombolysis in Myocardial Infarction Flow, ACUITY: Acute Catheterization and Urgent Intervention Strategy.

Allen's test. Operators had to perform at least 50 radial interventions in the previous year to be eligible to participate as a means to ensure competency. Patients were then randomized 1:1 to either radial or femoral access. Choices of antithrombotic medications and VCDs were at the discretion of the performing physician.

The primary outcome of this trial was the combined endpoint of death, MI, or non-CABG-related major bleeding within 30 days. Major bleeding was defined as any of the following: mortality, transfusion of 2 or more units of blood, hypotension requiring inotropes or surgery, disabling sequelae, symptomatic intracranial hemorrhage, or intraocular leading to vision loss. Post hoc analysis was also performed with the ACUITY[31] definition of bleeding. Initial sample size was estimated to be 4,000 patients based on 80% power for the detection of a 25% relative risk reduction with radial access assuming a 10% rate of the primary outcome. However, during the trial, the actual event rate was much lower, so a new sample size of 7,000 was recalculated based on an observed rate of 6% in the femoral group.

In total, 7,021 patients (3,507 randomized to radial and 3,514 to femoral) were enrolled from 158 hospitals in 32 countries, with only 23% being from North America. The average age was 62 years, 73% were male, and indication for PCI was STEMI (28%), NSTEMI (27%), and unstable angina (45%). Antithrombotic and antiplatelet use were similar between groups: aspirin (99%), clopidogrel (96%), LMWH (52%), glycoprotein IIb/IIIa inhibitors (25%), heparin (21%), fondaparinux (11%), and bivalirudin (2.6%). After randomization, 99.8% underwent catheterization; however, only 66% had a stent implanted, and almost 9% underwent CABG.

PCI success rates were similar between the groups (95.4% vs. 95.2%), but the radial group required significantly more crossover to femoral access (7.6% vs. 2.0%, $P < 0.0001$). Reasons for crossover from radial to femoral access included radial spasm, radial artery loop, and subclavian tortuosity. Reasons for crossover from femoral to radial access included iliac tortuosity or peripheral vascular disease.[22]

Cumulatively, these trials have shown similar success rates between radial and femoral access; however, the radial group did require more frequent crossover. It is important to stress again that the interventionalists performing radial artery access in these trials were proficient in this technique, and once one is comfortable with radial access, data support its use in the ACS setting. (The high crossover rate to femoral suggests that there were some inexperienced operators. Furthermore, it is also likely that if the change were from right to left radial, there would be a lower crossover rate. This is clearly more cumbersome than changing from right to left femoral, particularly in an emergency setting.)

Transradial Procedural Times and Door-to-Balloon Times

The initial hesitation with TRA for acute myocardial infarctions, especially STEMI, was the concern that it would lead to a delay in door-to-balloon (D2B) times. In fact, early studies did show that TRA was associated with an average increase in D2B times of 6 minutes, which was primarily due to increased time in obtaining access.[51–52,66] However, subsequent studies (Figures 10.4 and 10.5) have shown that TRA can be performed with comparable procedural and door-to-balloon times. In almost all trials, radial access was only attempted by those proficient in this method, again highlighting the importance of competency with radial access prior to utilizing in ACS patients where procedural time is of utmost importance.

Outcomes and Bleeding Events Associated with Transradial Access

The above trials show similar success rates without negatively affecting D2B times in ACS. This section will focus on the effect of radial access on actual outcomes and bleeding events. Observational studies are best designed to look at radial success rates, procedural times, and frequency for crossover to femoral access. However, several of these studies also attempted to compare hard endpoints such as death and MACE between access methods. One has to be careful drawing conclusions on these hard endpoints due to the nonrandomized design and significant possibility of selection bias. The data from

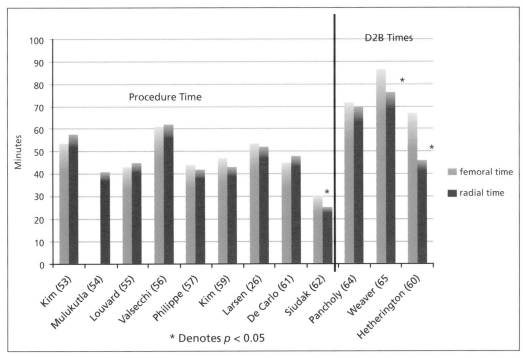

Figure 10.4 Summary of procedure and door-to-balloon times from observational studies.

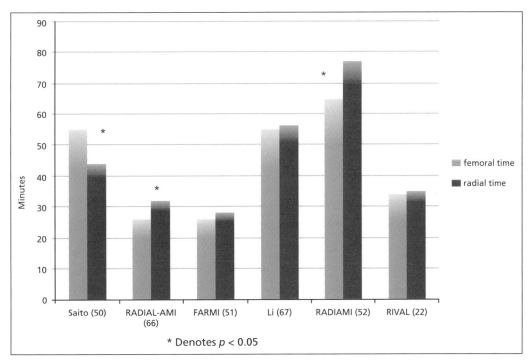

Figure 10.5 Summary of procedure times from randomized clinical trials.

these observational studies were useful and provided the framework for further randomized trials better designed to study outcomes of death, stroke, and MACE.

Table 10.4 summarizes the randomized clinical trials comparing radial access with femoral access. Mann et al conducted the first randomized trial comparing radial and femoral access and found that no patients in either group died, required emergent CABG, or had a procedural MI. However, 4% of patients in the femoral group had an access site–related hematoma prolonging hospital stay. Due to this, the radial group had a shorter hospital length of stay (3.0 vs. 4.5 days, $P < 0.01$) and lower total hospital costs ($20,476 vs. $23,389, $P < 0.01$).[49]

The TEMPURA trial found that both in-hospital (5.2% vs. 8.3%, $P = 0.444$) and 90-day MACE (17.8% vs. 24.2%, $P = 0.351$) were statistically no different between groups. Major bleeding occurred in 3% of patients in the femoral access group and 0% in the TRA group.[50] Brasselet et al found that radial access was associated with decreased time to ambulation and decreased peripheral arterial complications (hematomas), but TIMI minor and major bleeding were statistically no different between groups.[51] Similarly, the RADIAMI trial found that in-hospital outcomes including mortality, stroke, and MI were alike between groups with radial access trending toward fewer episodes of major bleeding.[52]

RIVAL Study. The primary outcome of death, MI, stroke, and non-CABG-related major bleeding occurred in 3.7% of patients in the radial group and 4.0% in the femoral group ($P = 0.50$). Secondary outcomes at 30 days of death, MI, stroke, and the combination were statistically no different between groups. PCI procedural time and hospital length of stay were similar between groups, but radial access was associated with greater fluoroscopy time (9.8 minutes vs. 8.0 minutes, $P < 0.0001$).

The unanticipated aspect of this trial was the lower-than-expected rates of bleeding and lack of correlation between bleeding and hard endpoints. Bleeding rates were compared between the groups using the RIVAL, TIMI, and ACUITY definitions because no standard definition exists. Comparing groups utilizing the RIVAL and TIMI definitions found no difference; however, the femoral access group did have higher rates of vascular complications (Table 10.5). The ACUITY definition of bleeding incorporates access site bleeding complications, and with this definition, radial access was superior to femoral access (1.9% vs. 4.5%, $P < .0001$). It is also important to note that in the femoral group, major access site bleeding occurred in 0.5% of patients while major bleeding not related to access site occurred in 1.6% of patients.

There was no significant difference between radial access and femoral access in the prespecified subgroups of age, sex, BMI, or radial volume by operator. There was a significant reduction in the primary outcome with radial artery access in the subgroups of patients presenting with STEMI and who underwent PCI at centers with the highest radial artery volume. This further supports the idea that outcomes are superior in centers with high radial access use where staff and physicians have higher proficiency and comfort.

Perhaps the most striking result of the trial was the benefit in the STEMI subgroup in which radial access reduced 30-day MACE

Table 10.5 Bleeding Outcomes from the RIVAL Study.

Outcome	Radial	Femoral	HR (95% CI)	P value
RIVAL major bleeding	0.7%	0.9%	0.73 (0.43–1.23)	0.23
TIMI major bleeding	0.5%	0.5%	1.00 (0.95–1.07)	1.00
ACUITY major bleeding	1.9%	4.5%	0.43 (0.32–0.57)	< 0.0001
Blood transfusions	1.1%	1.3%	0.87 (0.56–1.33)	0.51
Minor bleeding	2.9%	3.4%	0.84 (0.65–1.10)	0.21
Large hematoma	1.2%	3.0%	0.40 (0.28–0.57)	< 0.0001
Pseudoaneurysm requiring repair	0.2%	0.6%	0.30 (0.13–0.71)	0.0006

(3.1% vs. 5.2%, HR 0.60 [95% CI 0.38–0.94], $P = 0.026$), and death (1.3% vs. 3.2%, HR 0.39 [95% CI 0.20–0.76], $P = 0.006$). Major non-CABG bleeding was similar between the groups, but major vascular complications were significantly lower with radial access.

This trial concludes that there is no difference between radial and femoral access in terms of the primary outcome of death/MI/stroke/major bleeding in all patients with ACS. However, it does support the idea that radial artery access can be performed with equal success rates, without prolonging the total procedure time, and with lower vascular access site complications. Specifically in patients presenting with STEMI and to centers with the highest radial volume, radial artery access was associated with lower rates of death.[22]

Meta-Analyses

Individually, the above trials did not show a benefit in mortality with radial access, and therefore data have been pooled into meta-analyses in an attempt to increase power. Two meta-analyses have been performed comparing radial access to femoral access,[22,69] and despite limitations of these meta-analyses, they do provide further insight into the benefits of radial access.

The first meta-analysis performed by the RIVAL authors includes patients who underwent PCI for both elective and ACS

indications. This meta-analysis has a broad inclusion and may underestimate the potential benefit of radial access for acute MIs given that these patients are at higher risk of bleeding compared to elective PCI. These authors combined trials to include nearly 11,000 patients and found a significant benefit with radial access in reducing non-CABG major bleeding, transfusions, and major vascular access site complications (Figure 10.6). There was, however, no benefit in reducing death, MI, or stroke except when performed by radial experts at the highest-tertile radial volume centers. This again stresses the importance of proficiency in this technique by both the operator and catheterization laboratory staff and stresses how it affects outcomes.[22]

The meta-analysis by Vorobcsuk et al only included patients undergoing PCI for ACS. A total of 3,324 patients from 12 observational and randomized trials were included, and the 3 primary outcomes looked at were death, MACE, and bleeding (Figures 10.7A–C). Based on pooled data, radial access was associated with a reduction in death (2.59% vs. 3.18%, OR 0.54 [95% CI 0.33–0.86], $P = 0.01$), MACE defined as death, MI, or stroke (3.65% vs. 6.55%, OR 0.56 [95% CI 0.39–0.79], $P = 0.01$), and major bleeding was reduced by 70% (0.77% vs. 2.61% [95% CI 0.16–0.55], $P = 0.001$). Radial access was associated with shorter hospital stays and similar procedural

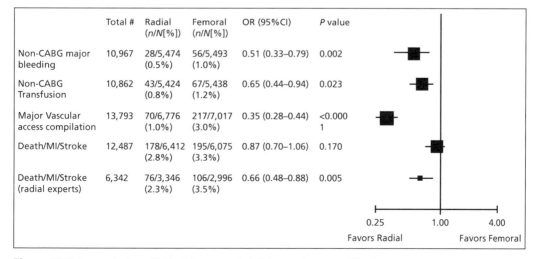

	Total #	Radial (n/N[%])	Femoral (n/N[%])	OR (95%CI)	P value
Non-CABG major bleeding	10,967	28/5,474 (0.5%)	56/5,493 (1.0%)	0.51 (0.33–0.79)	0.002
Non-CABG Transfusion	10,862	43/5,424 (0.8%)	67/5,438 (1.2%)	0.65 (0.44–0.94)	0.023
Major Vascular access compilation	13,793	70/6,776 (1.0%)	217/7,017 (3.0%)	0.35 (0.28–0.44)	<0.0001
Death/MI/Stroke	12,487	178/6,412 (2.8%)	195/6,075 (3.3%)	0.87 (0.70–1.06)	0.170
Death/MI/Stroke (radial experts)	6,342	76/3,346 (2.3%)	106/2,996 (3.5%)	0.66 (0.48–0.88)	0.005

0.25   1.00   4.00
Favors Radial   Favors Femoral

Figure 10.6 Forest plot from RIVAL trial meta-analysis.[22] *Source:* Courtesy of Elsevier.

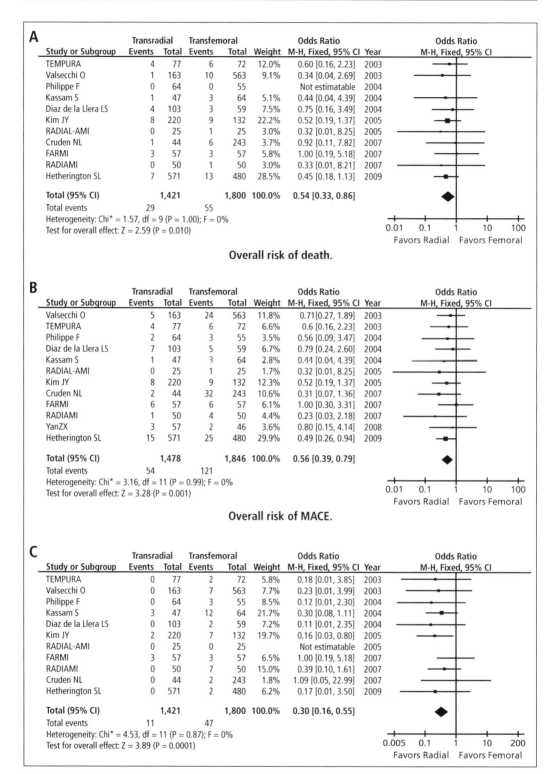

Figure 10.7 Odds ratio for death (**A**), major adverse cardiac events (**B**), and bleeding (**C**) for transradial percutaneous intervention versus femoral access.[69] *Source:* Courtesy of Elsevier.

times, but increased need for access site crossover and fluoroscopic time.[69]

These meta-analyses further support a trend toward a benefit in hard endpoints such as death and MACE with radial access, especially in the ACS setting. This is especially true in the hands of proficient operators. Despite combining multiple studies, these meta-analyses are limited by the small number of studies published on this topic. Other limitations of these meta-analyses are the fact that several studies included are observational studies, anticoagulation strategies varied greatly between trials, and some trials included rescue PCI after failed thrombolytic therapy. Although further studies are warranted, these meta-analyses further support the benefits of radial access.

■ GROUPS THAT MAY FURTHER BENEFIT FROM RADIAL ACCESS

Certain groups of patients are at higher risk of bleeding following PCI in the ACS setting and therefore at higher risk for adverse events.[33] Radial access is appealing in the elderly, women, and those undergoing rescue PCI after failed thrombolytics as a strategy to lower bleeding and improve outcomes. However, because these subgroups of patients were not well represented in the above trials, the safety and efficacy of radial access are not clear. Therefore, small observational and randomized studies have specifically attempted to evaluate these subgroups.

Elderly

Older patients are at increased risk of vascular complications, bleeding, and poor outcomes with PCI in the ACS setting.[16,70,71] Therefore, the ability to lower bleeding is very appealing as a means to improve outcomes. However, age over 75 years was a predictor of procedural failure when attempting transradial PCI in 1 study[72] and therefore raises concern of its safety in this population.

The OCTOPLUS study was the first to prospectively randomize elderly patients

presenting for angiography at 4 European centers to either femoral or radial access. Operators were well experienced in both forms of access and were required to have performed greater than 500 cases with each form of access. The primary outcome included any of the following vascular events: complication requiring surgical intervention, blood transfusion, hemoglobin drop > 3 g/dL, distal extremity ischemia, or delay in discharge due to bleeding. A total of 377 patients were randomized (192 radial and 185 femoral); however, only 10% of patients presented with an acute coronary syndrome/STEMI, making firm conclusions in this subgroup not possible. Both groups had high rates of success (95.8% vs. 96.6%) and equal need for crossover (8.9% vs. 8.1%). (This appears to be a high rate of crossover particularly for experienced operators. Frequently when an operator fails from the right radial, the crossover is to femoral rather than to left radial. When there is failure from right femoral, frequently the operator will switch to left femoral, and no crossover is recorded. Nevertheless, the crossover rate appears to be high for both groups.) However, radial artery access was associated with a reduction in the primary outcome of bleeding (0.5% vs. 7.5%, $P = 0.0001$).[73]

Subsequent randomized and observational trials have specifically looked at radial access for STEMI in the elderly. The next randomized study assigned 103 patients over the age of 65 with STEMI to either radial or femoral access. All patients were pretreated with aspirin and clopidogrel 600 mg prior to catheterization and received unfractionated heparin and tirofiban during the procedure. The average age was 70 years, and 74% were male. Procedural success and total procedure time were similar between access site groups. Radial access was associated with significantly fewer vascular complications such as major bleeding and hematoma (1.8% vs. 13.1%, $P < 0.05$) and a shorter hospital length of stay (7.2 days vs. 10.1 days, $P < 0.05$); however, death at 30 days was similar between groups (5.3% vs. 6.5%, $P > 0.05$). This trial supported that primary PCI in the setting of STEMI was feasible and associated with fewer vascular complications and shorter hospital stays in the elderly population.[74]

Two other retrospective observational trials compared outcomes in patients with STEMI stratified by age and access site from a single center in Germany[75] and Canada.[76] A total of 115 patients at a single center in Germany were analyzed with 34% undergoing PCI by radial access. Patients over the age of 75 had higher mortality rates (13.0% vs. 6.4%, $P = 0.03$) and bleeding compared to a cohort of younger patients despite having similar rates of success. Radial access in the elderly when compared to femoral access was associated with lower rates of transfusion and bleeding (0% vs. 6.6%, $P = 0.04$).[75] The observational study from Canada included patients over the age of 70 and found similar success rates, door-to-balloon times, and in-hospital MACE rates between radial and femoral access. Radial access was associated with fewer access site complications (0% vs. 2.9%, $P < 0.05$).[76]

Although larger randomized clinical trials looking at safety and efficacy of radial artery catheterization for ACS in the elderly are still necessary, these few studies suggest that radial access is equally successful and reduces bleeding.

Women

The role of gender in outcomes with ACS is still being evaluated. When women undergo PCI for ACS, they are at higher risk of adverse events compared to men,[16,78] in part because they tend to present later, have more comorbidities, and are less likely to be referred for invasive procedures.[77] Therefore, the ability to decrease adverse events by lowering bleeding is attractive in this group.

Women tend to compose only a minority in the above studies as seen in Tables 10.3 and 10.4; therefore, limited data exist in this group. In a retrospective observational manner, Pristipino et al reviewed their data from a single hospital in Italy and identified 2,919 patients, of which 838 were women who underwent PCI over a 2-year span. Of these women, 30% presented with ACS, and 33% underwent PCI through radial access. When compared to men, women were older

(66 years vs. 63 years), but had similar risk factors. PCI in women had equal success rates compared to men, but women did require more frequent crossover to femoral access (14% vs. 1.7%, $P = 0.00001$). Femoral access in women was associated with higher rates of major (4.1% vs. 1.5%, $P = 0.0001$) and minor bleeding (39.4% vs. 10.4%, $P = 0.0001$) compared to men. Major bleeding was defined as retroperitoneal bleed, death, requiring surgical intervention, blood transfusion, drop in hemoglobin of > 5 g/dL, or large hematoma. All other access site bleeds were considered minor. Despite the significant limitations of this study and possibility for confounders, it does provide some insight into the benefits of radial access in women.[79]

In the RIVAL trial as mentioned above, gender was a prespecified subgroup. In this large randomized trial, no difference in outcomes of death/MI/stroke/bleeding was found in women compared to men.[22] There are limited data specifically looking at outcomes in women, and further studies are necessary.

Rescue PCI

Thrombolysis is indicated for patients presenting with STEMI to facilities without a cardiac catheterization laboratory or when transfer times would prohibit achieving a 90-minute door-to-balloon time. Although thrombolysis can be an effective therapy, nearly 40% of patients fail this initial therapy. Studies have found that after thrombolytic failure, urgent PCI is superior compared to repeat administration of thrombolytics or medical therapy.[80–81] This invasive strategy is favored to reduce ischemic events but does increase the risk of bleeding,[80,82] and therefore radial access may be of utility.

The role of radial access in this setting is again limited to a few studies. Kassam et al describe their experience in 111 patients after failed thrombolysis that required rescue PCI. Radial access was attempted in 47 (42%) of these cases, with 4% requiring crossover to femoral access. Radial access was associated with fewer blood transfusions (4% vs. 19%, $P < 0.05$) and less access site–related major bleeding (0% vs. 9%, $P < 0.05$), but after excluding patients requiring balloon pumps, this difference was no longer significant.[83]

Cruden et al described their experience of 287 consecutive patients undergoing rescue PCI in which 15% were performed by radial access with baseline characteristics being similar between groups. The radial and femoral groups had similar primary access site success (97%), procedure times (71 minutes vs. 65 minutes, $P = 0.17$), and MACE rates (5% vs. 13%, $P = 0.13$). However, radial access was associated with fewer vascular complications (0% vs. 13%, $P < 0.01$) and shorter hospital length of stay (7.0 days vs. 7.9 days, $P < 0.005$).[84]

The only randomized trial on this topic is the RADIAL-AMI trial, in which 50 patients with STEMI randomized to either radial or femoral access, and 66% of these patients underwent PCI after failed thrombolysis. Procedural success was similar in both groups (88%), but the radial group required crossover in 4% of cases. The femoral access group had more hematomas (28% vs. 8%, $P = 0.07$) and a trend toward requiring more transfusions.[66]

Again, limited data exist on the role of radial artery access for rescue PCI, and although larger studies are necessary, radial access does appear to reduce bleeding.

■ SUMMARY

The approach to treating acute coronary patients with the combination of medical therapy and revascularization has improved mortality in the ACS setting. However, despite these remarkable advances, these patients are among those at highest risk for bleeding complications following interventional procedures. Furthermore, considerable recent evidence suggests that bleeding in the ACS setting increases MACE and death, and reducing bleeding should now be made a priority. As such, we recommend that the approach to care of patients with ACS further evolve with efforts to reduce bleeding.

Our approach to revascularization in the ACS setting is to consider all patients eligible for TRA and have a thoughtful process behind choosing radial access. Transradial PCI has

been shown in multiple trials to achieve equal success rates without prolonging door-to-balloon times in the setting of STEMI. Despite trends toward lower rates of mortality by radial access utilization, further trials are still necessary to precisely define the benefit. Nonetheless, improved patient satisfaction and the potential for decreased bleeding complications are compelling reasons to increase utilization of transradial PCI in this clinical population.

Certainly, several studies have shown that there is a learning curve with TRA, and we recommends that operators be proficient with TRA in the elective setting prior to attempting in ACS patients. In addition, we advocate for identifying patients at risk of bleeding using the predictive models discussed in this chapter. This will help to identify those patients who are at highest risk for bleeding and those who may benefit the most from bleeding-avoidance strategies such as TRA.

■ REFERENCES

1. Kushner FG, Hand M, Smith SC, et al. 2009 focused updates: ACC/AHA guidelines for the management of patients with ST-elevation myocardial infarction (updating the 2004 guidelines and 2007 focused update) and ACC/AHA/SCAI guidelines on percutaneous coronary intervention (updating the 2005 guidelines and 2007 focused update): a report of the American College of Cardiology Foundation/American Heart Association Task Force on Practice Guidelines. *J Am Coll Cardiol.* 2009;54:2205–2241.

2. Anderson JL, Adams CD, Antman EA, et al. ACC/AHA 2007 guidelines for the management of patients with unstable angina/non ST-elevation myocardial infarction: a report of the American College of Cardiology/American Heart Association Task Force on Practice Guidelines (writing committee to revise to 2002 guidelines for the management of patients with unstable angina/non ST-elevation myocardial infarction) developed in collaboration with the American College of Emergency Physicians, the Society of Cardiovascular Angiography and Interventions, and the Society of Thoracic Surgeons endorsed by the American Association of Cardiovascular and Pulmonary Rehabilitation and the Society for Academic Emergency Medicine. *Circulation.* 2007;116:803–877.

3. Lincoff AM, Bittl JA, Harrington RA, Feit F, et al. Bivalirudin and provisional glycoprotein IIb/IIIa blockade compared with heparin and planned

glycoprotein IIb/IIIa blockade during percutaneous coronary intervention: REPLACE-2 randomized trial. *JAMA*. 2003;289:853–863.

4. The PARAGON A Investigators. International, randomized, controlled trial of lamifiban (a platelet glycoprotein IIB/IIIa inhibitor), heparin, or both in unstable angina. *Circulation*. 1998;97:2386–2395.

5. The PURSUIT Trial Investigators. Inhibition of platelet glycoprotein IIb/IIIa with eptifibatide in patients with acute coronary syndromes: platelet glycoprotein IIb/IIIa in unstable angina: receptor suppression using integrillin therapy. *N Engl J Med*. 1998;339:436–443.

6. Kleiman NS, Lincoff AM, Flaker GC, et al; the PURSUIT Investigators. Early percutaneous coronary intervention, platelet inhibition with eptifibatide, and clinical outcomes in patients with acute coronary syndromes. *Circulation*. 2000;101:751–757.

7. Mukherjee D, Mahaffey KW, Moliterno DJ, et al. Promise of combined low-molecular-weight heparin and platelet glycoprotein IIb/IIIa inhibition: results from Platelet IIb/IIIa Antagonist for the Reduction of Acute coronary syndrome events in a Global Organization Network B (PARAGON B). *Am Heart J*. 2002;144:995 1002.

8. The PARAGON B Investigators. Randomized, placebo-controlled trial of titrated intravenous lamifiban for acute coronary syndromes. *Circulation*. 2002;105:316–321.

9. White HD, Kleiman NS, Mahaffey KW, et al. Efficacy and safety of enoxaparin compared with unfractionated heparin in high-risk patients with non-ST-segment elevation acute coronary syndrome undergoing percutaneous coronary intervention in the Superior Yield of the New Strategy of Enoxaparin, Revascularization and Glycoprotein IIb/IIIa Inhibitors (SYNERGY) trial. *Am Heart J*. 2006;152:1042–1050.

10. The GUSTO IIb Investigators. A comparison of recombinant hirudin with heparin for treatment of acute coronary syndromes. *N Engl J Med*. 1996;335:775–782.

11. Steg PG, Goldberg RJ, Gore JM, Fox KAA, Eagle KA, Flather MD, Sadiq I, Kasper R, Rushton-Mellor SK, Anderson FA; for the GRACE Investigators. Baseline characteristics, management practices, and in-hospital outcomes of patients hospitalized with acute coronary syndromes in the Global Registry of Acute Coronary Events (GRACE). *Am J Cardiol*. 2002;90:358–363.

12. Roger VL, Go AS, Lloyd-Jones DM, et al. Heart disease and stroke statistics—2011 update: a report from the American Heart Association. *Circulation*. 2011;123:e18–e209.

13. Yeh RW, Sidney S, Chandra M, et al. Population trends in the incidence and outcomes of acute myocardial infarction. *N Engl J Med*. 2010;36: 2155–2165.

14. Kadakia MB, Desai NR, Alexander KP, et al. Use of anticoagulant agents and risk of bleeding among patients admitted with myocardial infarction: a

report from the NCDR ACTION Registry–GWTG (National Cardiovascular Data Registry Acute Coronary Treatment and Intervention Outcomes Network Registry—Get with the Guidelines). *J Am Coll Cardiol Intv*. 2010;3:1166–1177.

15. Peterson ED, Shah BR, Parsons L, et al. Trends in quality of care for patients with acute myocardial infarction in the National Registry of Myocardial Infarction from 1990 to 2006. *Am Heart J*. 2008;156:1045–1055.

16. Rao SV, Ou FS, Wang TY, et al. Trends in the prevalence and outcomes of radial and femoral approaches to percutaneous coronary intervention: a report from the National Cardiovascular Data Registry. *J Am Coll Cardiol Intv*. 2008;1:379–386.

17. Caputo RP, Tremmel JA, Rao S, et al. Transradial arterial access for coronary and peripheral procedures: executive summary by the transradial committee of the SCAI. *Catheter Cardiovasc Interv*. 2011.

18. Ball WT, Sharieff W, Jolly SS, et al. Characterization of operator learning curve for transradial coronary interventions. *Circ Cardiovasc Interv*. 2011;4: 336–341.

19. Spaulding C, Lefevre T, Funchk F, et al. Left radial approach for coronary angiography: results of a prospective study. *Cathet Cardiolog Diagn*. 1996;39:365–370.

20. Schiahbasi A, Romagnoli E, Trani C, et al. Evaluation of the "learning curve" for left and right radial approach during percutaneous coronary procedures. *Am J Cardiol*. 2011;108:185–188.

21. Hildick-Smith DJ, Lowe MD, Walsh JT, et al. Coronary angiography from the radial artery-experience, complications and limitations. *Int J Cardiol*. 1998;64:231–239.

22. Jolly SS, Yusuf S, Cairns J, et al. Radial versus femoral access for coronary angiography and intervention in patients with acute coronary syndromes (RIVAL): a randomized, parallel group, multicenter trial. *Lancet*. 2011;377:1409–1420.

23. Hamon M, Rasmussen LH, Manoukian SV, et al. Choice of arterial access site and outcomes in patients with acute coronary syndromes managed with an early invasive strategy: the ACUITY trial. *EuroIntervention*. 2009;5:2156–2164.

24. Stone GW, McLaurin BT, Cox DA, et al. Bivalirudin for patients with acute coronary syndromes. *N Engl J Med*. 2008;158:2203–2216.

25. Stone GW, Witzenbichler B, Guagliumi G, et al. Bivalirudin during primary PCI in acute myocardial infarction. *N Engl J Med*. 2008;358:2218–2230.

26. Larsen P, Shah S, Waxman S, et al. Comparison of procedural times, success rates, and safety between left versus right radial artery access in primary percutaneous coronary intervention for acute ST-segment elevation myocardial infarction. *Catheter Cardiovasc Interv*. 2011;78:38–44.

27. Bertrand OF, Rao SV, Pancholy S, et al. Transradial approach for coronary angiography and interventions: results of the first international transradial practice survey. *J Am Coll Cardiol Int*. 2010;3: 1022–1031.

28. Bell BP, Ali IF, Pyne CT. Impella assisted transradial coronary intervention in patients with acute coronary syndromes and cardiogenic shock: case series. *Catheter Cardiovasc Interv.* 2011;78:880–885.

29. Fifth Organization to Assess Strategies in Acute Ischemic Syndromes Investigators; Yusuf S, Mehta SR, Chrolavicius S, Afzal R, Pogue J, Granger CB, Budaj A, Peters RJ, Bassand JP, Wallentin L, Joyner C, Fox KA. Comparison of fondaparinux and enoxaparin in acute coronary syndromes. *N Engl J Med.* 2006;354:1464–1476.

30. Eikelboom JW, Mehta SR, Anand SS, et al. Adverse impact of bleeding on prognosis in patients with acute coronary syndromes. *Circulation.* 2006;114:774–782.

31. Manoukian SV, Feit F, Mehran R, et al. Impact of major bleeding on 30-day mortality and clinical outcomes in patients with acute coronary syndromes: an analysis from the ACUITY trial. *J Am Coll Cardiol.* 2007;49:1362–1368.

32. Rao SV, O'Grady K, Pieper KS, et al. Impact of bleeding severity on clinical outcomes among patients with acute coronary syndromes. *Am J Cardiol.* 2005;96:1200–1206.

33. Fox KAA, Carruthers K, Steg G, et al. Has the frequency of bleeding changed over time for patients presenting with an acute coronary syndrome? The global registry of acute coronary events. *Eur Heart J.* 2010;31:667–675.

34. Rao SV, O'Grady K, Pieper KS, et al. A comparison of the clinical impact of bleeding measured by two different classifications among patients with acute coronary syndromes. *J Am Coll Cardiol.* 2006;47:809–816.

35. Yang X, Alexander KP, Chen AY, et al; CRUSADE Investigators. The implications of blood transfusions for patients with non-ST-segment elevation acute coronary syndromes: results from the CRUSADE National Quality Improvement Initiative. *J Am Coll Cardiol.* 2005;46:1490–1495.

36. Wiviott SD, Braunwald E, McCabe CH, et al. Prasugrel versus clopidogrel in patients with acute coronary syndromes. *N Engl J Med.* 2007;357:2001–2015.

37. Alexander KP, Chen AY, Wang TY, et al. Transfusion practice and outcomes in non-ST-segment elevation acute coronary syndromes. *Am Heart J.* 2008;155:1047–1053.

38. Pinto DS, Stone GW, Shi C, et al. Economic evaluation of bivalirudin with or without glycoprotein IIb/IIIa inhibition versus heparin with routine glycoprotein IIb/IIIa inhibition for early invasive management of acute coronary syndromes. *J Am Coll Cardiol.* 2008;52:1758–1768.

39. Aronow HD, Peyser PA, Eagle KA, et al. Predictors of length of stay after coronary stenting. *Am Heart J.* 2001;142:799–805.

40. Bassand JP. Impact of anemia, bleeding and transfusions in acute coronary syndromes: a shift in the paradigm. *Eur Heart J.* 2007;28:1273–1274.

41. Spencer FA, Moscucci M, Granger CB, et al. Does comorbidity account for excess mortality in patients with major bleeding in acute myocardial infarction? *Circulation.* 2007;116:2793.

42. Nikolsky E, Aymong ED, Halkin A, et al. Impact of anemia in patients with acute myocardial infarction undergoing primary percutaneous coronary intervention: analysis from the controlled abciximab and device investigation to lower late angioplasty complications (CADILLAC) Trial. *J Am Coll Cardiol.* 2004;44:547–555.

43. Subherwal S, Bach RG, Chen AY, et al. Baseline risk of major bleeding in non-ST-segment elevation myocardial infarction: the CRUSADE (can rapid risk stratification of unstable angina patients suppress adverse outcomes with early implementation of the ACC/AHA guidelines) bleeding score. *Circulation.* 2009;119:1873–1882.

44. Mehta SK, Frutkin AD, Lindsey JB, et al. Bleeding in patients undergoing percutaneous coronary intervention: the development of a clinical risk algorithm from the national cardiovascular data registry. *Circ Cardiovasc Intervent.* 2009;2:222–229.

45. Nikolsky E, Mehran R, Halkn A, et al. Vascular complications associated with arteriotomy closure devices in patients undergoing percutaneous coronary procedures: a meta-analysis. *J Am Coll Cardiol.* 2004;44:1200–1209.

46. Koreny M, Riedmuller E, Nikfardjam M, et al. Arterial puncture closing devices compared with standard manual compression after cardiac catheterization: systematic review and meta-analysis. *JAMA.* 2004;291:350–357.

47. Sanborn TA, Ebrahimi R, Manoukian SV, et al. Impact of femoral vascular closure devices and antithrombotic therapy on access site bleeding in acute coronary syndromes: the acute catheterization and urgent intervention triage strategy (ACUITY) trial. *Circ Cardiovasc Interv.* 2010;3:57–62.

48. Mann T, Cubeddu G, Bowen J, et al. Stenting in acute coronary syndromes: a comparison of radial versus femoral access sites. *J Am Coll Cardiol.* 1998;32:572–576.

49. Kiemeneij F, Laarman GJ, de Melker E. Transradial artery coronary angioplasty. *Am Heart J.* 1995;129:1–7.

50. Saito S, Tanaka S, Hiroe Y, et al. Comparative study on transradial approach vs. transfemoral approach in primary stent implantation for patients with acute myocardial infarction: results of the test for myocardial infarction by prospective unicenter randomization for access sites (TEMPURA) trial. *Catheter Cardiovasc Interv.* 2003;59:26–33.

51. Brasselet C, Tassan S, Nazeyrollas P, et al. Randomized comparison of femoral versus radial approach for percutaneous coronary intervention using abciximab in acute myocardial infarction: results of the FARMI trial. *Heart.* 2007;93:1556–1561.

52. Chodor P, Krupa H, Kurek T, et al. Radial versus femoral approach for percutaneous coronary interventions in patients with acute myocardial infarction (RADIAMI): a prospective, randomized, single-center clinical trial. *Cardiol J.* 2009;16:332–340.

53. Kim MH, Cha KS, Kim HJ, et al. Primary stenting for acute myocardial infarction via the transradial approach: a safe and useful alternative to the transfemoral approach. *J Invasive Cardiol.* 2000;12: 292–296.

54. Mulukutla SR, Cohen HA. Feasibility and efficacy of transradial access for coronary interventions in patients with acute myocardial infarction. *Catheter Cardiovasc Interv.* 2002;57:167–171.

55. Louvard Y, Ludwig J, Lefevere T, et al. Transradial approach for coronary angioplasty in the setting of acute myocardial infarction: a dual-center registry. *Catheter Cardiovasc Interv.* 2002;55:206–211.

56. Valsecchi O, Musumeci G, Vassileva A, et al. Safety, feasibility and efficacy of transradial primary angioplasty in patients with acute myocardial infarction. *Ital Heart J.* 2003;4:329–334.

57. Philippe F, Larrazet F, Meziane T, et al. Comparison of transradial vs. transfemoral approach in the treatment of acute myocardial infarction with primary angioplasty and abciximab. *Catheter Cardiovasc Interv.* 2004;61:67–73.

58. Diaz de la Llera LS, Fournier Andray JA, Gomez Moreno S, et al. Transradial approach for percutaneous coronary stenting in the treatment of acute myocardial infarction. *Rev Esp Cardiol.* 2004;57:732–736.

59. Kim JY, Yoon J, Jung HY, et al. Feasibility of radial artery as a vascular access route in performing primary percutaneous coronary intervention. *Yonsei Med J.* 2005;46:503–510.

60. Hetherington SL, Adam Z, Morley R, et al. Primary percutaneous coronary intervention for acute ST-segment elevation myocardial infarction: changing patterns of vascular access, radial versus femoral artery. *Heart.* 2009;95:1612–1618.

61. De Carlo M, Borelli G, Gistri R, et al. Effectiveness of the transradial approach to reduce bleedings in patients undergoing urgent coronary angioplasty with GPIIb/IIIa inhibitors for acute coronary syndromes. *Catheter Cardiovasc Interv.* 2009;74: 408–415.

62. Siudak Z, Zawislak B, Dziewierz A, et al. Transradial approach in patients with ST-elevation myocardial infarction treated with abciximab results in fewer bleeding complications: data from EUROTRANSFER registry. *Coronary Artery Disease.* 2010;21:292–297.

63. Sciahbasi A, Pristipino C, Ambrosio G, et al. Arterial access-site-related outcomes of patients undergoing coronary procedures for acute coronary syndromes (from the comparison of early invasive and conservative treatment in patients with non-ST-elevation acute coronary syndromes [PRESTO-ACS] vascular substudy). *Am J Cardiol.* 2009;103:796–800.

64. Pancholy S, Patel T, Sanghvi K, et al. Comparison of door-to-balloon times for primary PCI using transradial versus transfemoral approach. *Catheter Cardiovasc Interv.* 2010;75:991–995.

65. Weaver AN, Henderson RA, Gilchrist IC, et al. Arterial access and door-to-balloon times for primary percutaneous coronary intervention in patients presenting with acute ST-elevation myocardial infarction. *Catheter Cardiovasc Interv.* 2010;75:695–699.

66. Cantor WJ, Puley G, Natarajan MK, et al. Radial versus femoral access for emergent percutaneous coronary intervention with adjunct glycoprotein IIb/IIIa inhibition in acute myocardial infarction: the RADIAL-AMI pilot randomized trial. *Am Heart J.* 2005;150:543–549.

67. Li WM, Li Y, Zhao JY, et al. Safety and feasibility of emergent percutaneous coronary intervention with the transradial access in patients with acute myocardial infarction. *Chin Med J.* 2007;120:598–600.

68. Current-Oasis 7 Investigators. Dose comparison of clopidogrel and aspirin in acute coronary syndromes. *N Engl J Med.* 2010;363:930–942.

69. Vorobcsuk A, Konyi A, Aradi D, et al. Transradial versus transfemoral percutaneous coronary intervention in acute myocardial infarction: systematic overview and meta-analysis. *Am Heart J.* 2009;158:814–821.

70. Batchelor WB, Anstrom KJ, Muhlbaier LH, et al. Contemporary outcome trends in the elderly undergoing percutaneous coronary interventions: results of 7,472 octogenarians. National Cardiovascular Network Collaboration. *J Am Coll Cardiol.* 2000;36:723–730.

71. Kobayashi Y, Mehran R, Mintz GS, et al. Comparison of in-hospital and one-year outcomes after multiple coronary arterial stenting in patients > 80 years old versus those < 80 years old. *Am J Cardiol.* 2003;92:443–446.

72. Deghani P, Mohammad A, Bajaj R, et al. Mechanism and predictors of failed transradial approach for percutaneous coronary interventions. *J Am Coll Cardiol Intv.* 2009;2:1057–1064.

73. Louvard Y, Benamer H, Garot P, et al. Comparison of transradial and transfemoral approaches for coronary angiography and angioplasty in octogenarians (the OCTOPLUS study). *Am J Cardiol.* 2004;94:1177–1180.

74. Yan ZX, Zhou YJ, Zhao YX, et al. Safety and feasibility of transradial approach for primary percutaneous coronary intervention in elderly patients with acute myocardial infarction. *Chin Med J.* 2008;121:782–786.

75. Zimmerman S, Ruthrof S, Nowak K, et al. Outcomes of contemporary interventional therapy of ST elevation infarction in patients older than 75 years. *Clin Cardiol.* 2009;32:87–93.

76. Ziakas A, Gomma A, McDonald J, et al. A comparison of radial and femoral approaches in primary or rescue percutaneous coronary intervention for acute myocardial infarction in the elderly. *Acute Card Care.* 2007;9:93–96.

77. Berger S, Sanborn TA, Sherman W, et al. Influence of sex on in-hospital outcomes and long-term survival after contemporary percutaneous coronary intervention. *Am Heart J.* 2006;151:1026–1031.

78. Chacko M, Lincoff AM, Wolski KE, et al. Ischemic and bleeding outcomes in women treated with bivalirudin during percutaneous

coronary intervention: a subgroup analysis of the Randomized Evaluation in PCI Linking Angiomax to Reduced Clinical Events (REPLACE-2) Trial. *Am Heart J.* 2006;151:e1–e7.

79. Pristipino PC, Pecciccia F, Granatelli A, et al. Comparison of access-related bleeding complications in women versus men undergoing percutaneous coronary catheterization using the radial versus femoral artery. *Am J Cardiol.* 2007;99:1216–1221.

80. Gershlick AH, Stephens-Lloyd A, Hughes S, et al. Rescue angioplasty after failed thrombolytic therapy for acute myocardial infarction. *N Engl J Med.* 2005;353:2758–2768.

81. Carver A, Rafelt S, Gershlick A, et al. Longer-term follow-up of patients recruited to the REACT (rescue angioplasty versus conservative treatment or repeat thrombolysis) trial. *J Am Coll Cardiol.* 2009;54:118–126.

82. Berry C, Kelly J, Cobbe SM, et al. Comparison of femoral bleeding complications after coronary angiography versus percutaneous coronary intervention. *Am J Cardiol.* 2004;94:361–363.

83. Kassam S, Cantor WJ, Patel D, et al. Radial versus femoral access for rescue percutaneous coronary intervention with adjuvant glycoprotein IIb/IIIa inhibitor use. *Can J Cardiol.* 2004;20:1439–1442.

84. Cruden NLM, Teh CH, Starkey IR, et al. Reduced vascular complications and length of stay with transradial rescue angioplasty for acute myocardial infarction. *Catheter Cardiovasc Interv.* 2007;70: 670–675.

85. Chesebro JH, Knatterud G, Roberts R, et al. Thrombolysis in myocardial infarction (TIMI) Trial, phase I: a comparison between intravenous tissue plasminogen activator and intravenous streptokinase. *Circulation.* 1987;76:142–154.

chapter 11

Transradial Approach to Peripheral Interventions

John T. Coppola, MD
Cezar Staniloae, MD

■ INTRODUCTION

Percutaneous peripheral interventions have historically been performed using a femoral artery approach. Due to mounting evidence from the coronary literature about the benefits of the transradial approach (TRA) when compared with the transfemoral approach (TFA),[1,2] there has been an increased interest in performing peripheral interventions using the radial artery as an access site.

■ ANATOMY

Whether for coronary or for peripheral interventions, it is mandatory that the radial operator be well aware of the radial artery anatomy and its anatomical variants. The radial artery in most people starts at the bifurcation of the brachial artery just below the bend of the elbow. It then passes along the radial side of the forearm to the wrist and terminates by passing between the 2 heads of the first interosseous dorsalis and into the palm. At this level, it loops across the metacarpal bones toward the ulnar side of the hand, uniting with the deep palmar branch of the ulnar artery.[3] There is extensive communication between the ulnar and radial branches that maintain blood flow to the hand in the event of radial occlusion.

Knowledge of anatomical variants is essential, as it allows for anticipation of problems as they may arise during the course of the procedure and facilitates appropriate measures to overcome difficult anatomy. Two large reviews demonstrated that anatomical variants, including tortuosities, stenoses, hypoplasias, and radioulnar loops, occur in up to 23% of transradial catheterizations.[4,5]

Transradial Access: Techniques for Diagnostic Angiography and Percutaneous Intervention
©2013 Howard A. Cohen (Editor). Cardiotext Publishing, ISBN 978-1-935395-41-6.

These abnormalities could significantly limit the procedural success.

It is also important to discern the caliber of the radial artery, as this factor has implications regarding equipment selection. Abnormally small caliber of the radial artery may be due to spasm, hypoplasia, or atherosclerosis. In regard to the latter, the radial artery is not protected from atherosclerotic disease; histopathologic studies examining the radial artery in patients with coronary artery disease have shown that up to 7% have severe plaque burden and near 21% have medial calcification.[6,7] These diseased arteries are more likely prone to spasm. Given that the long sheaths used during peripheral interventions must traverse the entire length of the upper extremity, particular attention must be devoted to the administration of appropriate spasmolytic cocktails and sedation. This is of even greater importance at the end of the case during sheath removal

because the prolonged exposure of the radial artery to the large-sized sheath may lead to significant spasm.

Anthropometric data, including arm and torso length, are important considerations in the TRA because there are limitations to equipment use in taller individuals. Depending on individual variability, different catheter lengths are required to reach various vascular beds as shown in Figure 11.1.

■ GENERAL TECHNICAL CONSIDERATIONS

The routine approach to the peripheral vascular intervention starts with gaining access to the radial artery of choice. When possible, the left radial artery is the first choice because it has the advantage of traversing a shorter distance to the descending aorta and not crossing the aortic arch and

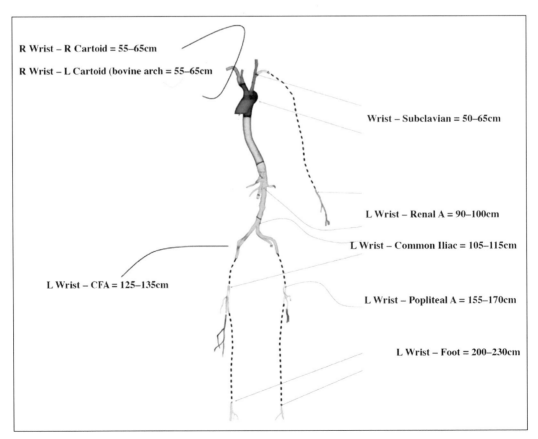

R Wrist – R Cartoid = 55–65cm

R Wrist – L Cartoid (bovine arch = 55–65cm

Wrist – Subclavian = 50–65cm

L Wrist – Renal A = 90–100cm

L Wrist – Common Iliac = 105–115cm

L Wrist – CFA = 125–135cm

L Wrist – Popliteal A = 155–170cm

L Wrist – Foot = 200–230cm

Figure 11.1 Anthropometric measurements in the vascular system.

cerebral vessels. The left subclavian artery most often directs the angiographer toward the descending aorta, so we usually begin the procedure with a 125-cm multipurpose catheter and an angle-tipped hydrophilic-coated 0.035-in wire. Occasionally, an internal mammary shape catheter may be required to negotiate the descending aorta due to a Type III aortic arch. Regardless of the wire used, it is mandatory to carefully monitor its passage via fluoroscopy to its destination in the lower abdominal aorta. Severe complications can result from "blind" advancement of the wire into tributaries of the thoracic or abdominal aorta.

Current stent and balloon platforms of all major manufacturers can be safely accommodated in 6-Fr-diameter sheaths, and there are stent platforms now available in 5 Fr.

■ SUBCLAVIAN ARTERY ANGIOPLASTY AND STENTING

Atherosclerotic subclavian artery stenosis is a recognized cause of various symptoms such as presyncope with upper extremity exercise, myocardial ischemia in patients with internal mammary bypasses, upper extremity claudications, or even embolic events.[8–10] The traditional revascularization method for subclavian artery obstruction was surgical bypass.[11] Over the last several years, balloon angioplasty and stenting of the subclavian artery have become the established therapy, and current recommendations suggest the endovascular approach as the first-line therapy for patients with symptomatic subclavian artery stenoses.

The technique of subclavian artery angioplasty using a transfemoral approach is well established. For the purpose of this review, we describe the transradial approach to subclavian artery stenting. The first step in preparation for the procedure is to document the patency of the ipsilateral radial artery. This should be done ideally by arterial duplex ultrasound because obstruction of the radial artery is encountered relatively frequently in this patient population, either due to embolization from the diseased subclavian artery or from prior use of the radial artery

for other revascularization purposes. Because most of the time the radial artery pulse is not easily palpable, the information provided by the duplex ultrasound is valuable in these situations. Once the patency of the radial artery is confirmed, the access is gained with relative ease, in spite of lack of a palpable pulse. A long, 5- or 6-Fr introducer sheath (55–65 cm) is then advanced just distal to the occlusion site, and a selective angiogram is performed (Figure 11.2). Various techniques could be used depending on the severity and the location of the obstruction. The majority of the time the lesion can be crossed with a 0.018-in wire. We predilate the lesion with an undersized balloon, which is then followed by stenting, with either a self-expandable or a balloon-expandable stent (Figure 11.3).[12] Should the lesion be located at the ostium of the subclavian artery, a balloon-expandable stent provides a better radial force, and it becomes preferable. Currently, most balloon-expandable stents fit a 5-Fr introducer sheath, and at least one manufacturer (Cook Medical, Bloomington, IN) has a self-expandable stent platform that can be accommodated in a 5-Fr introducer sheath. One should be aware that all the low-profile stent platforms require 0.014-in or 0.018-in guidewires.

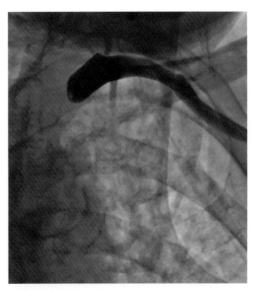

Figure 11.2 Subclavian angiogram via radial approach.

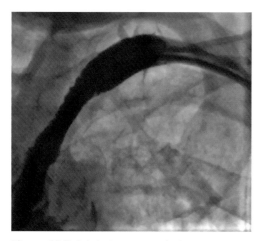

Figure 11.3 Subclavian stenting demonstrating excellent support for stent delivery.

The radial approach is particularly useful for situations where the subclavian artery is completely occluded. Although a classical wire technique could be used to cross the totally occluded subclavian arteries, newer technologies could be used to ensure intra-luminal location of the wire. One should be aware that most of the new crossing devices require a 6-Fr access. The major advantages of the radial approach are particularly relevant when facing totally occluded subcla-vian arteries. In these situations, the support offered by the radial access is significantly better than using the femoral approach. In our experience, once radial access is achieved, the success of subclavian artery angioplasty is close to 100%.

■ TRANSRADIAL STENTING OF THE CAROTID ARTERIES

Safe and successful stenting of the carotid arteries requires excellent positioning of the shuttle sheath. Therefore, we use the right radial approach for the carotid stenting in 2 circumstances: first, stenting of the left internal carotid artery when the left common carotid artery arises from the innominate artery and, second, stenting of the right internal carotid artery in the face of severe Type III aortic arch. In these circumstances, the access to the common carotid artery is much easier coming from the right radial approach than from the femoral access (Figure 11.4).

■ TECHNIQUE OF THE CAROTID ARTERY STENTING

The 6-Fr shuttle sheath is advanced from the right radial artery into the right subclavian artery, and the common carotid artery is accessed with a 0.035-in hydrophilic wire, which is guided by a 5-Fr internal mammary shape catheter (for the right carotid) or a vertebral shape (for the left carotid). Once the guidewire is positioned in the external carotid artery, the shuttle sheath is telescoped over the 5-Fr catheter and positioned in the common carotid artery (Figure 11.5). From this point on, the rest of the procedure is performed in the routine fashion.

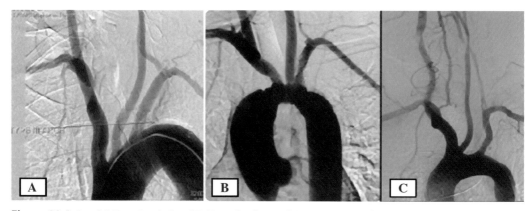

Figure 11.4 **Panel A:** Type 3 arch. **Panel B:** Normal arch. **Panel C:** Bovine arch (left carotid arising from right carotid).

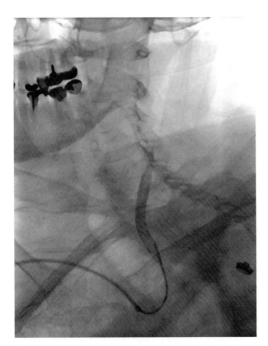

Figure 11.5 Use of telescoping catheter for shuttle sheath placement.

Stenting of the left carotid artery arising normally from the aortic arch is technically difficult from either radial artery.[13] Therefore, we do not advise using a radial approach in these situations.

■ TRANSRADIAL INTERVENTIONS FOR RENAL ARTERY STENOSIS

Renal artery disease is a common form of peripheral vascular disease seen in 6.8% of the population above the age of 65 years.[14] It is more common in patients with coronary artery disease or documented carotid or lower extremity disease and coexisting hypertension.[15,16]

Currently, the American College of Cardiology/American Heart Association (ACC/AHA) clinical guidelines recommend intervention in hemodynamically significant renal artery stenosis in patients with accelerated hypertension; resistant hypertension defined as therapy with 3 drugs, 1 of which is a diuretic; malignant hypertension; hypertension with a unilateral small kidney; or intolerance to medication.[17] Patients with flash pulmonary edema and renal stenosis, and the absence of any other etiology for heart failure, are the only group with a Class Ia recommendation for intervention. Renal intervention to preserve renal function is controversial and currently is a Class IIa recommendation in patients with progressive dysfunction and bilateral disease or disease in an artery to a solitary kidney.

Catheterization-based treatment for renal artery disease involves stenting, because balloon angioplasty results have been suboptimal. Renal atherosclerotic lesions are aorto-ostial lesions with high rates of recurring restenosis after balloon dilation. Patients undergoing renal stenting are usually pretreated with aspirin, and heparin is used during the procedure. Despite the lack of randomized data, most interventionists will use clopidogrel for 4–6 weeks after stenting.

An attractive benefit of performing renal interventions from the upper extremity is that the majority of renal arteries are oriented in a superior direction, making coaxial cannulation easier from the upper extremity. We have found that the radial approach offers several other benefits. Generally, patients undergoing renal intervention are hypertensive, making hemostasis after the procedure more difficult; using the radial artery eliminates this problem.

We have found that in elderly hypertensive patients, the abdominal aorta is often tortuous, making selective coaxial cannulation difficult from the groin (Figure 11.6) but straightforward from the arm (Figure 11.7). In addition, the presence of an abdominal aortic stent graft (Figure 11.8) makes cannulation of the renal artery difficult from the femoral approach.

We normally use the left radial artery for all of our peripheral procedures because this eliminates the need to cross the aortic arch and extends the distance the catheter will reach in the distal aorta.

With the use of the left radial artery, the renal arteries are reached in patients up to 190 cm tall with standard cardiac guiding catheters of 100 cm in length. In the majority of cases, we have found the Judkins Right

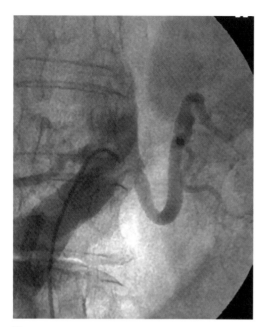

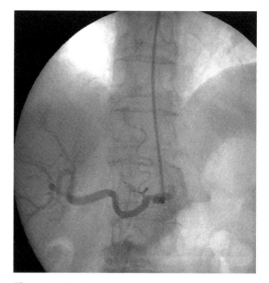

Figure 11.7 Same case as in Figure 11.6, approached from the radial approach.

Figure 11.6 Difficult engagement of the renal artery in elderly patient with tortuous aorta.

to be an ideally shaped catheter; if the renal artery is extremely up-looking, then a multi-purpose catheter may serve better.

A 6-Fr guiding catheter is of sufficient internal diameter to allow for a 6-mm-diameter balloon-expandable stent passing. At the head of the first lumbar vertebral body, the 0.035-in guidewire is removed, and the catheter is vigorously aspirated prior to cannulation of the renal artery. It is of importance to be able to identify the ostium of the renal artery; as a general rule, a shallow left anterior oblique (LAO), 10°–20°, will often show both ostia. Once the control angiogram is performed, a standard coronary guidewire is used to cross the lesion. We avoid hydrophilic wires because they have a slightly greater risk of distal wire perforation. Our practice is to predilate all lesions; this helps with sizing, judging the position of the ostium, and judging the character of the renal plaques. After predilation, an appropriately sized stent is chosen. We try to avoid overdilation or very-high-pressure deployment. If the patient complains of back pain, the balloon is deflated immediately and contrast is given to check for aorto-ostial damage.

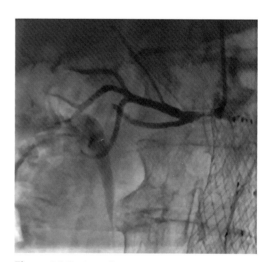

Figure 11.8 Coaxial engagement of renal artery with JR4.

We have found that engaging the renal artery from the arm provides excellent support; no difficulty has been encountered with stent delivery. At the completion of stenting, a final angiogram is obtained. The catheter is removed over a 0.035-in guidewire. Hemostasis is obtained by local compression at the wrist, and the patients may be discharged the same day if, after urination, there is no hematuria, back pain, or unexpected problems.

As an alternative to the 6-Fr guiding catheter, one could use a 5-Fr 110 Ansel-1 shape introducer sheath. The procedure is being performed in the same manner, but there are 2 advantages: first, it allows for reaching the renal ostia, even in very tall subjects; second, it accommodates stents with diameter larger than 6 mm, which would otherwise not fit a 6-Fr guiding catheter.

■ TRANSRADIAL INTERVENTION OF THE ILIAC ARTERY STENOSIS

Current ACC/AHA guidelines support endovascular intervention with stenting of most symptomatic iliac stenosis after a trial of medical therapy.[17] However, iliac disease may be less responsive to medical therapy alone compared to superficial femoral artery stenoses.[18] Surgical revascularization of the iliac lesions carries a significant morbidity and should be reserved for patients with low surgical risks and for lesions not amenable to percutaneous therapy. Symptoms of iliac arterial insufficiency may be atypical for classic lower extremity claudication; in fact, some patients present only with lower limb weakness. Exercise ankle-brachial index may be necessary to unmask aortoiliac occlusive disease, as robust collaterals may provide adequate lower extremity perfusion at rest.

■ ADVANTAGES OF TRANSRADIAL APPROACH FOR ILIAC ANGIOPLASTY

The transradial approach is particularly beneficial for patients undergoing peripheral interventions for multiple reasons. First, these patients frequently present with bilateral disease that makes them more susceptible to local vascular complications. Frequently, the crossover technique is hampered by severe tortuosity; this situation is particularly difficult when dealing with distal external iliac disease. The close proximity of the stenosis makes an ipsilateral approach difficult for distal external iliac interventions. A second benefit of the radial approach is to eliminate

the need to compress the common femoral artery after the procedure, which in the presence of occlusive disease may lead to ischemia or even thrombosis. Third, this approach facilitates same-day discharge, even in the presence of aggressive antithrombotic treatment.

■ ANATOMICAL CONSIDERATIONS

For obvious reasons, transradial intervention of the lower extremities, including the iliac arteries, may be more difficult in taller people and those with longer upper extremities, due to limitations of the length of equipment. Using the left versus the right radial artery for access has the advantage of a shorter distance to the descending aorta and allows the operator to avoid crossing the aortic arch and cerebral vessels. The left subclavian artery most often directs the angiographer toward the descending aorta, so we usually begin the procedure with a multipurpose catheter and standard 0.035-in J-wire. If needed due to tortuosity or Type III aortic arch, a soft, angle-tipped hydrophilic 0.035-in wire may be used with the aid of an internal mammary artery diagnostic catheter to facilitate entry into the descending aorta. Regardless of the wire used, it is mandatory that its passage be carefully followed with fluoroscopy to its destination in the lower abdominal aorta. Severe complications relating to renal, mesenteric, or even spinal vessel (artery of Adamkiewicz) injury can result from "blind" advancement of the wire into tributaries of the thoracic or abdominal aorta.

We recommend that in most cases, angiography of the aortoiliac system begin with a pigtail "power" injection of the lower abdominal aorta (typically 20 cc over 1 second in the anteroposterior projection). This initial scout film may help define any aortic aneurysms, collateral vessels, and presence of ostial disease of the common iliac arteries. This initial view may be forgone only in the presence of renal insufficiency with the backup of excellent noninvasive imaging. Selective angiography of each iliac artery may be performed with 5-Fr, 125-cm multipurpose catheters. Infrainguinal anatomy and internal iliac disease are important to assess not only for the appropriateness of endovascular intervention but also to assess postprocedure complications.

Once the decision to proceed with stenting is made, the 5-Fr diagnostic catheter is exchanged over a long (260-cm) 0.035-in guidewire for a long introducer sheath. Usually, we use 5-Fr, 110-cm-long straight introducers (Cook Medical, Bloomington, IN). The only time we use a 6-Fr, 110-cm sheath is in the situation where we anticipate the use of specific crossing devices (ie, chronic total occlusions). We routinely use long (300-cm) 0.014-in or 0.018-in wires. Once the sheath is positioned in the proximity of the iliac artery, the procedure is performed in the same fashion as from the groin (Figure 11.9, Figure 11.10).

■ SAFETY AND EFFICACY OF TRANSRADIAL ILIAC INTERVENTIONS

We reviewed procedural data and outcomes from 80 consecutive aortoiliac interventions treated either via transradial ($n = 33$) or trans-femoral ($n = 47$) approach.[19] Both the TRA and TFA groups showed similar mean baseline Rutherford category (2.9 vs. 2.6, respectively) and preintervention ankle-brachial index (0.64 vs. 0.67, respectively). However, lesion parameters differed, as the TRA group was characterized by a 3-fold higher presence of total occlusions (27.3% vs. 8.5%, $P = 0.03$) and a greater baseline-diameter stenosis (89.2% vs. 82.3%, $P = 0.003$). Despite this inequality in lesion types, there was no difference in mean procedural time (TRA: 97.9 minutes vs. TFA: 83.4 minutes, $P = 0.08$) or contrast volume requirement (TRA: 238.7 mL vs. TFA: 213.1 mL, $P = 0.35$). Interestingly, during the course of the study, the procedural time became shorter by an average of 25 minutes in the TRA group (112.3 minutes to 87.6 minutes, $P = 0.07$), suggesting a positive learning curve. In addition, the primary and secondary procedural success rates were similar between the TRA and TFA groups (87.9% vs. 97.8%, $P = 0.15$,

and 93.9% vs. 100%, $P = 0.17$, respectively). Postintervention hemodynamics, as measured by ankle-brachial index, showed similar degrees of improvement (TRA: 0.64 to 0.77 and TFA: 0.67 to 0.85, $P = 0.77$).

Our experience with TRA in aortoiliac interventions clearly demonstrated that despite the worse case mix that was present in the TRA group, this technique could be as successful as the TFA. Furthermore, radial access can be a viable option, even for more complex peripheral lesion types, as the prevalence of TASC C and D lesions in our study approached 40%. There are 2 additional issues that concern beginner radial operators. The first has to do with the anticipated need for larger balloon and stent sizes requiring bigger delivery sheaths, given the larger vessel diameters of the iliac arteries, and the second has to do with the longer distance from the puncture site to the target lesion. In our study, we were able to perform all aortoiliac interventions via a 6-Fr introducer sheath. Recently, most necessary equipment fits in 5-Fr introducers, and we shifted our approach to using preferentially 5-Fr introducers. Finally, the distance to the target lesion was never an indication to abort the TRA and resort to the TFA in order to complete the procedure.

■ SUMMARY

Peripheral vascular interventions can be safely performed using the radial artery as an access point. This approach is particularly beneficial because the patients with severe peripheral arterial disease are at higher risk for access site complications. The main limitation to this approach is the lack of equipment that could easily access every vascular bed, particularly at the level of superficial femoral artery and tibial vessels.

■ REFERENCES

1. Agostoni P, Biondi-Zoccai GG, de Benedictis ML, Rigattieri S, Turri M, Anselmi M, et al. Radial versus femoral approach for percutaneous coronary diagnostic and interventional procedures: systematic overview and meta-analysis of randomized trials. *J Am Coll Cardiol.* 2004;44(2):349–356.

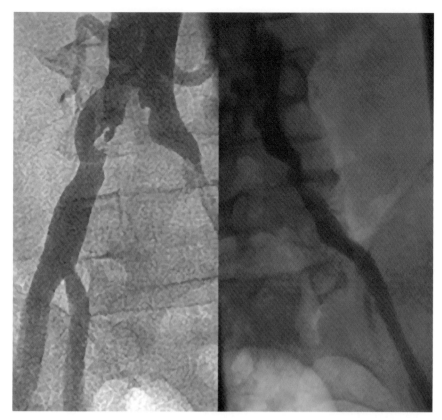

Figure 11.9
Iliac intervention
using a long
6-Fr sheath from
the left radial
approach.

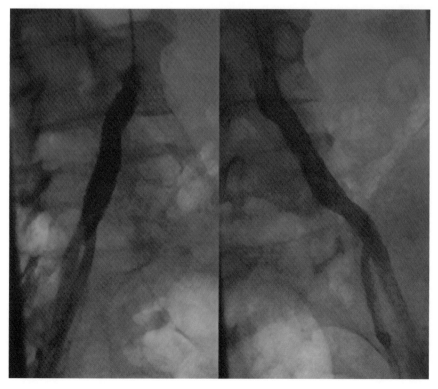

Figure 11.10
Excellent support
offered by radial
approach to
deliver stent.

2. Cox N, Resnic FS, Popma JJ, Simon DI, Eisenhauer AC, Rogers C. Comparison of the risk of vascular complications associated with femoral and radial access coronary catheterization procedures in obese versus nonobese patients. *Am J Cardiol.* 2004;94(9):1174–1177.

3. Elgharib NZ, Shah UH, Coppola JT. Transradial cardiac catheterization and percutaneous coronary intervention: a review. *Coron Artery Dis.* 2009;20(8):487–493.

4. Valsecchi O, Vassileva A, Musumeci G, Rossini R, Tespili M, Guagliumi G, et al. Failure of transradial approach during coronary interventions: anatomic considerations. *Catheter Cardiovasc Interv.* 2006;67(6):870–878.

5. Nie B, Zhou YJ, Li GZ, Shi DM, Wang JL. Clinical study of arterial anatomic variations for transradial coronary procedure in Chinese population. *Chin Med J (Engl).* 2009;122(18):2097–2102.

6. Oshima A, Takeshita S, Kozuma K, Yokoyama N, Motoyoshi K, Ishikawa S, et al. Intravascular ultrasound analysis of the radial artery for coronary artery bypass grafting. *Ann Thorac Surg.* 2005;79(1):99–103.

7. Staniloae CS, Mody KP, Sanghvi K, Mindrescu C, Coppola JT, Antonescu CR, et al. Histopathologic changes of the radial artery wall secondary to transradial catheterization. *Vasc Health Risk Manag.* 2009;5(3):527–532.

8. Bryan AJ, Hicks E, Lewis MH. Unilateral digital ischaemia secondary to embolisation from subclavian atheroma. *Ann R Coll Surg Engl.* 1989;71(2):140–142.

9. Sueoka BL. Percutaneous transluminal stent placement to treat subclavian steal syndrome. *J Vasc Interv Radiol.* 1996;7(3):351–356.

10. Olsen CO, Dunton RF, Maggs PR, Lahey SJ. Review of coronary-subclavian steal following internal mammary artery-coronary artery bypass surgery. *Ann Thorac Surg.* 1988;46(6):675–678.

11. Edwards WH Jr, Tapper SS, Edwards WH Sr, Mulherin JL Jr, Martin RS III, Jenkins JM. Subclavian revascularization. A quarter century experience. *Ann Surg.* 1994;219(6):673–677; discussion 677–678.

12. Yu J, Korabathina R, Coppola J, Staniloae C. Transradial approach to subclavian artery stenting. *J Invasive Cardiol.* 22(5):204–206.

13. Patel T, Shah S, Ranjan A, Malhotra H, Pancholy S, Coppola J. Contralateral transradial approach for carotid artery stenting: a feasibility study. *Catheter Cardiovasc Interv.* 75(2):268–275.

14. Hansen KJ, Edwards MS, Craven TE, Cherr GS, Jackson SA, Appel RG, et al. Prevalence of renovascular disease in the elderly: a population-based study. *J Vasc Surg.* 2002;36(3):443–451.

15. Weber-Mzell D, Kotanko P, Schumacher M, Klein W, Skrabal F. Coronary anatomy predicts presence or absence of renal artery stenosis: a prospective study in patients undergoing cardiac catheterization for suspected coronary artery disease. *Eur Heart J.* 2002;23(21):1684–1691.

16. Olin JW, Melia M, Young JR, Graor RA, Risius B. Prevalence of atherosclerotic renal artery stenosis in patients with atherosclerosis elsewhere. *Am J Med.* 1990;88(1N):46N-51N.

17. Hirsch AT, Haskal ZJ, Hertzer NR, Bakal CW, Creager MA, Halperin JL, et al. ACC/AHA guidelines for the management of patients with peripheral arterial disease (lower extremity, renal, mesenteric, and abdominal aortic): a collaborative report from the American Associations for Vascular Surgery/Society for Vascular Surgery, Society for Cardiovascular Angiography and Interventions, Society for Vascular Medicine and Biology, Society of Interventional Radiology, and the ACC/AHA Task Force on Practice Guidelines (writing committee to develop guidelines for the management of patients with peripheral arterial disease): summary of recommendations. *J Vasc Interv Radiol.* 2006;17(9):1383–1397; quiz 1398.

18. White CJ, Gray WA. Endovascular therapies for peripheral arterial disease: an evidence-based review. *Circulation.* 2007;116(19):2203–2215.

19. Staniloae CS, Korabathina R, Yu J, Kurian D, Coppola J. Safety and efficacy of transradial aortoiliac interventions. *Catheter Cardiovasc Interv.* 75(5):659–662.

chapter 12

Right Heart Catheterization and Transradial Access

Ian C. Gilchrist, MD

■ BACKGROUND

Transradial arterial access has evolved into an elegant technique, but without the ability to perform a complementary right heart or central venous catheterization, the technique is incomplete. The apparent inability to do right heart catheterization has been used as an indication, or excuse, to revert back to groin access. But the technique to access the central venous system from the arm has been known since the very first human cardiac catheterization, when Werner Forssman passed a ureteral ("uretic") catheter up from his forearm vein[1]—for which he was awarded the Nobel Prize in Medicine along with Dickinson Richards and Andre Cournand. With the advent of percutaneous techniques that allowed routine puncture of the femoral vessels, and further understanding of anatomical landmarks to allow central venous

access through the great veins of the neck, techniques of central venous access from the arm almost became lost in history.

Starting in the late 1990s, about a decade after the first modern transradial artery had been reported, several groups from diverse locations around the globe resurrected and improved central venous access techniques using peripheral veins to both take advantage of modern equipment and fulfill a greater potential for transradial techniques. Gilchrist et al, in 2002, published their initial experience obtaining central venous access through peripheral arm veins at the time of transradial catheterization.[2] Using extra-long 125-cm, balloon-tipped catheters, attempts were made by the operators with tourniquets to percutaneously enter peripheral veins that ran on the surface or that accompanied deeper arteries such as the radial artery. Although there was success many times, the technique was limited by the ability to reliably find distal veins and ultimately by the inability to secure a continued source of 125-cm catheters. Subsequently, the technique evolved so that the venous access was obtained initially outside the catheterization laboratory by IV teams placing heparin-well venous access anywhere between the antecubital fossa and the wrist. This temporary access was then exchanged in the laboratory for a vascular sheath that would then subsequently permit passage of a central venous catheter. This approach resulted in reliable central venous access[3] that has been reported by several different groups using analogous techniques.[4–6]

■ PERIPHERAL VENOUS ANATOMY AND PHYSIOLOGY

There are several distinguishing features of the peripheral venous system that distinguishes it from the arterial system and must be considered by the radial operator. These are outlined in Table 12.1. The venous system is low in pressure and reacts differently than the arterial system. Veins are more distensible and far less likely to respond with spasm compared to the arterial system. Although conceptually, catheterization in the venous system that is far more anatomically complex than the arterial tree appears difficult, the realities are that most who venture into the venous system find it relatively easy compared to the arterial tree and far more forgiving.

Although variability is the rule, there are some general anatomical principles that forearm veins follow, as shown in Figure 12.1.

All veins below the antecubital fossa eventually drain into the subclavian vein by coursing up either the lateral system of the cephalic vein or the medial system of the axillary/basilic vein. Medial (ulnar) side veins form the most direct route to the central system passing up the basilic, then the axillary vein, and subsequently the subclavian vein. The basilic and axillary veins may be quite large with diameters of > 1 cm. Veins on the lateral (radial) side of the arm below the antecubital fossa tend to pass either medially or laterally in a 50/50 distribution above the antecubital fossa.[7] The lateral veins of the hind arm join to form the cephalic vein that is usually significantly smaller in diameter than the axillary vein. The cephalic vein makes a right-angle turn at its junction with the axillary vein defining the origin of the subclavian vein as pictured in Figure 12.2. This junction, also referred to as a "T" junction, may represent a technical challenge that should be recognized but is easily met with forethought.

The physiology of veins is slightly different from that of arteries, and in particular, the forearm veins represent vessels that are significantly smaller in diameter than the femoral venous structures. Veins in general are significantly less muscular and have much thinner walls than arteries. Although they are less muscular than arteries, veins are still capable of spasm, especially when an indwelling catheter diameter is similar in size to the vein. Venospasm was historically a hazard reported in the literature when venous cutdowns were common and catheters were larger (8 Fr) and stiffer compared to present equipment. Modern experience with smaller

Table 12.1 Anatomical Comparison and Pharmacophysiology of Arterial and Venous System of the Forearm.

Feature	Arterial System	Venous System
Anatomic Variability	+	+++
Collaterals/Redundancy	+	+++
Distensibility	–	++
Risk of Spasm	+++	–
Pharmacoreactivity		
Prophylactic antispasm medications required	Yes	No
Calcium channel blocker responsive	Yes	No
Nitrates responsive	Yes	Yes

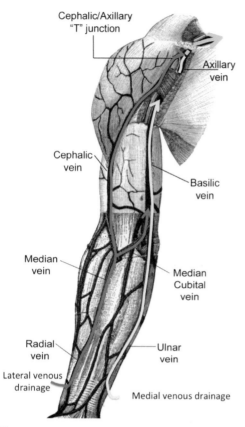

Figure 12.1 Schematic diagram of arm veins with relative drainage patterns of medial (yellow) and lateral (blue) veins. Lateral forearm drainage is distributed in a 50/50 proportion between the cephalic and basilic venous systems that meet at the "T" junction forming the subclavian vein (green). *Source:* Modified from public domain: Gerrish FH (ed). *A Text-book of Anatomy by American Authors,* 2nd ed. Philadelphia, PA: Lea Brothers & Co, 1902:483-484.

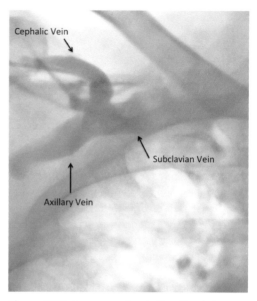

Figure 12.2 Venogram of cephalic-axillary vein junction. This is known as the "T" junction because the cephalic vein intersects at a 90° angle. This combination forms the subclavian vein that continues into the central venous system.

and more flexible balloon-tipped catheters is remarkably free of venospasm. Routine antispasm medications are not needed. If venospasm does occur, it is far more likely to respond to nitrates and warmth than to the calcium channel blockers that work so well as arterial dilators.[8]

■ PRACTICAL APPROACH TO CENTRAL VENOUS ACCESS FROM THE FOREARM

Planning for Venous Access

Although veins tend to run next to the radial artery, and can be accessed to reach the central system, their utility is limited by their inconsistent location and size. There is also the practical reality that industry does not produce devices long enough to reliably reach from such distal locations. Peripheral venous access from the arm will almost always be not as close to the radial arterial access site as what one experiences with venous access during a femoral procedure. This presents both challenges and opportunities to redefine how catheterization services are delivered.

If there is a need for central venous access, access will need to be found in an area that will be accessible at the same time the forearm is positioned for radial artery access. Although veins on the back of the forearm will provide access to the central system, their location is usually impractical for use with ipsilateral radial artery access. Realistically, peripheral venous access is best obtained in the area defined by the antecubital fossa down the palmar aspect of the forearm to the wrist. Alternatively, venous access in the contralateral arm of the arterial access can increase the options for access in patients with limited superficial veins.

Preprocedural staff can facilitate the procedure by obtaining the initial venous access prior to arrival in the catheterization laboratory. If venous access is obtained in the forearm and reserved with a heparin lock or similar device in a setting of warmth and comfort, it avoids the need to find de novo access in a busy catheterization laboratory. These devices can be placed both in patients requiring a right heart catheterization and in patients who might require rapid central venous access such as those with acute myocardial infarction or perhaps those requiring interventions that may require temporary transvenous pacing.

■ VASCULAR SHEATH PLACEMENT IN THE CATHETERIZATION LABORATORY

Venous Access in the Catheterization Laboratory

If venous access is not obtained prior to arrival, access will need to be done in the laboratory. The room should not be cold, and the patient needs to be relaxed. At times, veins will be readily visible and may even be entered directly with a micropuncture needle without a tourniquet. If a tourniquet is used, it needs to be released after access is obtained to allow free passage of catheters up the veins. Once wire access has been successful, the placement of an appropriately sized vascular sheath can be accomplished similar to arterial access. Local anesthesia at the entry site prevents pain from sheath passage. If skin laceration

with a scalpel is needed, be careful to not lacerate the very superficial venous structures. At times, it may be difficult to obtain venous access, and other techniques such as venous ultrasound or levophase angiograms[9] may be necessary to be successful.

Exchange of Heparin Lock/IVs Placed Outside of Laboratory

If venous access is already present on arrival to the catheterization laboratory, exchange to a vascular sheath can be done sterilely and efficiently. The venous access site should be isolated and cleaned with a Food and Drug Administration (FDA)-approved alcohol-based bactericidal wash. Alcohol-based chlorhexidine antiseptic solutions are far more bactericidal than iodine-based solutions, especially in situations where blood or protein may potentially be present on the heparin lock in the sterile field. Once clean and dry, a wire compatible with both the indwelling venous catheter and the vascular sheath is passed through the latex cap of the heparin lock using an introducer needle, as shown in Figure 12.3. The wire should pass without resistance. The previously placed heparin lock with the introducer needle still impaled in the latex cap can be grasped in a block with sterile gauze and slid off the wire that remains in the venous system. The extracted heparin lock/introducer needle complex is then passed off the sterile field. If done right, there will be no need for contact

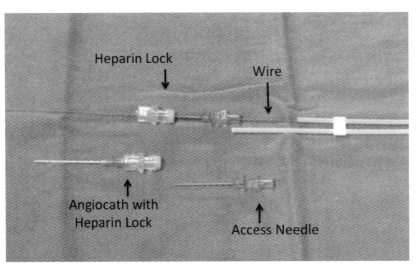

Figure 12.3
Heparin locks, angiocaths, access needles, and vascular wires used to exchange peripheral intravenous access for vascular sheaths in the cardiac catheterization laboratory.

Heparin Lock

Wire

Angiocath with Heparin Lock

Access Needle

between sterile work gloves and the chemically treated intravenous device (heparin lock) placed outside the laboratory. The vascular sheath is then placed on the wire and slid into the venous system with subsequent removal of the wire and sheath's associated dilator.

Venous "Cocktails" for the Vascular Sheath

Venospasm is rare. Many operators do not use preemptive antispasm medication in the venous system. If an antispasm cocktail is desired or needed due to spasm, nitrates should be used in dosages similar to those used in the arterial tree. Calcium channel blockers are less effective in contradistinction to the arterial system's response to these agents. Whether or not an antispasm cocktail is added, the side arm of the vascular sheath should be flushed to reduce the risk of thrombosis. Due to the low vascular pressure in the peripheral veins, there may be no drawback of blood on aspiration of the sheath. As long as the sheath flushes without resistance or patient pain, the lack of blood aspiration is not indicative of poor venous position.

■ PASSAGE TO THE CENTRAL VENOUS AND PULMONARY CIRCULATION

Right heart catheters from several manufacturers are available in a variety of sizes from 4 to 8 Fr. These can be obtained in balloon-tipped, both single-lumen and multilumen devices with thermodilution capabilities depending on the operator's preference. Industry has failed to manufacture catheters beyond the 110-cm length, although access to long lengths such as 125 cm would be helpful in individuals with long arms, especially if more distal extremity venous access is used.

Initially, the catheter should be passed up the arm with the flow-directing balloon tip deflated. As long as no resistance is encountered, one does not have to watch this under fluoroscopy. When the catheter reaches the level of the shoulder, it is often useful to spot-check the location under fluoroscopy. This fluoroscopy is needed to confirm whether the catheter has passed up the basilica/axillary system or the lateral cephalic venous system.

If the catheter is in the subclavian vein or proximal axillary vein, the balloon can be inflated and continue through the right heart, often just under pressure monitoring.

If the catheter has passed up the cephalic vein, its crossing into the axillary-subclavian junction needs visual supervision. The cephalic vein enters in a 90° fashion, and the balloon should be inflated only when it is clear that the tip of the catheter is freely in the subclavian and heading toward the heart. Difficulty maneuvering the "T" junction can be remediated with the help of a deep breath by the patient or through the use of a wire in the catheter to redirect the device. Once the catheter is correctly positioned in the subclavian, it can be advanced under pressure monitoring through the right heart unless fluoroscopy is needed to confirm location of the catheter tip. Overall, once the peripherally placed devices reach the subclavian vein, they behave very similarly to those placed in any central chest vein and can be advanced to their desired location using standard approaches.

■ POSTPROCEDURAL ACCESS SITE MANAGEMENT

At the conclusion of the procedure, the central venous catheter should be removed from the central system with the balloon deflated. The side arm of the introducer sheath is once again flushed, noting that blood return may still not be possible on aspiration due to venous collapse, and a vasodilator cocktail is not normally needed. The vascular sheath can then be removed and pressure applied to prevent bleeding without waiting for any periprocedural anticoagulation to dissipate. Due to the low venous pressure, relatively low external pressure is required to obtain hemostatic control. The venous site can typically be managed with sterile pressure dressing and no specific hemostasis device. If the venous site is in close proximity to the radial arterial site, the hemostatic device for the artery may also be used to control the venous site. Venous hemostasis usually is readily obtained and occurs before arterial hemostasis.

A summary of the venous procedure is outlined in Table 12.2, as discussed in the

Table 12.2 Steps to Forearm Venous Catheterization of the Heart.

Preprocedural
Identify potential need for venous access
Establish venous access and cap intravenous catheter (heparin lock)
Do prior to entry in the catheterization laboratory for greatest efficiency
Place in the catheterization laboratory as an alternative
Cardiac Catheterization Laboratory
Vascular Sheath Placement
Sterile prep of venous access line site
Puncture cap of heparin lock with wire insertion needle
Pass vascular wire through introducer wire up vein without resistance
Slide heparin lock with insertion needle off the wire and dispose off field
Place vascular sheath over vascular wire
Remove dilator and wire from vascular sheath
Flush sheath; no specific vasodilator required
Central Venous/Right Heart Catheter Placement
Pass equipment up arm without resistance watching under x-ray at the cephalic-axillary "T" junction
Flow-directing balloon can be inflated in the subclavian vein
Pass equipment to central location as indicated
After Procedure
Remove catheter with flow-directed balloon deflated
Flush remaining vascular sheath; no specific vasodilator required
Remove vascular sheath and apply appropriate pressure
Bandage site to maintain pressure suitable for venous stasis

Source: Adapted in part: Gilchrist IC. Radial approach to right heart catheterization and intervention: state of the art paper. *Indian Heart J.* 2010;62:245–250.

preceding section. Using this type of approach to right heart catheterization, it is possible to get procedural results consistent with those using the femoral vein without the risks of femoral trauma. The potential complications of directly puncturing a central vein in the neck are also avoided, and the benefits from the safety and convenience of the transradial approach remain with this addition to the transradial toolbox. As noted in Figure 12.4, procedural times and x-ray times[3] are similar when the forearm approach is compared to the femoral approach for central venous and right heart catheterization. [*Editor's note*: In

patients with severe pulmonary hypertension, particularly in the presence of tricuspid regurgitation, procedural time is probably shorter from the arm.]

■ OVERCOMING POTENTIAL CHALLENGES

Difficult Venous Access

Several different techniques have been used to help find concealed forearm veins. Ultrasound equipment can also be helpful to map out the

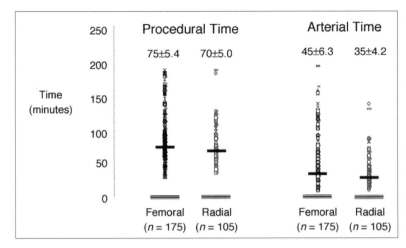

Figure 12.4 Comparison of procedural times and arterial times of bilateral cardiac catheterizations done at a single center using either radial or femoral approaches at the discretion of the operators.

location of deeper veins such as the axillary vein or deep antecubital veins. Even at the level of the wrist, a vein usually accompanies both the radial and the ulnar artery similar to the femoral artery and its vein. Whether a vein lies lateral or in a medial position to that of the artery is patient specific, but a vascular ultrasound device can localize the vein in relationship to the arterial pulse. The operator can then approximate the venous position by palpating the arterial pulse and often obtain venous access in patients who otherwise appear to have little hope for peripheral access.

An alternative approach, when radial artery access is available, is a levophase angiogram.[9] In this case, diluted contrast is injected into the radial artery and observed during the venous phase. The venous system can then be visualized. If a tourniquet is placed to trap the contrast, the operator can have some time to further localize the vein. This technique works best in the antecubital region where the veins pass superficially in front of the elbow bones. Care needs to be taken to not puncture a neighboring artery or nerve in this region.

Finally, if one arm does not have a reasonable vein, the contralateral arm may work. Patients typically would rather have venous and arterial access in opposing arms versus being subjected to the risks of either neck or groin access. Once removed, the venous site care is not much greater than removal of any superficial venous access and does not add significantly to the postprocedural morbidity.

Resistance to Forward Passage of Catheter

Resistance is a sign of either venospasm, entrapment in a side branch, a venous valve sinus, or venous obstruction. Using the modern hydrophilic-coated, flexible catheters, true venospasm is rare. If venospasm does occur, intravenous nitroglycerine in 100- to 200-µg dosages is the best approach, although it is rarely needed. Nitrates can also be delivered cutaneously or sublingually. Further manipulation of the vein should be minimized while pharmacologic or other changes are made to reduce the tone of the vein. Other causes of spasm that should be corrected include patient anxiety and cold ambient temperatures. Finally, changing brand of catheter may help as coatings differ by manufacturer and at times may make a difference.

If resistance occurs with passage of a catheter or wire, it is especially important not to push. Pushing will cause perforation or tearing of the vein that is less resilient than the artery. A small contrast injection can often define the issue of whether there is spasm, perforation of the vein, or perhaps another route to the heart that may be better, as the venous system often has redundant systems that lead to the central system.

Congenital Venous Anomalies

Left arm approaches can be potentially challenged by a persistent left-sided superior vena cava. This results in left-sided arm blood draining into the coronary sinus and then right atrium. With modern flow-directed catheters, passage through the right heart and out into the pulmonary artery may still occur, although the course will appear radiographically unusual. If a persistent left-sided superior vena cava is encountered and cannot be passed due to tortuous vascular course, an alternative right-sided approach will need to be found.

Electrophysiological Devices

The leads on electrophysiological devices may obstruct the venous system, and even without arm swelling, extensive collaterals may be present (Figure 12.5). Whether thrombosis is present is difficult to predict. Transit past the site of lead entry may require extra manipulation with a wire in the hemodynamic catheter. The option to use the contralateral side is also reasonable.

Previous Upper Extremity/Shoulder Trauma

Prior procedures or major trauma to the ipsilateral shoulder or upper arm, even decades earlier, can be problematic. Prior cardiac

catheterization by cutdown at the brachial site may have resulted in surgical destruction of the venous system and resulting collaterals that cannot be transversed. Brachial arteriotomies were usually repaired, but venotomies were usually ligated with the vein's integrity sacrificed. In such instances, contralateral access may be required.

Motor vehicle and other traumatic injuries of the upper arm and chest need to be considered because venous trauma may have also rendered the central venous system damaged even without overt signs of chronic venous obstruction (Figure 12.6). If resistance to passage occurs, a limited angiogram may define whether there is an insurmountable challenge for which an alternative venous approach will be needed.

Another group of patients who are occasionally problematic includes those who have received chemotherapy or radiation to the chest. These patients may have had long-term indwelling central venous ports for chemotherapy, and extensive sclerosis may impede catheter passage to the central venous system. Likewise, high-dose radiation may have similarly resulted in obstructive changes to the normal venous channels. A limited

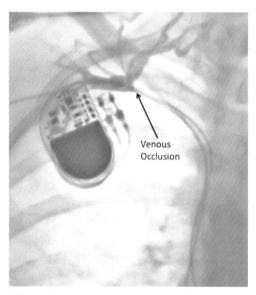

Figure 12.5 Venogram of right subclavian system taken by injection dilute contrast through right heart catheter in distal subclavian vein showing occlusion at site of pacemaker electrodes (arrow) and multiple collaterals extending to the jugular venous system.

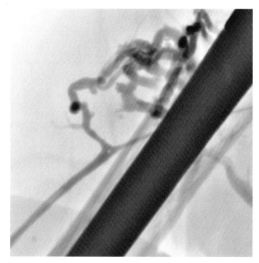

Figure 12.6 Trauma resulting in humerus fracture and subsequent repair with rod 10 years prior to attempt to do right heart catheterization from the forearm. Venogram of upper arm taken through right heart catheter that failed to advance without resistance. Extensive venous collaterals are seen at site of occlusion.

angiogram will provide information critical in deciding whether one can continue to use this particular access site. Finally, patients who have had breast cancer are another group that may have had significant surgical manipulation of the venous structures or have been instructed to not have procedures done in the ipsilateral arm. An alternative site should be sought in this subgroup of cancer patients.

■ ADVANCE TECHNIQUES

The need for routine right heart catheterization has been obviated by the advances in echocardiography and other noninvasive testing. Although this tends to leave invasive evaluation primarily for problematic patients, there is also a need for central venous access that extends beyond simple hemodynamics. Central venous access techniques, similar to those described above, can be adapted to provide for temporary transvenous pacing and endomyocardial biopsy[10] along with a potential portal for a variety of interventional venous techniques. Because the brachial/axillary venous route provides the straightest course to the central venous system, this is the preferred route for such advanced nonhemodynamic procedures. The greatest challenge encountered in extending the list of interventional procedures possible from the arm rests with the lack of appropriate-length catheters to reach the target of intervention from the arm.

■ SUMMARY

Central venous access can actually be readily obtained using forearm veins. Whether needed for catheter-based hemodynamic monitoring or diagnosis, for temporary pacing during periods of iatrogenic bradycardia from interventional techniques, or for a transvenous interventional procedure, forearm venous access can provide a reliable and safe entry site to complement or complete the transradial procedure. Venous access from the forearm can be accomplished efficiently and without compromise by avoiding otherwise riskier anatomical approaches. Understanding venous techniques and recognizing this

important adjunct to transradial interventions completes the operator's radial skills and further advances the potential of transradial interventions.

■ REFERENCES

1. Forssmann W. Die Sondierung des rechten Herzens. *Klin Wochenschr*. 1929;8:2085.
2. Gilchrist IC, Kharabsheh S, Nickolaus MJ, et al. Radial approach to right heart catheterization: early experience with a promising technique. *Cathet Cardiovasc Intervent*. 2002;55:20–22.
3. Gilchrist IC, Moyer CD, Gascho JA. Trans-radial right and left heart catheterization: a comparison to traditional femoral approach. *Cathet Cardiovasc Intervent*. 2006;67:585–588.
4. Cheng NJ, Ho WC, Ko YH, et al. Percutaneous cardiac catheterization combining direct venipuncture of superficial forearm veins and transradial arterial approach: a feasible approach. *Acta Cardiol Sin*. 2003;19:159–164.
5. Yang C-H, Guo B-F, Yip H-K, et al. Bilateral cardiac catheterization: the safety and feasibility of a superficial forearm venous and transradial arterial approach. *Int Heart J*. 2006;47:21–27.
6. Lo TSN, Buch AN, Hall IR, et al. Percutaneous left and right heart catheterization in fully anticoagulated patients utilizing the radial artery and forearm vein: a two-center experience. *J Intervent Cardiol*. 2006;19:258–263.
7. Chun HJ, Byun JY, Yoo S-S, et al. Tourniquet application to facilitate axillary venous access in percutaneous central venous catheterization. *Radiol*. 2003;226:918–920.
8. Low RI, Takeda P, Mason DT, et al. The effects of calcium channel blocking agents on cardiovascular function. *Am J Cardiol*. 1982;49:547–553.
9. Pancholy SB, Sweeney J. A technique to access difficult to find upper extremity veins for right heart catheterization: the Levogram technique. *Cathet Cardiovasc Intervent*. First published online: May 3, 2011, DOI:10.1002/ccd.23037.
10. Moyer CD, Gilchrist IC. Transradial bilateral-cardiac catheterization with endomyocardial biopsy: a feasibility study. *Cathet Cardiovasc Intervent*. 2005;64:134–137.

chapter 13

The Learning Curve for Transradial Access

Yves Louvard, MD

Hakim Benamer, MD

Thierry Lefèvre, MD

■ INTRODUCTION

The transradial approach to interventional cardiology procedures is by no means a novel technique. The first nonselective coronary angiograms were carried out during and after the Second World War by a member of the prestigious Swedish School of Radiology, Dr. Radner, who used the proximal cutoff technique followed by ligation of the radial artery at the elbow level (1945).[1] This technique was supplanted in 1953 by the percutaneous femoral approach proposed by Dr. Seldinger, another member of the Swedish School.[2] In 1964, Campeau developed the proximal radial denudation technique followed by suturing.[3] The first femoral introducers became available during the following year. In 1989, Campeau performed distal percutaneous transradial coronary angiography followed by compression.[3,4] In 1992, the first transradial balloon coronary angioplasty[5] and, in 1993, the first transradial percutaneous coronary intervention (PCI) with stent implantation was carried out by Kiemeneij.[6]

Initially, the implantation of coronary stents via femoral access combined with extreme anticoagulation therapy generated a very high percentage of vascular complications; this led to the development of the radial approach, which almost completely eliminated such complications. A steady increase in the use of the transradial route was observed in Europe and Japan during this period, despite the advent (very early on in France)[7] of antiplatelet treatments, encouraged by the first angioplasty courses. In some countries (France, Spain, United Kingdom, Norway, Taiwan, Japan), the percentage of transradial procedures rose sharply, becoming

Transradial Access: Techniques for Diagnostic Angiography and Percutaneous Intervention
©2013 Howard A. Cohen (Editor). Cardiotext Publishing, ISBN 978-1-935395-41-6.

often higher than transfemoral interventions between 2000 and 2010. In many countries,[8] however, the acceptance of this strategy was more selective (Canada, United States, Germany, Switzerland . . .)[9] or was linked to the growing use of PCI (China).

The attested relationship between the occurrence of bleeding vascular complications and the rate of short-term and midterm mortality in patients undergoing PCI[10–12] has stimulated the progression of the transradial technique in the United States and in several European countries (Germany, Switzerland) over the past few years.

Establishing how the transradial technique should be taught and learned is crucial in ensuring that this vascular access strategy meets its objectives and results in a reduction in mortality, morbidity, overall cost, and improved patient comfort.

The objective of this review is to describe the learning curve of the transradial coronary angiography and angioplasty as well as the predictive factors of failure and difficulty in order to define appropriate learning and teaching methods. The present analysis of transradial-related issues applies only to the field of coronary interventional cardiology.

■ HOW TO ASSESS THE LEARNING CURVE

In order to best describe the learning curve associated with the transradial approach, one should analyze the activity of isolated operators, who are not under the guidance of experienced colleagues, from their first transradial procedures in an unselected population of patients. Such a description has never been published.

It seems feasible to evaluate the progress achieved by a single operator or a group of operators by analyzing the success rate of coronary angiography procedures (selective and appropriate visualization of the coronary vessels) or the success rate and procedural time of coronary angioplasty procedures.

For both types of procedure (diagnostic and interventional), such an assessment process involves factors nonspecifically related to the vascular access: quality of injection for coronary angiography, and achievement of an appropriate result in the treatment of more or less complex coronary lesions with respect to coronary angioplasty.

One must also take into account the fact that an experienced operator in left main or chronic total occlusion angioplasty may not achieve the same results in terms of quality or safety via the transradial approach if he or she is just beginning to use this vascular route. Consequently, the learning curve of the transradial approach may be more accurately analyzed by focusing on the success rate of puncture or introducer insertion or by evaluating a more specific component of the learning curve such as the rate of catheter penetration into the ascending aorta.[13,14]

The appropriateness of the criteria used to assess the learning curve varies according to patient selection criteria, which influence the degree of procedural difficulty (size of the artery, size of the patient, age, gender, diabetes, previous coronary artery bypass graft [CABG], etc). It might also be appropriate to assess the leaning curve by adding the exclusion rate to the failure rate.

Procedural duration and x-ray time are conventional assessment criteria for analyzing the efficacy of a given technique or operator.

Transradial percutaneous coronary interventions are not complication-free. The occurrence of complications is obviously related to the expertise of the operator.

Finally, the learning curve of the transradial approach cannot be analyzed without taking into account the characteristics of the population and/or the presence of a proctor guiding the beginner operator. The learning curve is probably also influenced by the availability of technical enhancements, the reading of publications, and participation in dedicated courses.

■ WHAT IS THE LEARNING CURVE OF THE RADIAL APPROACH?

Success Rate

Contemporary success rate of transradial approach for diagnosis or intervention is higher than 98% in very experienced operator hands. Previous as well as current publications report preliminary or low-volume personal experiences. The large series of transradial procedures that could potentially be reported is currently performed in countries where this vascular route has gained wide acceptance. As a consequence, the procedures are no longer submitted and/or accepted for publication.

The first author of the present review recorded the clinical and procedural characteristics as well as complications associated with more than 2,400 separate, consecutive, diagnostic, and/or interventional procedures he carried out between 1994 and 1999.[8] The success criterion of the transradial procedure was the achievement of catheter penetration into the ascending aorta. The rate of failure is shown in Figure 13.1. It was close to 5% after 100 procedures, which supports the frequently mentioned observation that 50 to 100 cases are sufficient to achieve an acceptable 95% rate of success. After performing 800 procedures, the rate of failure is 3% and decreases to 1.5% after 2,400 procedures. However, in 1994, the first 100 transradial procedures accounted for 51% of all interventions whereas in the last 800 patients, 81% of procedures were performed via the transradial route.

This tends to show that the 5% rate of failure after 50 to 100 procedures is an artifact associated with an intuitive or recommended selection of patients. Kiemeneij's recommendation in 1994 was to begin with big, young male patients with a simple coronary anatomy.

This is further supported by a study performed in 2003 in our institution (Institut Cardiovasculaire Paris Sud, Massy, France) by 3 interventional cardiology fellows[8] who had no experience in the transradial approach but were able to perform transfemoral angiography on their own, and 3 senior operators with wide experience in transradial diagnosis and PCI. Figure 13.2 shows the rate of success achieved in the first 90 transradial procedures performed without assistance from junior operators (higher panel), and the final rate of success of procedures carried out with the help of senior operators (lower panel) in a nonselected population of patients (> 95% of procedures). This study showed the actual rate of procedural success achieved in a nonselected population and underlined the

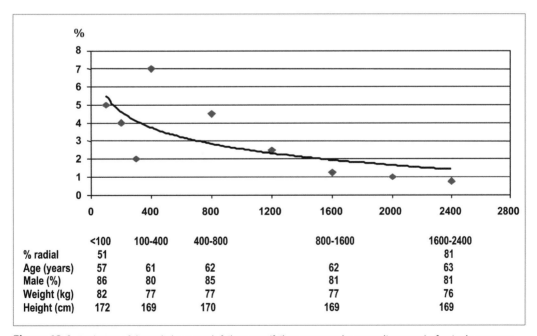

Figure 13.1 Evolution of the radial approach failure rate (failure to enter the ascending aorta) of a single operator in 2,400 consecutive patients from the first one in 1994 to 1999. Evolution of certain clinical factors and rate of radial approach attempt in the same population.

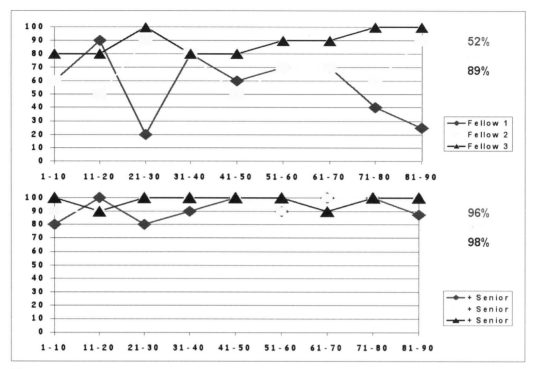

Figure 13.2 Radial approach success rate (catheterization of the ascending aorta) achieved by 3 fellows (upper panel), and with the help of a senior radial operator (lower panel) in the first 90 transradial cases performed by the fellows.

variability between operators, as well as the excellent rate of success achieved by the senior operator following failed attempts by the fellow (no disadvantage for the patient).

In a large population of consecutive patients ($N = 1,826$) referred for angiography and/or angioplasty in 2005–2007, 2 operators with wide experience, Guédès and Dangoisse,[15] implemented the same strategy as for the femoral approach (ie, first attempt on one side, then on the other side in cases of failure). They achieved a 98.8% rate of approach success (the failure rate for the first attempt was 6.8%, and 4.9% when patients with previous CABG were excluded; the rate of failure was shown to regress by about 40% per year and was 3.2% in the last year of the study).

Procedural Duration

The total duration of a coronary angioplasty procedure has often been reported in randomized trials as similar for transfemoral and transradial procedures alike.[16,17]

This does not mean that procedural duration does not decrease with experience; it means only that comparisons involve seasoned operators with wide experience in transradial angiography. Moreover, there are few specific differences between transfemoral and transradial PCI procedures. The vascular access route, therefore, does not seem to be a discriminating factor.

However, the findings associated with coronary angiography are different. Indeed, the duration of a coronary angiogram decreases with operator experience. Analysis of the first 1,000 transradial coronary angiograms (no graft, 2 left ventricular angiographies) by the same operator[18] showed that the procedural duration decreased from 23.3 minutes for the first 100 angiograms to 13.1 minutes for the last 100 (Figure 13.3). The analysis of this reduction in procedural time takes into account the various catheterization strategies implemented: from the initial use of one catheter for each artery to the systematic quest for an ideal multipurpose catheter. It is,

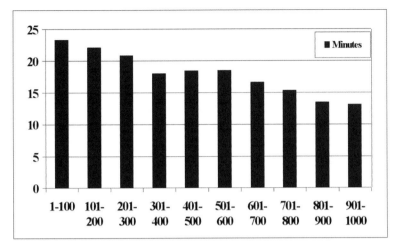

Figure 13.3 Procedural time of the first 1,000 transradial coronary angiographies (no graft, 2 left ventricle angiographies), performed by a single operator.

however, difficult to distinguish between the effect of operator experience and the advantages provided by new catheter shapes that have not yet been adequately evaluated. In an early dual-center study involving 4 operators, Spaulding[19] reported a decrease in procedure duration from 25.7 ± 12.9 minutes after 80 cases (20 per operator) to 17.48 ± 4.71 minutes in the last 100 cases. One of the main reasons for this improvement is the reduction in radial cannulation time (10.2 ± 7.6 minutes to 2.85 ± 2.53 minutes) whereas the rate of failure decreased from 14% to 2%.

X-ray Exposure

X-ray exposure has often been reported as nondifferent between transradial and transfemoral procedures in high-volume randomized angioplasty studies.[16,17] The influence of the operator seems to be more significant than the influence of the vascular route.[20]

A higher duration of x-ray exposure has been observed in transradial angiography.[17,21,22] Such a difference generally decreases with growing operator experience.

A study reported by Pezzano et al[23] showed that although procedural duration is similar with both routes, the x-ray duration and the area exposure product are higher in transradial procedures, due exclusively to fluoroscopy (catheter handling, guiding of the catheter all along the route, systematic antebrachial angiography, etc). Lange[22] underlined the fact that despite similar duration of x-ray exposure

and dose area product, radiation received by transradial operators is 2-fold compared with transfemoral procedures. This can probably be attributed to correctable factors such as the distance between the operator and the x-ray source, which should be increased during transradial procedures, or to the inadequacy or inappropriate positioning of protective equipment. With appropriate shielding, there should be little difference between femoral and radial access because when the arm is placed next to the body, the wrist is exactly at the same level as the femoral artery. In some instances, however, there are anatomic and technical issues in transradial access that may prolong fluoroscopy time and therefore radiation exposure.

Complications

No systematic analysis was carried out on the evolution of the rate of transradial procedural complications in relation to increasing operator experience. However, in the series published by the first author of the present review, 2 forearm compartment syndromes requiring surgical repair occurred in 1995, and no complications of this nature have been reported since.

The meta-analysis performed by Jolly underlined a difference in terms of frequency between radial experts and nonradial experts with respect to the occurrence of major bleeding.[24]

The data of the Swedish Coronary Angiography and Angioplasty Register

(SCAAR)[25] initially pointed out an excess incidence of stroke in the transradial group at a time when use of the radial route was still infrequent. This finding was invalidated 2 years later by the first author (B. Lagerqvist, MD, personal communication, June 2005, Massy transradial course) and was not observed in the meta-analysis by Jolly[24] or in the more recent French registry.[26]

The influence of experience was confirmed in RIVAL,[27] a large randomized study in which the primary endpoint (death, myocardial infarction [MI], stroke, and non-CABG bleeding) failed to demonstrate the superiority of the transradial route. However, in centers with a high volume of transradial procedures, the superiority of the radial route was demonstrated as well as the combined endpoint of death, MI, or stroke with a clear trend in favor of the most experienced operators (assessment based on the average number of procedures per center). The prerequisite for operators taking part in this study was to have performed 50 transradial procedures during the year prior to the beginning of the study. During the course of the study, one-third of operators performed fewer than 70 transradial angioplasties over a 1-year period and the remaining two-thirds fewer than 142. Although the total number of transradial angioplasties performed by each individual operator prior to the study was not reported, it was probably very low (< 100, for example) given the 40% rate of transradial procedures in the year prior to the study and the 7.6% rate of crossover from the radial to the femoral route. This may be attributed to lack of experience or the absence of any selection process.

A strong trend toward reduced mortality also has been observed in centers where a high volume of transradial procedures is carried out. Such a reduction was reported in all centers in the subgroup of ST-segment elevation myocardial infarction (STEMI) patients at higher risk for vascular and bleeding complications. A post hoc analysis of access site major bleeding events showed that none of these bleeding events was associated with actual transradial procedures but that all of them occurred in the radial to femoral crossover group. No compartment syndrome was reported. Finally, the alleged lack of experience of transradial operators in the femoral approach was not confirmed by the findings of the study.

Thus, it appears clearly that the rate of transradial procedures and the rate of transradial success, which are both related to operator experience, may play a major role in reducing the complication and mortality rates associated with coronary angioplasty.

Differences between the Left and the Right Transradial Routes

The randomized study CARAFE[21] comparing right radial ($n = 70$), left radial ($n = 70$), and femoral approaches ($n = 70$) for standardized coronary angiography (no graft, 1 left ventricular angiography), performed by 2 experienced operators, showed a procedural duration of 12.4 ± 5.8 minutes, 14.2 ± 3.3 minutes, and 11.2 ± 5.8 minutes, respectively. The left transradial approach was found to be significantly more time-consuming than the other 2 (single-catheter strategy associated with the right radial approach). X-ray exposure was 3.8 ± 2.2 minutes, 4.2 ± 1.7 minutes, and 3.1 ± 1.7 minutes, respectively, in favor of the transfemoral route.

The TALENT randomized trial analyzed the comparative efficiency of the left and right transradial routes for angiography and angioplasty procedures, using fluoroscopy time as an endpoint.[28] With respect to left transradial angiography ($n = 735$), x-ray time was 149 seconds (interquartile range [IQR] 95–270) and dose area product [DAP] for fluroscopy 10.7 Gy.cm^2 (IQR 6–20.5) versus 168-second x-ray time (IQR 110–277; $P = 0.0025$) and 12.1 Gy.cm^2 DAP (IQR 7–23.8 Gy cm^2, $P = 0.004$) for right transradial angiography ($n = 732$). No difference was observed regarding DAP for x-ray acquisition, possibly due to the extra difficulties associated with catheter manipulation on fluoroscopy when using the right transradial route. No significant differences emerged between left and right transradial angioplasty procedures ($n = 344$). The predictors of prolonged x-ray duration were operator experience and advanced patient age.

Most interestingly, this study analyzed the evolution in x-ray time during procedures carried out by fellows, according to experience.[29] In 532 and 935 angioplasty procedures performed by 6 fellows and senior operators, respectively, x-ray exposure times were compared and divided into 3 periods: < 100 procedures, between 100 and 200 procedures, and > 200 procedures for the right and the left transradial approach, respectively. X-ray exposure duration did not vary in senior operators, whereas it decreased with experience in fellows. After more than 200 procedures performed by fellows, the difference in x-ray time for left radial approach was borderline compared with senior operators, whereas it remains considerable for right transradial procedures. DAP did not vary in right transradial procedures and was significantly reduced in left transradial procedures performed by fellows. In both operator groups, radial cannulation time was identical and rapidly decreased with experience.

As a consequence, it appears clear that transradial catheterization following sheath insertion is more difficult to learn via the right radial route. This is probably mainly related to the anatomy, which is more favorable through the left approach (fewer subclavian tortuosities, etc). Coronary engagement from the left radial approach is similar to the femoral approach and requires little manipulation of the catheter as with the Judkins technique as compared to angiography from the right radial approach that is similar to the Sones technique.

Differences Compared with the Learning Curve of the Transfemoral Approach

There are no reports in the literature on the learning curve associated with transfemoral interventional cardiology procedures, nor are there any randomized or nonrandomized comparisons other than the experience-related decrease in the crossover rate between the radial and femoral routes observed in the RIVAL trial.[27] However, any interventional cardiologist with wide experience in the transfemoral approach who undertook transradial procedures would confirm the greater difficulty posed by the transradial route.

Systematic use of the transradial route in all patients requires a long learning curve, well beyond 50 to 100 procedures, before a 95% success rate can be obtained. However, 50 procedures are probably enough for an operator to be able to reach this reasonable objective in selected patients. Except for radial artery cannulation (no difference), the left radial approach is easier to learn than the right radial route.

■ WHAT DOES THE LEARNING PERIOD INVOLVE?

Clinical Predictors of Failure

The predictors of failure were identified by Barbeau et al[30] in a multivariate analysis involving 6,962 coronary procedures with a 7% rate of failure. By decreasing order of importance, these predictors were female gender, operator experience, advanced age, and low body mass index. The univariate analysis of the first 2,400 procedures performed by a single operator in our center identified the following predictors of failure: low patient weight, small patient size, more advanced age, and female gender.[8] The presence of diabetes was found to be a predictor of failure in female patients. Hypertension also emerged as a predictor of failure in the first 1,677 angioplasties carried out by a single operator.[8]

After exclusion of patients with previous CABG, Guédès[15] identified four predictors of failed transradial approach: operator experience, as assessed by the year of the procedure ($P < 0.001$), history of peripheral arterial disease ($P = 0.016$), "small radial artery size" ($P = 0.003$), and "difficult access" by clinical evaluation ($P = 0.006$). By univariate analysis of the prespecified clinical characteristics, only gender was predictive of the need for a nonradial access (procedural failure in female patients: 2.1% vs. 0.9%; $P = 0.036$); there was also a trend for diabetes ($P = 0.099$).

In a consecutive series of 1,052 transradial procedures, Pristipino[31] did not identify any clinical predictor of the selection of transradial cardiac catheterization (no patient selection). However, high-volume centers and high-volume radial operators were predictors of the choice of transradial route. Predictors of failure were found to be the presence of peripheral obstructive vascular disease and lower use of the transradial approach (failure for > 85% radial approaches: 3.8% vs. 33% when < 25%, $P < 0.001$).

Difficulties and Technical Predictors of Failure

In the series reported by Guédès,[15] failed attempts at radial puncture accounted for 52.6% of all failures. It was 69% in the series of Barbeau et al.[30] Other failed attempts involved the crossing of the brachial, axillary, or innominate arteries (11.1%); selective catheterization of a coronary artery or bypass graft (9.6%); and catheterization of the controlateral mammary artery (26.7%).

In 2,211 consecutive patients undergoing transradial coronary angiography, Valsecchi et al[32] conducted a systematic analysis of the anatomic variations and their influence on the rate of failure. Anatomic variations of upper limb arteries were noted in 22.8% and included tortuous configurations (3.8%), stenosis (1.7%), hypoplasia (7.7%), radio-ulnar loop (0.8%), abnormal origin of the radial artery (8.3%), and retro-esophageal right subclavian artery (0.45%). Patients with anatomic variations of radial artery had a significantly lower puncture (96.2% vs. 99.7%, $P < 0.0001$) and procedural (93.1% vs. 98.8%, $P < 0.0001$) success rate. The procedural failure rates were 1.2% for tortuous configurations, 3.3% for radial coming from axillary origin, 6.1% for hypoplastic radial arteries, 8.1% for radial stenosis, 16.7% for radio-ulnar loops, and 40% for retro-esophageal right subclavian artery.[33]

In a study involving 1,540 consecutive transradial procedures where retrograde transradial angiography was systematically performed,[34] the observed frequency of radial artery abnormality was 13.8%: 7.0% of high radial takeoff, 2.3% of complete loops, 2.0% of extreme radial tortuosities, and 2.5% of various abnormalities such as atherosclerosis or accessory branches. Instances of

failed transradial catheterization were more frequent in the presence of radial anatomical variations (14% vs. 0.9%, $P < 0.0001$). Procedural failure was 4.6% with high radial bifurcation, 23.3% with severe radial tortuosity, 37.1% with radial loop, and 12.9% with other anomalies.

The presence of subclavian tortuosities (10.8% in right subclavian arteries in the series reported by Cha) is also a predictor of transradial failure (4%).[35] Tortuosities are a much less frequent occurrence in left subclavian arteries, 0 in 232, compared to the right, 20 in 205 (9.8%), in the series reported by Kawashima.[36] Such a difference seems to account for prolonged procedural duration and higher x-ray exposure when using the right radial approach.

Anticipating Technical Difficulties

In the study by Guédès,[15] bedside clinical evaluation identified the radial access of 253 patients (13.8%) as "difficult" due to a weak pulse, "small vessel" size, or both. This assessment was more frequent for females (28.3% vs. 7.6%; $P < 0.001$), diabetics (19.5% vs. 12.4%; $P = 0.001$), patients with peripheral artery disease (17.4% vs. 12.6%; $P = 0.012$), and hypertensive patients (17.8% vs. 10.5%; $P < 0.001$). Puncturing was actually less difficult than anticipated.

Radial tortuosities have been shown to be associated with arterial hypertension[37] and right subclavian tortuosities with hypertension, advanced age, and higher body mass index.[38] Small radial arteries are more frequent in women[39] and diabetic patients.[40] Radial calcifications are also found in diabetic patients.[40] There is no predictor for the presence of a radio-ulnar loop,[41] but they can be identified by systematic echography, which complicates the procedure and reduces the cost-effectiveness associated with transradial catheterization.[42] Although angiographic identification of any unfamiliar anatomical variation hindering catheter advancement does not result in a reduction of the failure rate, it may allow a reduction in the occurrence of complications.

■ HOW TO BEST TEACH AND LEARN THE TRANSRADIAL APPROACH

Teaching the Transradial Approach

It can be accomplished using multiple tools, such as dedicated textbooks,[43,44] websites,[45,46] dedicated courses, and virtual bench or radial sessions held during major interventional cardiology courses. However, practical learning is irreplaceable, hence the hands-on workshops organized in centers where the rate of transradial coronary procedures is more than 90%. Regular practice of the transradial approach in an adequate number of cases is the most efficient means of learning. However, this must be combined with the tools mentioned above in order to be able to identify and overcome difficulties that are less frequently encountered.

Fellowship. In a high-volume radial center, fellowship enables beginners to learn transradial catheterization in a population of unselected patients. Fellows can be gradually introduced to cases of increasing complexity. Overcoming difficulties by learning established tips and tricks can be achieved with the help of several experienced senior operators. This learning method is indeed efficient, though it requires both a significant investment in terms of availability and the ability to take time off from one's own cardiac catheterization laboratory.

Self-teaching. An option that was successfully adopted by the pioneers of transradial catheterization is self-teaching. This relies on two principles: the volume of transradial procedures and the selection of patients (see Figures 13.4, 13.5, and 13.6). Appropriate patient selection results in an acceptable success rate of transradial angiography and angioplasty in a reasonable procedural time, in accordance with x-ray protection standards, in the best interest of patients, operators, cath-lab staff, and cath-lab management (in the event of conflicts, beginning operators are supported by the rest of the team). Patient selection, as well as crossover to the trans-femoral route, relies on the analysis of various previously described predictors of failure: clinical, technical (vessel route abnormality, lesion issues for PCI), and practical factors (pulse, radial artery size, tortuosities). It is possible to "manage the learning curve" by gradually introducing new operators to increasingly complex cases, based on previously collected data in a prospective database.[15] Each new difficulty encountered can be overcome with the help of various media sources and by seeking the advice of experienced colleagues. Several simple tips and tricks may prove extremely efficient, such as the successful crossing of nearly any obstacles in the right subclavian artery by using the deep breathing maneuver. The use of the left radial route, with puncture on the left side of the patient,

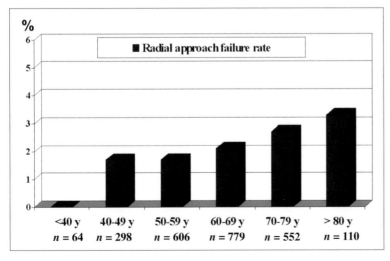

Figure 13.4 Failure rate of the radial approach for diagnosis and intervention in a population of 2,400 consecutive cases in different age groups.

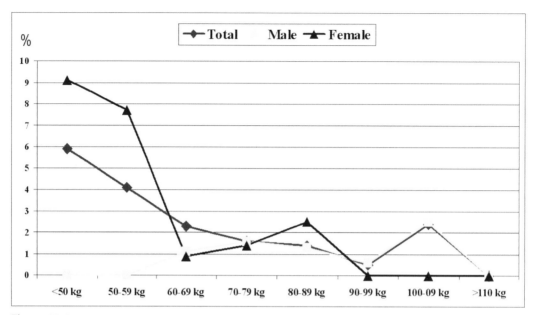

Figure 13.5 Failure rate of the radial approach for diagnosis and intervention in a population of 2,400 consecutive cases in different weight groups.

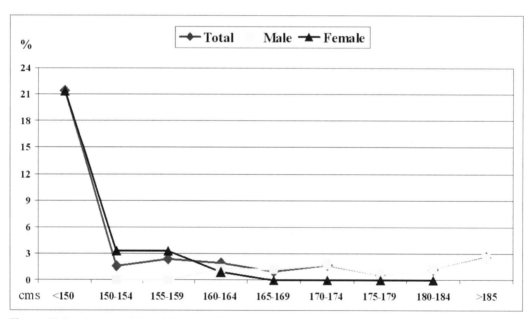

Figure 13.6 Failure rate of the radial approach for diagnosis and intervention in a population of 2,400 consecutive cases in different height groups.

enables the operator to learn the puncture process and cardiac catheterization maneuvers separately in a limited period of time (the left approach delivers more x-ray to the operator closer to the source and is also responsible for back pain for the operator). Even when the access is left radial, most operators prefer to work from the right side, as that is the way the catheterization laboratory is usually set up. When the patient is not obese, the left arm can usually be pulled to the right side with a "sling" that obviates the need to lean over the patient to reach the left radial access site. Alternatively, the operator can work on the left side by reversing the monitors and the shielding in the laboratory. This is usually, however, not very efficient.

Simultaneous teaching of the transfemoral and transradial approaches. In centers dedicated to the teaching of cardiac catheterization, it is recommended that the less demanding transfemoral approach be taught in a limited number of cases.

■SUMMARY

Use of the transradial route in interventional cardiology procedures may practically eradicate the occurrence of arterial access complications with their subsequent effects on mortality, morbidity, disability, and the need for transfusion or vascular surgery. In addition, the elimination of these complications reduces health care costs. Such improvements may be achieved with a modest increase in x-ray exposure for coronary angiography, but without any increase in procedural time, or operator irradiation for coronary angioplasty, and without any differences in terms of efficiency in almost all patients and all clinical and technical settings.

However, these results can only be achieved after completion of a long learning curve. Thanks to the multiple training opportunities available and after appropriate patient selection, a good command of clinical and technical predictors of failure allows transradial operators to obtain rapidly acceptable success rates, procedural durations, and x-ray exposure. This may encourage colleagues, coworkers, paramedics, patients, and hospital managers to support widespread use of this vascular approach.

■REFERENCES

1. Radner S. Thoracal aortography by catheterization from the radial artery. *Acta Radiol.* 1948;29:178–180.
2. Seldinger S. Catheter replacement of the needle in percutaneous arteriography: a new technique. *Acta Radiologica.* (Stockholm). 1953;39:368–376. Reproduced in *AJR* 1084;142:5–7.
3. Campeau L. Entry sites for coronary angiography and therapeutic interventions: from the proximal to the distal radial artery. *Can J Cardiol.* Mar 2001;17(3):319–325. Review.
4. Campeau L. Percutaneous radial artery approach for coronary angiography. *Cathet Cardiovasc Diagn.* Jan 1989;16(1):3–7.
5. Kiemeneij F, Laarman GJ, de Melker E. Transradial artery coronary angioplasty. *Am Heart J.* 1995;129:1–7.
6. Kiemeneij F, Laarman GJ. Percutaneous transradial artery approach for coronary stent implantation. *Am Heart J.* 1995;128:167–174.
7. Barragan P, Sainsous J, Silvestri M, Bouvier JL, Comet B, Siméoni JB, Villain P, Pietri P, Quatre JM, Bayet G. Pilot study of the efficacy of ticlopidine in early patency of coronary endoprostheses. *Arch Mal Coeur Vaiss.* 1994;87(11):1431–1437.
8. Louvard Y, Kumar S, Lefèvre T. Percentage of transradial approach for interventional cardiology in the world and learning the technique. *Ann Cardiol Angeiol.* (Paris). 2009;58(6):327–332.
9. Rao SV, Ou FS, Wang TY, Roe MT, Brindis R, Rumsfeld JS, Peterson ED. Trends in the prevalence and outcomes of radial and femoral approaches to percutaneous coronary intervention: a report from the National Cardiovascular Data Registry. *JACC Cardiovasc Interv.* Aug 2008;1(4):379–386.
10. Doyle BJ, Rihal CS, Gastineau DA, Holmes DR Jr. Bleeding, blood transfusion, and increased mortality after percutaneous coronary intervention: implications for contemporary practice. *J Am Coll Cardiol.* 2009;53:2019–2027.
11. Rao SV, Eikelboom JA, Granger CB, Harrington RA, Califf RM, Bassand JP. Bleeding and blood transfusion issues in patients with non-ST-segment elevation acute coronary syndromes. *Eur Heart J.* 2007;28:1193–1204.
12. Chase AJ, Fretz EB, Warburton WP, et al. Association of the arterial access site at angioplasty with transfusion and mortality: The M.O.R.T.A.L

study (Mortality benefit Of Reduced Transfusion after percutaneous coronary intervention via the Arm or Leg). *Heart.* 2008;94:1019–1025.

13. Louvard Y, Lefevre T, Morice MC. Radial approach: what about the learning curve? *Cathet Cardiovasc Diagn.* Dec 1997;42(4):467–468.

14. Louvard Y, Pezzano M, Scheers L, Koukoui F, Marien C, Benaim R, Goy P, Lardoux H. Coronary angiography by a radial artery approach: feasibility, learning curve: one operator's experience. *Arch Mal Coeur Vaiss.* 1998;91(2):209–215.

15. Guédès A, Dangoisse V, Gabriel L, Jamart J, Chenu P, Marchandise B, Schroeder E. Low rate of conversion to transfemoral approach when attempting both radial arteries for coronary angiography and percutaneous coronary intervention: a study of 1,826 consecutive procedures. *J Invasive Cardiol.* 2010;22(9):391–397.

16. Kiemeneij F, Laarman GJ, Odekerken D, Slagboom T, van der Wieken R. A randomized comparison of percutaneous transluminal coronary angioplasty by the radial, brachial and femoral approaches: the Access study. *J Am Coll Cardiol.* 1997;29:1269–1275.

17. Louvard Y, Benamer H, Garot P, Hildick-Smith D, Loubeyre C, Rigattieri S, Monchi M, Lefèvre T, Hamon M. Comparison of transradial and trans-femoral approaches for coronary angiography and angioplasty in octogenarians (the OCTOPLUS study); OCTOPLUS Study Group. *Am J Cardiol.* Nov 2004 1;94(9):1177–1180.

18. Louvard Y, Krol M, Pezzano M, Sheers L, Piechaud JF, Marien C, Benaim R, Lardoux H, Morice MC. Feasibility of routine transradial coronary angiography: a single operator's experience. *J Invasive Cardiol.* Sep 1999;11(9):543–548.

19. Spaulding C, Lefèvre T, Funck F, Thébault B, Chauveau M, Ben Hamda K, Chalet Y, Monségu H, Tsocanakis O, Py A, Guillard N, Weber S. Left radial approach for coronary angiography: results of a prospective study. *Cathet Cardiovasc Diagn.* 1996;39(4):365–370.

20. Larrazet F, Dibie A, Philippe F, Palau R, Klausz R, Laborde F. Factors influencing fluoroscopy time and dose-area product values during ad hoc one-vessel percutaneous coronary angioplasty. *Br J Radiol.* Jul 2003;76(907):473–477.

21. Louvard Y, Lefèvre T, Allain A, Morice M. Coronary angiography through the radial or the femoral approach: the CARAFE study. *Catheter Cardiovasc Interv.* Feb 2001;52(2):181–187.

22. Lange H, von Boetticher H. Randomized comparison of operator radiation exposure during coronary angiography and intervention by radial or femoral approach catheterization and cardiovascular interventions. *Catheter Cardiovasc Interv.* 2006;67:12–16

23. Pezzano M, Louvard Y, Lefèvre T et al. Radiation dose and arterial approach for coronary angiography. *Am J Cardiol.* 2001;88(Suppl 5A):111G (TCT 2001).

24. Jolly SS, Amlani S, Hamon M, Yusuf S, Mehta SR. Radial versus femoral access for coronary angiography or intervention and the impact on major bleed-

ing and ischemic events: a systematic review and meta-analysis of randomized trials. *Am Heart J.* Jan 2009;157(1):132–140.

25. Lagerqvist B, Albertsson P, James S, Nilsson T. Increased risk of complications with a transradial approach in coronary procedures: a report from the Swedish coronary angiography and angioplasty registry. AHA meeting, 2004.

26. Blanchard D. TIA or stroke during PCI: is the radial route a risk factor? Results from 2 large nationwide registries in France: PACIFIC and FAR registries. European Society of Cardiology meeting, 2007.

27. Jolly SS, Yusuf S, Cairns J, Niemelä K, Xavier D, Widimsky P, Budaj A, Niemelä M, Valentin V, Lewis BS, Avezum A, Steg PG, Rao SV, Gao P, Afzal R, Joyner CD, Chrolavicius S, Mehta SR. Radial versus femoral access for coronary angiography and intervention in patients with acute coronary syndromes (RIVAL): a randomised, parallel group, multicentre trial. RIVAL trial group. *Lancet.* Apr 23 2011;377(9775):1409–1420. Erratum in: *Lancet.* Apr 23 2011;377(9775):1408. *Lancet.* Jul 2 2011;378(9785):30.

28. Sciahbasi A, Romagnoli E, Burzotta F, Trani C, Sarandrea A, Summaria F, Pendenza G, Tommasino A, Patrizi R, Mazzari M, Mongiardo R, Lioy E. Transradial approach (left vs. right) and procedural times during percutaneous coronary procedures: TALENT study. *Am Heart J.* Jan 2011;161(1): 172–179.

29. Sciahbasi A, Romagnoli E, Trani C, Burzotta F, Pendenza G, Tommasino A, Leone AM, Niccoli G, Porto I, Penco M, Lioy E. Evaluation of the "learning curve" for left and right radial approach during percutaneous coronary procedures. *Am J Cardiol.* Jul 15 2011;108(2):185–188.

30. Barbeau G, et al. Predictors of failure of transradial approach for coronary angiography and intervention. American Heart Association meeting, 1999.

31. Pristipino C, Roncella A, Trani C, Nazzaro MS, Berni A, Di Sciascio G, Sciahbasi A, Musarò SD, Mazzarotto P, Gioffrè G, Speciale G. Identifying factors that predict the choice and success rate of radial artery catheterisation in contemporary real world cardiology practice: a sub-analysis of the PREVAIL study data. Prospective Registry of Vascular Access in Interventions in Lazio region (PREVAIL) study group. *EuroIntervention.* 2010;6(2):240–246.

32. Valsecchi O, Vassileva A, Musumeci G, Rossini R, Tespili M, Guagliumi G, Mihalcsik L, Gavazzi A, Ferrazzi P. Failure of transradial approach during coronary interventions: anatomic considerations. *Catheter Cardiovasc Interv.* Jun 2006;67(6):870–878.

33. Abhaichand RK, Louvard Y, Gobeil JF, Loubeyre C, Lefevre T, Morice MC. The problem of arteria lusoria in right transradial coronary angiography and angioplasty. *Catheter Cardiovasc Interv.* Oct 2001;54(2):196–201.

34. Lo TS, Nolan J, Fountzopoulos E, Behan M, Butler R, Hetherington SL, Vijayalakshmi K, Rajagopal R,

Fraser D, Zaman A, Hildick-Smith D. Radial artery anomaly and its influence on transradial coronary procedural outcome. *Heart.* Mar 2009;95(5): 410–415.

35. Cha et al. *Cathet Cardiovasc Intervent.* 2003;56:abst 29 (SCAI meeting).

36. Kawashima O, Endoh N, Terashima M, Ito Y, Abe S, Ootomo T, Ogata K, Honda H, Takizawa K, Miyazaki Y, Sugawara D, Komatsu M, Sawazi Y, Ozaki T, Uchimuro T, Meguro T, Isoyama S. Effectiveness of right or left radial approach for coronary angiography. *Catheter Cardiovasc Interv.* Mar 2004;61(3):333–337.

37. Yoo et al. *Am J Cardiol.* 2002;90(Supp 6A):167H, TCT meeting.

38. Cha et al. *Cathet Cardiovasc Intervent.* 2002;56:abst 69 (SCAI meeting).

39. Saito S, Ikei H, Hosokawa G, Tanaka S. Influence of the ratio between radial artery inner diameter and sheath outer diameter on radial artery flow after transradial coronary intervention. *Catheter Cardiovasc Interv.* Feb 1999;46(2):173–178.

40. Nicolosi AC, Pohl LL, Parsons P, Cambria RA, Olinger GN. Increased incidence of radial artery calcification in patients with diabetes mellitus. *J Surg Res.* Jan 2002;102(1):1–5.

41. Louvard Y, Lefèvre T. Loops and transradial approach in coronary diagnosis and intervention. *Catheter Cardiovasc Interv.* Oct 2000;51(2):250–252.

42. Yokoyama N, Takeshita S, Ochiai M, Koyama Y, Hoshino S, Isshiki T, Sato T. Anatomic variations of the radial artery in patients undergoing transradial coronary intervention. *Catheter Cardiovasc Interv.* Apr 2000;49(4):357–362.

43. Hamon M, McFadden E, ed. *Trans-radial Approach for Cardiovascular Interventions.* ESM Editions. France: Carpiquet, 2003.

44. Patel T. *Atlas of Transradial Intervention: The Basics.* www.transradialWORLD.org. France: Carpiquet, 2003.

45. Patel T. www.transradialWORLD.org.

46. Amor M. www.incathlab.com.

47. Bertrand O. http://www.aimradial.org

chapter 14

Transradial Arterial Access: Economic Considerations

Ronald P. Caputo, MD

The shift toward increased utilization of transradial arterial access (TRA) for cardiac and peripheral vascular procedures has been propelled both by a demonstrated decrease in complications (mainly vascular access and bleeding complications) and by improved patient satisfaction as compared to transfemoral arterial access (TFA).[1-11] Another important advantage of TRA is the opportunity for economic benefit compared to TFA. These benefits are related to a lower incidence of bleeding and vascular complications as well as more rapid and safe mobility compared to TFA (Table 14.1). Changes in the US health care system have led to the linking of reimbursement to quality and appropriateness of care. This increases the importance of these economic considerations.

■ ECONOMIC BENEFIT OF TRA RELATED TO REDUCED COMPLICATIONS

Small randomized studies, large registries, meta-analysis, and now one major randomized study have demonstrated that TRA significantly reduces the incidence of complications compared to TFA.[1-11] Early randomized single-center experiences by Kiemeneij (0% vs. 2.0%; $P = 0.03$) and Mann (0% vs. 4.0%; $P < 0.01$) reported lower vascular complications/bleeding with TRA compared to TFA, even at a time when transradial techniques were still being refined.[2,3] One large registry analysis (the M.O.R.T.A.L study; $N = 32,822$), after adjusting for pertinent variables, demonstrated a reduction in mortality at 30 days (OR 0.71 [95% CI 0.61–0.82]; $P < 0.001$)

Transradial Access: Techniques for Diagnostic Angiography and Percutaneous Intervention
©2013 Howard A. Cohen (Editor). Cardiotext Publishing, ISBN 978-1-935395-41-6.

and 1 year (OR 0.68 [95% CI 0.71–0.92]; $P < 0.001$).[10] A large ($N = 7,020$) meta-analysis of 23 randomized studies comparing TRA to TFA reported a trend toward decreased occurrence of death/myocardial infarction/stroke with TRA (2.5% vs. 3.8%; OR 0.71 [95% CI 0.49–1.01; $P = 0.058$].[8] The incidence of death/myocardial infarction was also lower for TRA ($n = 307$) compared to TFA ($n = 863$) (4.9% vs. 8.3%; $P = 0.05$) 1 year postprocedure in the PRESTO-ACS study.[9] Bleeding and net clinical outcomes were also lower in the TRA group (0.7% vs. 2.7%; $P = 0.03$ and 5.5% vs. 9.9%; $P = 0.03$). The recently reported large randomized RIVAL study ($N = 7,021$) compared TRA to TFA for patients with acute coronary syndromes treated by PCI and demonstrated a significant decrease in vascular complications for the overall TRA group (1.4% vs. 3.7%; $P < 0.0001$). In the high-risk subgroup of ST-elevation myocardial infarction (STEMI) patients, both major adverse cardiac events (MACE) and bleeding were lower in the TRA group (3.1% vs. 5.2%; $P < 0.0001$).[11]

Although TRA may result in lower MACE events post-percutaneous coronary intervention (PCI) compared to TFA, there is stronger evidence to support the conclusion that TRA is associated with lower incidence of vascular access/bleeding complications. Reducing these complications provides a large economic advantage for TRA. Examination of the multiple additional cost events occurring after a significant vascular/bleeding complication helps to illustrate the economic burden (Table 14.2). The cumulative costs of bleeding and vascular complications following PCI have been calculated in several studies.[13–25] Rao et al examined the GUSTO IIb data and found increasing length of stay (LOS) and hospital costs commensurate with severity of GUSTO IIb–defined bleeding following PCI for an indication of non-STEMI (Table 14.3). After adjusting for baseline patient differences, each bleeding event and transfusion was determined to add $3,770 and $2,080 to costs, respectively. LOS was the main component leading to increased cost.[12] An analysis of the ACUITY trial revealed that a minor bleeding event increased costs by $2,822 and a major bleeding event increased costs by $8,658. Furthermore, the investigators determined that a hematoma, a clinically significant bleed, and a pseudoaneurysm translated into incremental costs of $1,399, $5,440, and $6,357 per event, respectively.[13] Jacobson and colleagues at the Mayo Clinic examined patients treated with PCI for a variety of indications between 1998 and 2003. In this study, incremental adjusted mean costs were $5,882 for a bleeding event and $15,437 for a bleeding event associated with a MACE event.[14] A series of 6,008 patients in the Christiana Care Health System were found to have increased costs due to GUSTO-defined post-PCI bleeding, which increased according to severity of bleeding, adding $4,037 for mild, $6,980 for moderate, and $14,006

Table 14.1 Economic Advantages Related to Transradial Arterial Access.

Cost Savings with Transradial Access
Decreased vascular and bleeding complications
Improved efficiency/room turnover
Enhanced same-day PCI opportunities
Lower nursing/technologist intensity
• Sheath removal (manual)
• Patient transfer
• Postprocedure care
Lower closure device costs
Universal catheter
• Lower catheter costs
Improved reimbursement (?)

Table 14.2 Cumulative Cost and Economic Burden After Singular Vascular/Bleeding Complication.

Item	Cost (US $)
Femoral vascular ultrasound	$243.00
CT of abdomen w/o contrast	$586.00
CT of pelvis w/o contrast	$586.00
Hemoglobin and hematocrit × 3	$103.86
Type and crossmatch, etc	$138.23
1 unit of PRBC/transfusion cost	$473.00
Thrombin injection for femoral artery pseudoaneursym	$667.00
Operating room charge (per 30 min)	$1,680.00
Acute nursing time (per hour) × 3	$124.17

Table 14.3 Cost of Bleeding/Vascular Complications by Severity.

		None	Any	Mild	Moderate	Severe
Rao et al[1]	LOS $	5.4 $14,282		6.9, $21,674	15, $45,798	16.4, $66,564
Pinto et al[2]	$			$2,822		$8,658
Jacobson et al[3]	$		$5,883		$5,883	
Kugelmass et al[4]	LOS $		1.8, $4,278			
Ewen et al[5]	$			$4,037		$14,006

LOS = length of stay (days)

$ = US dollars

[1] Rao SV, Kaul PR, Liao L, et al. Association between bleeding, blood transfusion, and costs among patients with non-ST segment elevation acute coronary syndromes. *Am Heart J.* 2008;155(2):369–374.

[2] Pinto DS, Stone GW, Shi C, Dunn ES, Reynolds MR, York M, Walczak J, Berezin RH, Mehran R, McLaurin BT, Cox DA, Ohman EM, Lincoff AM, Cohen DJ. Economic evaluation of bivalirudin with or without glycoprotein IIb/IIIa inhibition versus heparin with routine glycoprotein IIb/IIIa inhibition for early invasive management of acute coronary syndromes. *J Am Coll Cardiol.* 2008;52(22):1758–1768.

[3] Jacobson KM, Hall Long K, McMurtry EK, et al. The economic burden of complications during percutaneous coronary intervention. *Qual Saf Health Care.* 2007;16(2):154–159.

[4] Kugelmass AD, Cohen DJ, Brown PP, et al. Hospital resources consumed in treating complications associated with percutaneous coronary interventions. *Am J Cardiol.* 2006;97(3):322–327.

[5] Ewen EF, Zhao L, Kolm P, et al. Determining the in-hospital cost of bleeding in patients undergoing percutaneous coronary intervention. *J Interv Cardiol.* Jun 2009;22(3):266–273. Epub 2009.

for severe events. When these investigators used thrombolysis in myocardial infarction (TIMI) bleeding definitions for this same patient group, minor bleeds translated into incremental costs of $4,310, and major bleeds increased costs by $8,794.[15] Kugelmass et al reviewed data from Medicare patients undergoing PCI ($N = 335,477$) and demonstrated adjusted incremental costs of $4,278 for those experiencing a vascular complication.[16]

Early single-center studies attempted to quantify the economic benefits of transradial PCI. The first, described by Kiemeneij et al in 1995, showed that stenting via TRA was associated with a 45% cost reduction compared to stenting via TFA. Savings were driven mainly by a significantly shorter length of hospital stay.[26] Mann et al also quantified the economic benefit of TRA in a study that randomized 142 patients to TRA PCI versus TFA PCI demonstrating a 15% decrease in hospital charges with the radial approach. In this study, total charges were significantly reduced with transradial access compared to the femoral approach ($20,476 ± $811 vs. $23,389 ± $1,180; $P < 0.01$) due both to a lower incidence of access site complications (0% vs. 4%; $P < 0.01$) and to shorter length

of hospital stay (1.4 ± 0.2 days vs. 2.3 ± 0.4 days).[27] Examination of the economic benefit of TRA versus TFA for diagnostic catheterization was performed by Cooper et al in a randomized single-center study. Significant reduction in hospital costs for transradial versus transfemoral diagnostic catheterization ($2,010 vs. $2,299, respectively; $P < 0.0001$) were related to reductions in LOS (3.6 hours vs. 10.4 hours), pharmacy, and total costs. It is notable that a difference was demonstrated even though vascular closure devices were not used in this study, minimizing equipment costs for the transfemoral group.[28]

Acknowledging that the definitions for major bleeding and vascular complications differ somewhat between studies, these events are generally reported to occur in < 1.5% of TR patients compared to 3%–7% of TFA patients. There is, as yet, no large published multicenter randomized data examining the cost benefit related to decreased bleeding and vascular complications comparing TRA with TFA. The information above, however, allows for a rough estimate of the cost savings. Assuming a reduction in vascular and bleeding complications provided by TRA of 4.5% and an incremental increased median cost of $4,328 for a mild/moderate bleeding event, this would translate into a savings of $194,760 per 1,000 treated patients or $194.76 per patient. This likely underestimates the savings per patient, as (1) the definitions of bleeding and vascular complications used in the above studies are strict, and therefore these events are likely underreported, and (2) the cost for severe complications is much higher.

■ ECONOMIC IMPACT OF POLICY CHANGES IN THE HEALTH CARE SYSTEM

Economic stress placed on modern health care systems has led to several new concepts that are now being applied in the clinical arena that are designed to aid in overall reduction of health care costs. In the United States, the Deficit Reduction Act of 2005 resulted in a policy change at the Centers for Medicare & Medicaid Services (CMS) whereby incremental payments following the occurrence of a hospital-acquired complication have been eliminated, thereby shifting the economic burden of that complication solely to the providing institution. Examples of these potentially preventable complications (PPCs) include "post operative hemorrhage and hematoma with/without hemorrhage control procedure," and "post hemorrhagic acute anemia with transfusion."[29] Using data standardized for case mix and severity of illness (All Patient Refined Diagnosis Related Group [APR-DRG] data) from the states of Maryland and California, the additional costs of these complications has been estimated to be $6,190 (MD)/$6,758 (CA), $11,602 (MD)/$16,481 (CA), and $4,513 (MD)/$7,604 (CA), respectively.[30] Lack of additional reimbursement for the care related to these complications obviously compounds the negative economic impact to the providing institution. Negative economic effects may also occur from cost control efforts at the state level. Maryland has initiated a Hospital Acquired Conditions Initiative assigning a financial penalty to hospitals that fail to meet targets set for PPCs.[31] Therefore, significant motivation exists for hospitals to minimize or eliminate these complications due to the negative financial implications at both the federal and state levels.

The concept of value-related reimbursement has been further expanded by the Affordable Care Act that ties reimbursement to a Value-Based Purchasing (VBP) Program. The VBP Program mandates that hospitals use the Hospital Inpatient Quality Reporting (IQR) Program to determine their clinical performance as compared to similar institutions. Institutions with good health care outcomes (low complications, high compliance with core measures, etc), compared to their peers with inferior outcomes, enjoy higher rates of reimbursement.[32,33] Initial measures of quality will include treatment of cardiovascular disease such as acute myocardial infarction. As demonstrated in the RIVAL study, improved outcomes in this patient group may be achieved by the choice of TRA.[11]

Public reporting of health care outcomes is a relatively recent phenomenon that developed concordantly with the widespread availability of information access via the Internet. Public reporting has been demonstrated to augment quality improvement in hospitals beyond the gains achieved by "pay for performance" programs.[34] The greatest improvements in quality tend to occur at hospitals with poor outcomes.[35] Negative public perception regarding poorly performing hospitals and the consequent decline in market share drive these quality improvement efforts. As PCI outcomes are reported by several states, improved outcomes realized by the utilization of TRA may potentially provide indirect economic benefit.

■ ECONOMIC BENEFITS OF TRA RELATED TO RECOVERY AND MOBILITY

Additional indirect economic benefits of TRA are related to the rapid and safe postprocedure mobility patients enjoy compared to TFA. This translates into several advantages, including (1) same-day or outpatient PCI, (2) more efficient patient transport, room turnover, and room utilization, and (3) decreased nursing intensity.

Outpatient PCI

The development of improved equipment, procedural techniques, and adjunctive pharmacology has resulted in significant improvement in the predictability of results following PCI, making same-day or outpatient PCI feasible. Same-day or outpatient PCI is a concept driven by the potential economic benefit for the health care system at large as well as the benefit of increased patient comfort and satisfaction. Rapid patient ambulation and the demonstrated reduction in access site complications make TRA a natural application for same-day or outpatient PCI. As demonstrated in the STRIDE study, all complications following transradial PCI occurred within 6 hours of the procedure. In this study, the incidence of access site/bleeding complications was only 2.4%, and all vascular events spontaneously resolved, bolstering the argument for safe outpatient PCI in uncomplicated patients.[36]

The safety of outpatient or same-day TRA PCI has been examined in several studies with reports as early as 2001.[37] Oh et al reported a small single-center experience with 230 patients undergoing PCI, of which 206 were discharged the same day with no adverse events/complications at both 1-day and 7-day follow-up. The reasons for overnight stay in this study included patient preference, complicated PCI, and suboptimal PCI result.[38] A subsequent single-center experience of low-risk patients undergoing elective PCI ($N = 150$) by Kumar et al also demonstrated a high success rate (80%).[39] Patients remained in the hospital post-PCI mainly due to unsuccessful radial access or suboptimal PCI outcomes. Wiper et al described a single-center experience with outpatient transradial stenting ($N = 442$) in which there was no occurrence of any vascular complication.[40] Cohen compared economic data from elective single-vessel transfemoral coronary stenting with a traditional overnight hospital stay to data from 100 consecutive patients treated by transradial single-vessel stenting and same-day discharge. Costs were decreased by the latter strategy by more than $1,000.[41] The EASY study randomized 1,005 patients to a strategy of outpatient PCI bolus-only abxicimab or PCI with standard bolus and infusion dosing of abxicimab and overnight hospitalization. There was no significant difference in outcomes between groups, and importantly, there was no difference in major bleeding (0.8% vs. 0.2%; $P = $ NS).[42] A subsequent analysis of the economic impact of outpatient PCI from the 1,005 patients enrolled in the EASY study was recently reported. This revealed a decrease in LOS with outpatient versus inpatient TRA PCI (8.9 hours vs. 26.5 hours; $P < 0.001$) and a decrease in 30-day costs per case of $1,141 ($1,117 ± $1,554 vs. $2,258 ± $1,328), helping to quantify the economic benefit of outpatient TRA PCI.[43]

Decreased Nursing Workload and Improved Throughput

Immediate hemostasis, early patient mobility, and the lack of required bed rest allow for advantages in regard to patient transport and postprocedure care. This results in improved patient flow efficiencies and decreases the workload for nursing personnel. Amoroso et al quantified the workload for both catheterization laboratory and recovery-area nurses following 260 consecutive transradial ($n = 208$) and transfemoral ($n = 52$) procedures. The workload was significantly reduced for transradial procedures (TR = 86 minutes vs. TF = 174 minutes; $P < 0.001$) and for transradial recovery (TR = 386 minutes vs. TF = 720 minutes). The workload benefit was related to the reduction in time required for sheath removal, early patient mobility, a shorter recovery time, and shorter time to ambulation.[44] Using the time savings for nursing workload reported in this study for the procedure (1.4 hours) and recovery (5.5 hours) and employing representative hourly wage plus benefits data from our institution, this translates into a savings of $53 and $232 per procedure for catheterization laboratory nurses and recovery nurses, respectively. A similar study comparing costs for TRA versus TFA with a vascular closure device revealed a significantly shorter postprocedure recovery interval (126 ± 36 minutes vs. 150 ± 48 minutes; $P < 0.05$) and 33% lower costs during recovery ($185 ± $52 vs. $208 ± $70.4; $P < 0.001$) with the transradial strategy.[45]

∎ OTHER POTENTIAL ECONOMIC BENEFITS

Patient Return to Productivity

Lost worker productivity is a large contributor to the economic burden of coronary artery disease with absenteeism, presenteeism, loss of income, and disability contributing to the estimated annual $273 billion in total indirect costs of cardiovascular disease in the United States.[46] Household income losses for workers with ischemic heart disease have been estimated to be $3,013 annually.[47] One study comparing triple-vessel coronary artery bypass to 3-vessel PCI demonstrated that faster recovery and improved mobility following the less invasive strategy was associated with reduced time out of work and fewer lost wages ($7,022 vs. $14,685; $P < 0.05$).[48] Although there are no published data, a secure access site and rapid postprocedure mobility following TRA for elective procedures provide the potential for a more rapid return to productivity compared to similar patients undergoing these procedures by the femoral approach.

Universal Catheters

The use of a single catheter to perform ventriculography, as well as right and left coronary angiography, originated with the brachial cutdown and Sones catheter. This concept has been successfully applied to the radial approach where several shapes of universal catheters are now employed.[49,50] Benefits of a universal catheter include minimizing catheter exchanges and the potential for trauma to the radial, brachial, and axillary arteries and reduced risk for resultant spasm and dissection. Other advantages may include shorter procedure durations and lower material costs resulting in minor economic benefit.

Lower Closure Device Costs

Although TRA is utilized in < 10% of cases in the United States, vascular closure devices are used in approximately 40% of femoral catheterization procedures in the United States.[51,52] Femoral vascular closure devices can cost more than $200 per unit. The most expensive radial artery compression device is approximately $40 per unit.[51] Conversion from TFA with a closure device to TRA with a compression device can be associated with net material cost savings of approximately $149 per case. The overall savings of course will be in proportion to case volume and the magnitude of the conversion from TFA to TRA.[53]

∎ NEGATIVE ECONOMIC CONSIDERATIONS RELATED TO TRA

Compared to TFA with manual compression, some minor additional expenses can accrue with TRA depending on the operator's choice of equipment and institutional agreements. Arterial access kits (micropuncture), routine administration of pharmacologic agents (heparin, nitroglycerin, calcium channel blockers), and radial artery compression devices are some examples. The routine use of ultrasound imaging to aid in arterial access has been adopted at some centers and may be associated with a significant initial capital equipment cost.

TRA is associated with a longer learning curve compared to TFA with operators potentially requiring ≥ 200 cases to maximize expertise.[54–57] During this learning period, case times are longer, resource utilization is higher, and patient throughput in the catheterization laboratory is less efficient with TRA compared to TFA.[54,55] However, these negative effects have been demonstrated to be temporary with differences in fluoroscopy and procedure times disappearing as operators become more proficient with TRA.[57,58]

∎ SUMMARY

Transradial arterial access for coronary and peripheral arterial procedures provides economic advantages compared to transfemoral arterial access. Significant benefit is realized through decreased vascular and bleeding complications that are associated with added expenses related to diagnosis, treatment, and, most impactful, prolonged length of stay. Decreasing vascular complications is especially relevant in today's health care environment, given the emergence of value-related reimbursement. Early and safe mobility following TRA also confers economic advantage by decreasing nursing requirements, improving patient flow efficiency, and facilitating safe outpatient PCI.

■ REFERENCES

1. Kiemeneij F, Laarman GJ, Odekerken D, Slagboom T, Van Der Wieken R. A randomized comparison of percutaneous transluminal coronary angioplasty by the radial brachial and femoral approaches: the Access study. *J Am Coll Cardiol.* 1997;29(6): 1269–1275.
2. Mann T, Cubeddu G, Bowen J, et al. Stenting in acute coronary syndromes: a comparison of radial versus femoral access sites. *J Am Coll Cardiol.* 1998;32(3):572–576.
3. Louvard Y, Lefevre T, Allain A, Morice M. Coronary angiography through the radial or the femoral approach: the CARAFE study. *Catheter Cardiovasc Interv.* 2001;52(2):181–187.
4. Cox N, Resnic FS, Popma JJ, Simon DI, Eisenhauer AC, Rogers C. Comparison of the risk of vascular complications associated with femoral and radial access coronary catheterization procedures in obese versus nonobese patients. *Am J Cardiol.* 2004;94(9):1174–1177.
5. Cruden NL, Teh CH, Starkey IR, Newby DE. Reduced vascular complications and length of stay with transradial rescue angioplasty for acute myocardial infarction. *Catheter Cardiovasc Interv.* 2007;70(5):670–675.
6. Eichhofer J, Horlick E, Ivanov J, Seidelin PH, Ross JR, Ing D, Daly P, Mackie K, Ridley B, Schwartz L, et al. Decreased complication rates using the transradial compared to the transfemoral approach in percutaneous coronary intervention in the era of routine stenting and glycoprotein platelet IIb/IIIa inhibitor use: a large single-center experience. *Am Heart J.* 2008;156(5):864–870.
7. Agostoni P, Biondi-Zoccai GG, de Benedictis ML, Rigattieri S, Turri M, Anselmi M, Vassanelli C, Zardini P, Louvard Y, Hamon M. Radial versus femoral approach for percutaneous coronary diagnostic and interventional procedures: systematic overview and meta-analysis of randomized trials. *J Am Coll Cardiol.* 2004;44(2):349–356.
8. Jolly SS, Amlani S, Hamon M, Yusuf S, Mehta SR. Radial versus femoral access for coronary angiography or intervention and the impact on major bleeding and ischemic events: a systematic review and meta-analysis of randomized trials. *Am Heart J.* 2009;157(1):132–140.
9. Sciahbasi A, Pristipino C, Ambrosio G, Sperduti I, Scabbia EV, Greco C, Ricci R, Ferraiolo G, Di Clemente D, Giombolini C, et al. Arterial access-site-related outcomes of patients undergoing invasive coronary procedures for acute coronary syndromes (from the ComPaRison of Early Invasive and Conservative Treatment in Patients with Non-ST-Elevation Acute Coronary Syndromes [PRESTO-ACS] Vascular Substudy). *Am J Cardiol.* 2009;103(6):796–800.
10. Chase AJ, Fretz EB, Warburton WP, Klinke WP, Carere RG, Pi D, Berry B, Hilton JD. Association of the arterial access site at angioplasty with transfusion and mortality: the M.O.R.T.A.L study (Mortality benefit Of Reduced Transfusion after percutaneous coronary intervention via the Arm or Leg). *Heart.* 2008;94(8):1019–1025.
11. Jolly SS, Yusuf S, Cairns J, Neimela K, Xavier D, Widimsky P, Budaj A, Neimela M, Valentin V, Lewis BS, Avezum A, Steg PG, Rao SV, Gao P, Afzal R, Hoyner CD, Chrolavicius S, Mehta SR. Radial versus femoral access for coronary angiography and intervention in patients with acute coronary syndromes (RIVAL): a randomized, parallel group, multicenter trial. *The Lancet.* Apr 23 2011;377(9775):1409–1420. Epub Apr 4 2011.

Cost of Bleeding

12. Rao SV, Kaul PR, Liao L, Armstrong PW, Ohman EM, Granger CB, Califf RM, Harrington RA, Eisenstein EL, Mark DB. Association between bleeding, blood transfusion, and costs among patients with non-ST-segment elevation acute coronary syndromes. *Am Heart J.* 2008;155(2):369–374.
13. Pinto DS, Stone GW, Shi C, Dunn ES, Reynolds MR, York M, Walczak J, Berezin RH, Mehran R, McLaurin BT, et al. Economic evaluation of bivalirudin with or without glycoprotein IIb/IIIa inhibition versus heparin with routine glycoprotein IIb/IIIa inhibition for early invasive management of acute coronary syndromes. *J Am Coll Cardiol.* 2008;52(22):1758–1768.
14. Jacobson KM, Hall Long K, McMurtry EK, et al. The economic burden of complications during percutaneous coronary intervention. *Qual Saf Health Care.* 2007;16(2):154–159.
15. Ewen EF, Zhao L, Kolm P, et al. Determining the in-hospital cost of bleeding in patients undergoing percutaneous coronary intervention. *J Interv Cardiol.* Jun 2009;22(3):266–273. Epub 2009.
16. Kugelmass AD, Cohen DJ, Brown PP, Simon AW, Becker ER, Culler SD. Hospital resources consumed in treating complications associated with percutaneous coronary interventions. *Am J Cardiol.* 2006;97(3):322–327.
17. Milkovich G, Gibson G. Economic impact of bleeding complications and the role of antithrombotic therapies in percutaneous coronary intervention. *Am J Health Syst Pharm.* 2003;60(14 Suppl 3):S15–S21.

18. Lincoff AM, Bittl JA, Harrington RA, Feit F, Kleiman NS, Jackman JD, Sarembock IJ, Cohen DJ, Spriggs D, Ebrahimi R, et al. Bivalirudin and provisional glycoprotein IIb/IIIa blockade compared with heparin and planned glycoprotein IIb/IIIa blockade during percutaneous coronary intervention: REPLACE-2 randomized trial. *JAMA.* 2003;289(7):853–863.

19. Mehta SR, Granger CB, Eikelboom JW, Bassand JP, Wallentin L, Faxon DP, Peters RJ, Budaj A, Afzal R, Chrolavicius S, et al. Efficacy and safety of fondaparinux versus enoxaparin in patients with acute coronary syndromes undergoing percutaneous coronary intervention: results from the OASIS-5 trial. *J Am Coll Cardiol.* 2007;50(18):1742–1751.

20. Stone GW, McLaurin BT, Cox DA, Bertrand ME, Lincoff AM, Moses JW, White HD, Pocock SJ, Ware JH, Feit F, et al. Bivalirudin for patients with acute coronary syndromes. *N Engl J Med.* 2006;355(21):2203–2216.

21. Yusuf S, Mehta SR, Chrolavicius S, Afzal R, Pogue J, Granger CB, Budaj A, Peters RJ, Bassand JP, Wallentin L, et al. Comparison of fondaparinux and enoxaparin in acute coronary syndromes. *N Engl J Med.* 2006;354(14):1464–1476.

22. Fitts J, Ver Lee P, Hofmaster P, Malenka D. Fluoroscopy-guided femoral artery puncture reduces the risk of PCI-related vascular complications. *J Interv Cardiol.* 2008;21(3):273–278.

23. Montalescot G, White HD, Gallo R, Cohen M, Steg PG, Aylward PE, Bode C, Chiariello M, King SB III, Harrington RA, et al. Enoxaparin versus unfractionated heparin in elective percutaneous coronary intervention. *N Engl J Med.* 2006;355(10):1006–1017.

24. Stone GW, McLaurin BT, Cox DA, Bertrand ME, Lincoff AM, Moses JW, White HD, Pocock SJ, Ware JH, Feit F, et al. Bivalirudin for patients with acute coronary syndromes. *N Engl J Med.* 2006;355(21):2203–2216.

25. Yusuf S, Mehta SR, Chrolavicius S, Afzal R, Pogue J, Granger CB, Budaj A, Peters RJ, Bassand JP, Wallentin L, et al. Comparison of fondaparinux and enoxaparin in acute coronary syndromes. *N Engl J Med.* 2006;354(14):1464–1476.

26. Kiemeneij F, Hofland J, Laarman GJ, van der Elst DH, van der Lubbe H. Cost comparison between two modes of Palmaz Schatz coronary stent implantation: transradial bare stent technique vs. transfemoral sheath-protected stent technique. *Cathet Cardiovasc Diagn.* Aug 1995;35(4):301–308, discussion 309.

27. Mann T, Cowper PA, Peterson ED, et al. Transradial coronary stenting: comparison with femoral access closed with an arterial suture device. *Catheter Cardiovasc Interv.* 2000;49(2):150–156.

28. Cooper CJ, El-Shiekh RA, Cohen DJ, et al. Effect of transradial access on quality of life and cost of cardiac catheterization: a randomized comparison. *Am Heart J.* 1999;199:430-436.

Health Care Policy

29. Hughes JS, Averill RF, Goldfield NI, Gay JC, Muldoon J, McCullough E, Xiang J. Identifying potentially preventable complications using a present on admission indicator. *Healthcare Financing Rev.* 2006;27:63–82.

30. Fuller RL, McCullough EC, Rao MI, Averill RF. Estimating the cost of potentially preventable hospital acquired complications. *Healthcare Financing Rev.* 2009;30:17–32.

31. www.cms.gov/Medicare/Medicare-Fee-for-Service Payment/HospitalAcqCond/downloads/hacfactsheet.pdf

32. Medicare program; hospital inpatient value-based purchasing program. A rule by the Centers for Medicare & Medicaid Services. May 6, 2011. www.federalregister.gov/articles/2011/05/06/2011–10568/medicare-program-hospital-inpatient-value-based-purchasing.

33. Casale PN, Thomas GS, Gillam LD. www.cardiosource.org/~/media/Files/Advocacy/Health%20Refrom/PaymentReformWhitePaper.ashx

34. Lindenauer PK, Remus D, Roman S, Rothberg MB, Benjami EM, Ma A, Bratzler DW. Public reporting and pay for performance in hospital quality improvement. *N Engl J Med.* 2007;356:486–496.

35. Hibbard JH, Stockard J, Tusler M. Hospital performance reports: impact on quality, market share, and reputation. *Health Affairs.* 2005;24:1150–1160.

Outpatient PCI

36. Jabara R, Gadesam R, Pendyala L, et al. Ambulatory discharge after transradial coronary intervention: preliminary US single-center experience (Same-day TransRadial Intervention and Discharge Evaluation, the STRIDE study). *Am Heart J.* 2008;156(6):1141–1146.

37. Slagboom T, Keimeneij F, Laarman GJ, et al. Actual outpatient PTCA: results of the OUTCLAS pilot study. *Cathet Cardiovasc Interven.* 2001;53:204–208.

38. Oh HL, Gwan H-C, Lee SM, Kim YH, Chean IS, Chean WJ, Choi JH. Safety of one day admission for transradial coronary intervention. *Korean Circ J.* 2004;34:647–654.

39. Kumar S, Anantharman R, Das P, et al. Radial approach to day case intervention in coronary artery lesions (RADICAL): a single centre safety and feasibility study. *Heart.* 2004;90:1340–1341.

40. Wiper A, Kumar S, MacDonald J, Robers DH. Day case transradial coronary angioplasty: a four-year single center experience. *Cathet Cardiovasc Interv.* 2006;68:445–453.

41. Cohen DJ. Outpatient transradial coronary stenting: implications for cost-effectiveness. *J Invasive Cardiol.* 1996;8(Suppl D):36D-39D.

42. Bertrand OF, De Larochelliere R, Rodes-Cabau J, et al. A randomized study comparing same-day

home discharge and abciximab bolus only to overnight hospitalization and abciximab bolus and infusion after transradial coronary stent implantation. *Circulation.* 2006;114(24):2636–2643.

43. Rinfret S, Kennedy WA, Lachrne J, Lemay A, Todes-Cabau J, Hohen DJ, Costerbusse O, Bertrand OF. Economic impact of same-day discharge after uncomplicated transradial percutaneous coronary intervention and bolus only absxicimab regimen. *JACC Cardiovasc Interv.* Oct 2010;3(10):1011–1019.

44. Amoroso G, Sarti M, Bellucci R, et al. Clinical and procedural predictors of nurse workload during and after invasive coronary procedures: the potential benefit of a systematic radial access. *Eur J Cardiovasc Nurs.* 2005;4(3):234–224.

45. Roussanov O, Wilson SJ, Henley K, Estacio G, Hill J, Dogan B, Henley WF, Jarmukli N. Cost-effectiveness of the radial versus femoral artery approach to diagnostic cardiac catheterization. *J Invasive Cardiol.* 2007;19(8):349–353.

46. Heidenreich PA, Torgdon JG, Khavjou OA, et al, for the Interdisciplinary Council on Quality of Care and Outcomes Research. Forecasting the future of cardiovascular disease in the United States: a policy statement from the American Heart Association. *Circulation.* 2011;123(8):933–944.

47. Herrin J, Cangialose CB, Boccuzzi SJ, Weintraub WS, Ballard DJ. Household income losses associated with ischaemic heart disease for US employees. *Pharmacoeconomics.* 2000;17:305–314.

48. Myler RK, Shaw RE, Sterter SH, Zapolanski A, Zipkin R, Murphy MC, Hecht H, Chan J, Mengarelli L, Cumberland DC. Triple vessel revascularization: coronary angioplasty versus coronary artery bypass surgery: initial results and five-year follow-up. Comparative costs and loss of working days and wages. *J Invasive Cardiol.* 1994;6(4):125–135.

Universal Catheter

49. Pancholy SB. Randomized comparison of Judkins and Tiger catheters for transradial catheterization. *Journal of Medicine.* 2008;1:101–104.

50. Lu R, Yao M, Qiao SB, Dai J, Yang YJ, Qin XW, Liu HB, Wu YJ, Yuan JQ, Chen J, et al. Coronary angiography by transradial approach with 5F universal catheter. *Zhonghua Xin Xue Guan Bing Za Zhi.* 2005;33(1):62–65.

51. *Global Vascular Closure Device Markets: U.S., Europe, Rest of World.* Huntington Beach, CA: Life Science Intelligence; 2008.

52. Caputo RP, Tremmel JA, Rao SV, et al. Transradial arterial access for coronary and peripheral procedures: Executive summary by the transradial committee of the SCAI. *Cathet Cardiovasc Interv.* 2011;78:823-839.

53. Gaskins-McClaine B. Transradial at Wake Med since 1994. *Cath Lab Digest.* (Suppl) Sept 2 2010;10.

54. Goldberg SL, Renslo R, Sinow R, French WJ. Learning curve in the use of the radial artery as vascular access in the performance of percutaneous transluminal coronary angioplasty. *Cathet Cardiovasc Diagn.* 1998;44(2):147–152.

55. Ball WT, Sharieff W, Jolly SS, Hong T, Kutryk MJ, Graham JJ, Fam NP, Chisholm RH, Cheema AN. Characterization of operator learning curve for transradial coronary interventions. *Circ Cardiovasc Interv.* 2011;4(4):336–341.

56. Sciahbasi A, Romangnoli E, Trani C, Burzotta F, Pendenza G, Tommasino A, Leone AM, Niccoli G, Porto I, Penco M, Lioy E. Evaluation of the "learning curve" for left and right radial approach during percutaneous coronary procedures. *Am J Cardiol.* 2011;108:185–188.

57. Looi JL, Cave A, El-Jack S. Learning curve in transradial coronary angiography. *Am J Cardiol.* Jul 26 2011 [Epub ahead of print].

58. Eccleshall SC, Banks M, Carroll R, et al. Implementation of a diagnostic and interventional transradial programme: resource and organizational implications. *Heart.* 2003;89(5):561–562.

chapter 15

Tips and Tricks for Transradial Access

Tejas Patel, MD, DM
Sanjay C. Shah, MD, DM
Samir B. Pancholy, MD

■ BACKGROUND

The purpose of this chapter is to provide a stepwise guide to deal with the issues related to transradial access, particularly for new as well as moderately experienced radial operators. In writing this chapter, we presume that the radial operator is determined and transradial approach (TRA) is a default approach with at least 50% diagnostic and interventional procedures in his or her cath lab.

The issues related to TRA can be divided into 4 categories:

1. Radial access-related issues

2. Issues related to radial and brachial regions

3. Issues related to subclavian, innominate, and aortic arch regions

4. Issues related to cannulation of coronary ostia

Issues 1 and 2 have already been discussed in detail in separate chapters of this book. Hence, we will confine ourselves to issues 3 and 4.

■ ISSUES RELATED TO RADIAL AND BRACHIAL REGIONS

Here is the normal anatomy of this region (Figure 15.1).

The authors are grateful to Mr. Yash Soni and Mr. Chidambaram Iyer for their extremely valuable support during preparation of this manuscript.

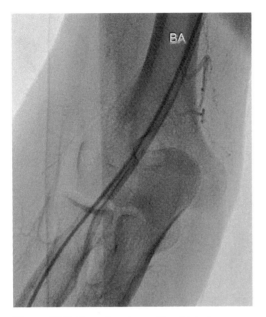

Figure 15.1 Normal anatomy of brachial artery.

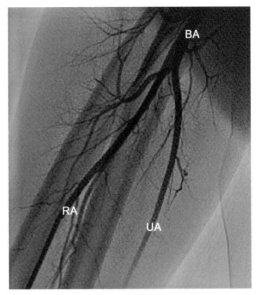

Figure 15.2 Normal anatomy of radial and ulnar branches. BA = brachial artery; RA = radial artery; UA = ulnar artery.

The artery that supplies the upper limb continues as a single trunk from its origin down to the elbow. But different parts of the artery have different names, depending on the regions through which they pass. The part of the artery that extends from its origin to the lateral border of the first rib is the subclavian artery. Beyond this point, to the lower border of the axilla, is the axillary artery. From that point, to the bend of the elbow, is the brachial artery (see Figures 15.1 and 15.2).

The radial artery (RA) commences at the bifurcation of the brachial artery, just below the bend of the elbow, and passes along the radial side of the forearm to the wrist. The RA extends from the neck of the radius to the front part of the styloid process. The upper (proximal) part lies on the medial side of the radius, and the lower (distal) part lies on the bone. The upper part is deep and lies below the muscle (brachioradialis). The lower part is superficial, covered by skin and superficial and deep fascia. In general, the RA is slightly smaller in caliber than the ulnar artery.

The following are the important relevant issues:

- RA spasm

- Tortuosity

- Perforation

- Loops and curvatures

- RA occlusion

The last issue has also been discussed extensively in a separate chapter in this book, so we will be discussing the first four issues.

RA Spasm

New radial converts are apprehensive to deal with this issue. The incidence varies between 5% and 15%.[3–7] In our series, it was found to be 5%, out of which 0.5% had severe spasm.[15] [*Editor's note:* Spasm, particularly severe spasm, is more common with inexperienced operators.]

It can be broadly classified into focal spasm and diffuse spasm.

Tips and Tricks for Identification and Management of RA Spasm.

- ■ RA spasm should be suspected when a patient complains of local pain or discomfort during passage of a guide-wire or catheter.

- ■ Radial angiogram done through the side port of an introducer sheath or through the catheter itself will differentiate between RA spasm and anatomical variation.

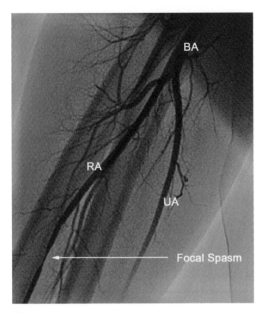

Figure 15.3 Example of focal spasm of RA.

- ◼ If RA spasm is confirmed, usually an additional dose of spasmolytic cocktail should resolve it (see Figure 15.3).

- ◼ If spasm develops in RA with a small caliber, downsizing the catheter (ie, 4-Fr instead of 5-Fr diagnostic catheter, 5-Fr instead of 6-Fr guide catheter) helps to complete the procedure successfully.

- ◼ If RA spasm leads to disappearance of the RA pulse as a result of multiple puncture attempts, subcutaneous injection of nitroglycerine should bring back the RA pulse in most instances (see Figure 15.4).[16]

- ◼ Anomalous origin of RA is most commonly being interpreted as RA spasm. Whenever RA has an anomalous origin (from high brachial or axillary artery), its caliber is almost invariably very small (Figure 15.5). This leads to significant resistance in catheter movement. Downsizing the catheter resolves this problem (see Figure 15.5).

Tortuosity

Tortuosity is an important issue, particularly when dealing with patients older than 70 years, long-standing diabetics, hypertensives, and females (see Figure 15.6).[1,4,7]

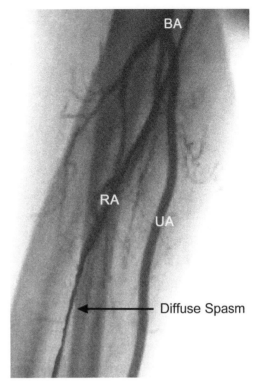

Figure 15.4 Example of diffuse spasm of RA.

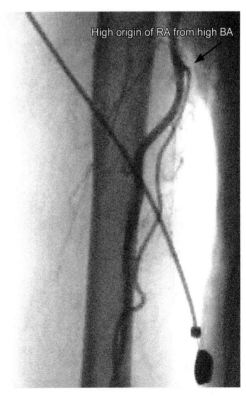

Figure 15.5 Example of high origin of RA from high BA.

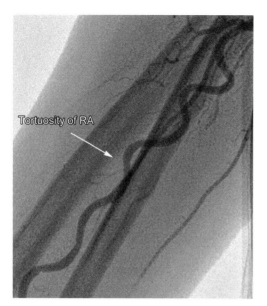

Figure 15.6 Example of tortuosity of RA.

Tips and Tricks for Identification and Management of Tortuosity.

■ It is an important cause of resistance to the movement of a guidewire or a catheter.

■ RA angiogram should define its severity and extent.

■ Once it is diagnosed, it should be crossed using a 0.025-in or 0.032-in J-shaped hydrophilic guidewire or a 0.014-in soft-tip percutaneous transluminal coronary angiography (PTCA) guidewire. The catheter should be negotiated slowly and carefully over the wire, using corkscrew movement under fluoroscopic guidance. Once the tortuous segment is crossed, the procedure can be completed in the usual fashion.

■ Sometimes, a repeat dose of cocktail helps with working through a tortuous segment in small RA, with or without spasm.[15]

Perforation

This complication should be identified and managed promptly, as it is the most common cause of large forearm hematoma.[2,4,8,15] In our series, the incidence is 0.1%.

Tips and Tricks for Identification and Management of Perforation. Resistance to the passage of a guidewire and/or a catheter felt by the operator associated with a complaint of significant local pain and discomfort in the radial and/or brachial region by a patient, with or without development of expanding forearm hematoma, makes this diagnosis.

• Immediate removal of the assembly and injection of diluted contrast through the side port of an introducer sheath confirms the site and size of perforation.

• A radial operator might have an appre-hension to work through it. In that case, we recommend that you abandon the procedure, reverse the effect of heparin, and apply manual compression at the local site for a time sufficient to prevent a larger hematoma. The sealing of the perforation can be confirmed by injecting diluted contrast through the side port of the introducer sheath. The procedure may be completed after several hours or the next day using the contralateral radial or a femoral route.

• We strongly recommend the following technique to work past the perforation.[8] The steps are as follows:

1. Identify the site and size of the perforation by injecting diluted contrast through the side port of the introducer sheath (see Figure 15.7A).

2. Use a floppy-tip 0.014-in PTCA wire and carefully cross the affected area. Park the wire higher in the brachial or axillary region (see Figure 15.7B).

3. Negotiate a diagnostic or a guide catheter over the wire, and stop when the tip of the catheter reaches the perforated segment (see Figure 15.7C).

4. Gently negotiate the catheter using a slow corkscrew movement (instead of the usual push), to reduce the friction in the perforated segment. Once the tip crosses the affected segment, the movement of the catheter becomes smooth, and the procedure can be completed in the usual fashion.

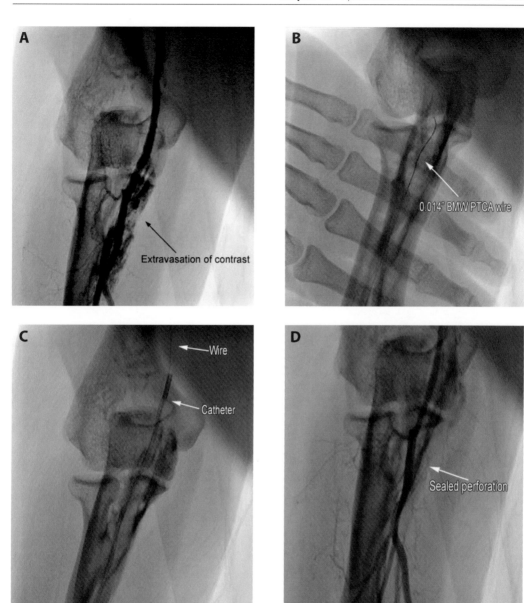

Figure 15.7 **Panel A**: Perforation of BA leading to extravasation of contrast. **Panel B**: The affected segment was crossed with 0.014-in BMW PTCA wire. **Panel C**: Catheter was carefully negotiated over-the-wire across the perforated segment. **Panel D**: Documentation of sealed perforation.

5. If there is resistance in the movement of the catheter tip at the perforation site, remove the catheter immediately and downsize it (ie, a 4-Fr diagnostic catheter instead of a 5-Fr, or a 5-Fr guide catheter instead of a 6-Fr). This strategy facilitates the successful crossing of affected segment with less friction.

Once the diagnostic or interventional procedure is over, the catheter is pulled back over the wire, which is parked higher up, so the catheter can be advanced again across the perforated segment, if required. An injection of diluted contrast is made through the catheter or the side port of introducer sheath, to confirm appropriate sealing of the perforated segment (see Figure 15.7D). *It is important to understand that the catheter functions as an internal hemostatic device that helps to seal the perforated segment.*

Loops and Curvatures

These are important anatomical variations to understand and manage.[1,4,6,7,15] In our experience, most of the time what we think is that RA spasm is actually an anatomical variation that presents in the form of tortuosity, loop, or curvatures. We strongly recommend to keep a low threshold for performing a radial artery angiogram to define the anatomy for working through the vast majority of loops and curvatures.

Tips and Tricks for Identification and Management of Loops and Curvatures. We have already developed a protocol to work through loops and curvatures.[15] It should reduce apprehension of a new radial operator and give additional confidence to an experienced operator (see Table 15.1).

The following are the important steps to remember:

1. Define the task. When you encounter resistance in the movement of a wire and/or a catheter, inject diluted contrast to define the anatomy. If a simple loop is identified, you can work through it under fluoroscopic guidance. If it is a complex loop, take multiple views (ie, right and

left anterior oblique, cranial or caudal angulations). Identify the view that best defines the loop. The view that is chosen can then be used as a "road map" for working through it (see Figure 15.8 A–C).

2. Downsize the guidewire. If you encounter resistance in the passage of a standard 0.032-in or 0.035-in guidewire while working through the loop, remove the wire because repeated attempts to negotiate it against the resistance can lead to perforation, spasm, and severe local pain. A flexible guidewire (ie, 0.014-in soft-tip PTCA guidewire or a 0.025-in hydrophilic guidewire) should be used in place of a standard guidewire to cross the loop. The tip of a guidewire (especially of a 0.014-in PTCA wire) can be shaped to the angle of the loop to facilitate crossing. When the guidewire crosses the loop, its tip is parked as high as possible (ie, high brachial, axillary, or subclavian region). Then the catheter can be advanced over it. Sometimes, when these guidewires may not provide adequate support for the advancement of the catheters, the strategy should be changed (mentioned in the later part of this discussion).

3. Use buddy wire(s). When a single 0.014-in PTCA guidewire provides inadequate support for a catheter to

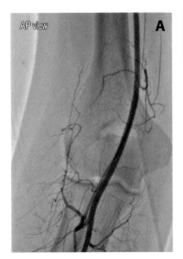
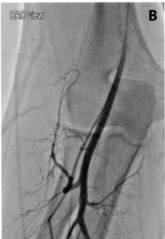
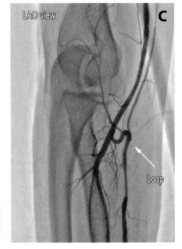

Figure 15.8 **Panel A**: Contrast injection in AP view does not reveal the anatomy properly. **Panel B**: RAO view reveals the loop and a communicating artery. **Panel C**: LAO view adequately defines the loop.

cross the loop, use of additional 1 or 2 such guidewires should facilitate the advancement of the catheter by adding an additional support.

4. Straighten the loop. Mostly, the catheter can easily be negotiated over the wire across a loop without disturbing the shape of the loop. When there is resistance in passage of the catheter while working through the loop, this technique is useful.

   Push the catheter as far as possible into the loop, keeping the wire tip as high as possible (ie, in high brachial, axillary, or subclavian region). Then pull

the entire assembly slightly back (ie, the catheter along with the guidewire). This maneuver opens up the loop and straightens it. At this stage, advancement of the catheter across the loop becomes easy.

5. Exchanging the guidewire is helpful in addressing the most difficult loops. It is used if the catheter is partly inside the loop, but has not crossed the entire loop, and it is difficult to advance it any farther.

   Advance the catheter into the loop as far as possible. Exchange the thin guidewire with another guidewire to

Table 15.1 Algorithm for Dealing with Loops

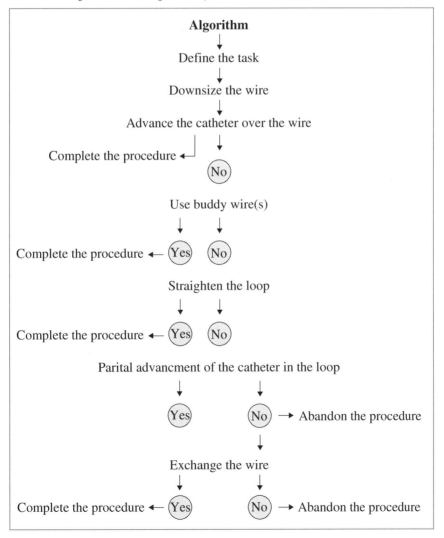

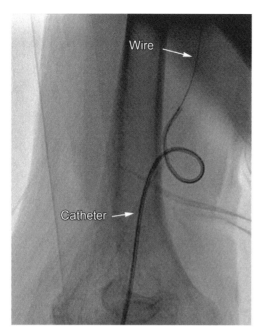

Figure 15.9 Catheter was negotiated across the loop over a 0.014-in BMW PTCA wire.

provide extra support (see Figure 15.9). A 0.014-in PTCA guidewire can be exchanged with a 0.025-in hydrophilic guidewire, and a 0.025-in hydrophilic guidewire can be exchanged with a standard 0.035-in guidewire, if necessary. Then, advance the catheter on the new wire. Avoid using a super-stiff guidewire unless you have crossed the loop and the catheter tip is well into the higher segment (ie, high brachial, axillary, or subclavian region). This technique is useful in working through a difficult radiocubital trunk and a 360° loop with very small diameter (see Figure 15.10 A–C, Figure 15.11 A–D, and Figure 15.12 A–D.

■ ISSUES RELATED TO SUBCLAVIAN, INNOMINATE, AND AORTIC ARCH REGIONS

The anatomy differs on the right and left sides as far as the subclavian artery is concerned. On the right side, the subclavian artery arises from the innominate artery (Figure 15.13). On the left side, it arises from the arch of the

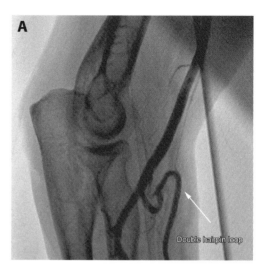

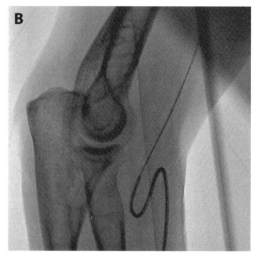

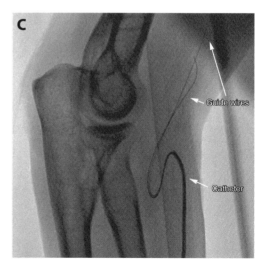

Figure 15.10 Panel A: Example of a complex double hairpin loop. **Panel B**: Demonstration of buddy wire technique (two PTCA wire). **Panel C**: Catheter crossed the loop successfully.

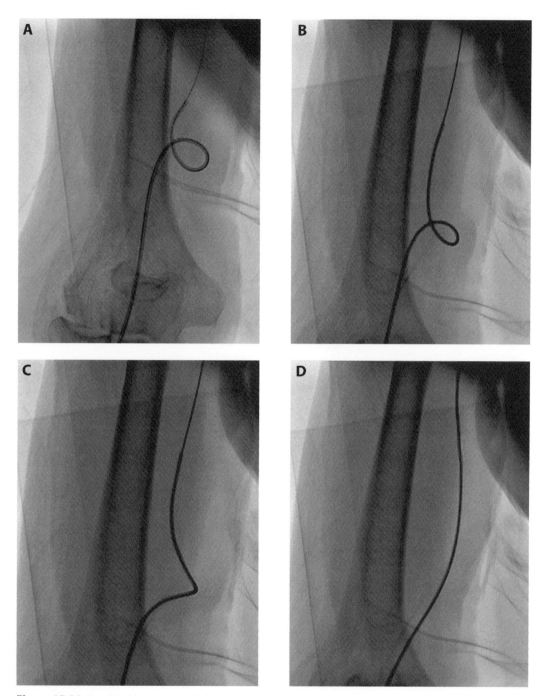

Figure 15.11 Panel A: After crossing the loop, the catheter refuses to advance farther. **Panel B**: Assembly (catheter and guidewire together) was carefully pulled back. **Panel C**: Demonstration of unfolding of the loop. **Panel D**: The loop has been straightened.

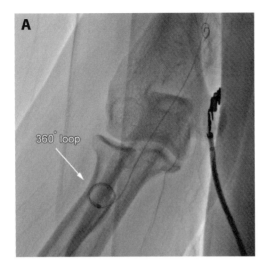

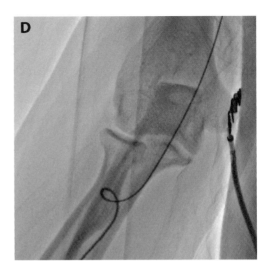

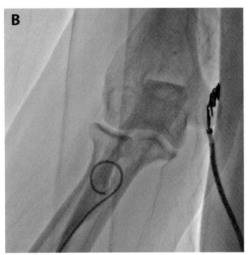

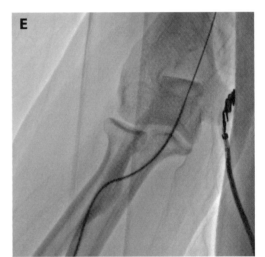

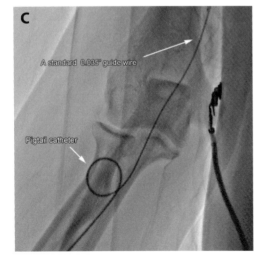

Figure 15.12 **Panel A**: 360° loop was crossed successfully with a PTCA wire; however pigtail catheter could not cross the last part. **Panel B**: PTCA wire was removed. **Panel C**: A standard 0.035-in guidewire was negotiated across the loop through pigtail catheter. **Panel D**: Whole assembly was carefully pulled back and loop started unfolding. **Panel E**: Loop was unfolded and catheter was negotiated easily.

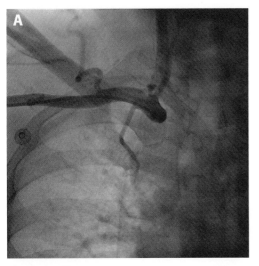
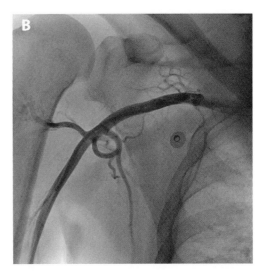

Figure 15.13 (**A**) Normal right subclavian and (**B**) axillary artery anatomy.

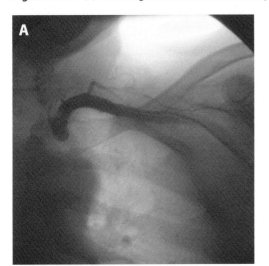
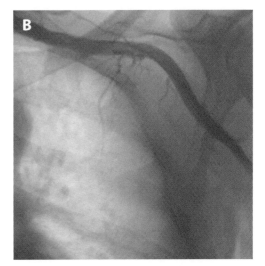

Figure 15.14 (**A**) Normal left subclavian and (**B**) axillary artery anatomy.

aorta (Figure 15.14). Therefore, they differ in length, direction, and relationship to neighboring structures in their proximal parts.

The innominate-arch junction is unique to transradial procedures. Here the catheters and guidewires must take an obtuse-angle turn to enter into the ascending aorta.

In cases of normal anatomy, the turn is smooth and does not pose challenges in performing diagnostic or interventional procedures. In cases of abnormal anatomy due to dilation or distortion of the aorta, the procedure requires judicious use of guidewires (0.025-in or 0.032-in hydrophilic guidewires, standard 0.035-in guidewires, and super-stiff guidewires) and catheters (unusual curves, if necessary) to complete the procedure.

Following are the important relevant issues:

- Tortuosity in subclavian region
- Severely dilated and distorted aortic route (pseudo-arteria lusoria)
- Arteria lusoria

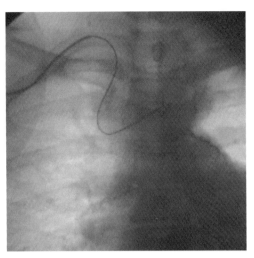

Figure 15.15 Example of mild subclavian tortuosity.

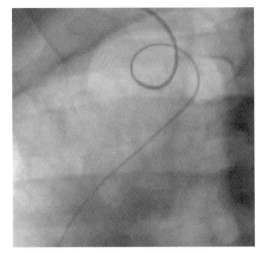

Figure 15.16 Example of severe subclavian tortuosity.

Tortuosity in Subclavian Region

Tortuosity in the subclavian region is divided into mild tortuosity (Figure 15.15) and severe tortuosity (Figure 15.16). Old age, female gender, long-standing diabetes, and hypertension are the predictors for this issue.[4,10,11,12,17]

Tips and Tricks for Identification and Management of Tortuosity.

■ Resistance to a guidewire and/or a catheter movement in this region is an important clue.

■ Gentle movement of assembly under fluoroscopic guidance leads to successful entry in the ascending aorta particularly for mild tortuosity.

■ Use of a super-stiff guidewire is avoided unless the ascending or descending aorta is entered, as it can lead to injury and dissection in this region.

■ At times, deep inspiration facilitates entry of a guidewire and catheter in the ascending aorta. [*Editor's note:* This is an excellent maneuver. Taking a deep breath elongates and straightens the artery, allowing for access of the wire or the catheter into the ascending aorta.]

■ At times, in a case of severe tortuosity, despite optimal position of a guidewire in the ascending aorta, there is severe resistance to the catheter movement at the subclavian-innominate junction. At

this stage, instead of pushing the catheter farther over the wire, pulling the whole assembly slightly back straightens the tortuosity and allows its smooth entry in the ascending aorta.

■ Always use fluoroscopic guidance while working through this region to prevent damage to origins of carotid, vertebral, or internal mammary artery (IMA). [*Editor's note:* We have also found that using a long hydrophilic sheath may help to overcome subclavian tortuosity just as it does when working from the femoral, and there is severe tortuosity of the iliac and abdominal aorta.]

Severely Dilated and Distorted Aortic Route (Pseudo-arteria Lusoria)

This is seen mainly in patients with advance-stage, uncontrolled hypertension and long-standing severe aortic valve lesions. Dilatation and distortion of the aorta lead to changes in the anatomy, particularly distances of origin of aortic arch branches and positions of coronary ostia.[4,10,11,12,17]

Tips and Tricks for Identification and Management of Pseudo-arteria Lusoria.

■ Entry in the ascending aorta is usually not so difficult; however, for coronary cannulation, wider catheter curves are required.

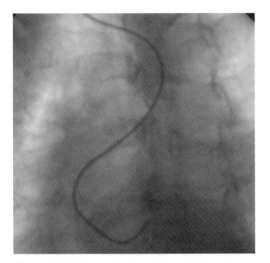

Figure 15.17 Example of pseudo-arteria lusoria.

- If the catheter has tendency to enter the descending aorta, deep inspiration helps entry in the ascending aorta.

- While working through a left radial approach, the catheter traverses through a wider angle, and at times it has a tendency to slip in the descending aorta. Deep inspiration helps with ascending aortic entry, and wider catheter curves help coronary cannulation.

Working Through Arteria Lusoria Using Right TRA

Arteria lusoria is a congenital anomaly of the right subclavian artery characterized topographically as follows: The artery originates below the left subclavian artery as the fourth main branch of the aortic arch and turns to the right behind the esophagus and in front of the vertebral column.[9,13,14,17,18] In more than 32,000 transradial procedures, we have objectively documented arteria lusoria only 45 stimes (0.14%). It is a rare anomaly. See Figure 15.17 for pseudo-arteria lusoria.

We have developed a protocol to work through this situation.[14] It is divided into two parts: (1) entering the ascending aorta through arteria lusoria and (2) the cannulation of the coronary arteries (see Figure 5.18).

Entering the Ascending Aorta.

■ Step 1

The catheter and guidewire have a tendency to enter the descending aorta. If this happens, withdraw the catheter and the guidewire together as an assembly.

After asking the patient to take a deep breath, gently push the 0.035-in standard guidewire. If the guidewire enters the ascending aorta effortlessly, you can then push the catheter over the guidewire.

■ Step 2

If Step 1 is not successful, keep the guidewire in the descending aorta. Remove the Judkins right or left catheter, or the first catheter you tried. Take a 5-Fr IMA diagnostic catheter, put it into the descending aorta over the guidewire, and try the same maneuver. In many cases, you will be successful in entering the ascending aorta.

■ Step 3

If the IMA catheter fails, then a 5-Fr Simmon catheter can be used to enter the ascending aorta.

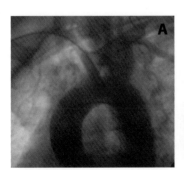
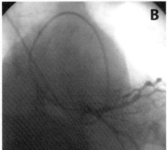
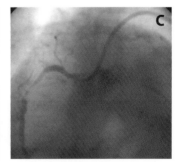

Figure 15.18 Panel A: Documentation of arteria lusoria. **Panel B**: LCA cannulation through arteria lusoria. **Panel C**: RCA cannulation through arteria lusoria.

■ Step 4

If the 0.035-in standard guidewire has a tendency to slip into the descending aorta, the second choice is a 0.032-in or a 0.025-in hydrophilic guidewire. The slippery character of a hydrophilic guidewire facilitates relatively easy entry into the ascending aorta in challenging situations.

Note:

- Prefer working in the 40° left anterior oblique view.

- Do not use super-stiff guidewires unless you have entered the ascending aorta.

Cannulation of the Coronary Arteries.
Once the guidewire and the catheter are in the ascending aorta, cannulate the left or right coronaries in the usual fashion. It is relatively easy to cannulate the coronaries. If there is a challenge, follow these steps:

■ Step 1

Remove the standard 0.035-in guidewire or the hydrophilic guidewire, keeping the catheter in the ascending aorta.

■ Step 2

Using a 0.035-in super-stiff guidewire, make a loop of wire in the ascending aorta, and slowly slide the catheter over it so that you can make a loop of the assembly (catheter and guidewire).

■ Step 3

Slowly pull the guidewire slightly inside the mouth of the catheter and pull the assembly back. This usually cannulates the left coronary artery.

For cannulation of the right coronary artery, slowly and gently rotate the assembly clockwise.

For diagnostic procedures, use a Judkins left, an Optitorque TIG, or an Amplatz left catheter to cannulate the left coronary ostium. Sometimes, a 5-Fr extra backup guide catheter is useful to cannulate the left coronary ostium. Use a Judkins right or an Amplatz left catheter to cannulae the right coronary ostium.

For intervention in the left coronary arteries, choose any extra backup guide catheter as your first choice. If this is not successful, use a Judkins left or an Amplatz left guide catheter.

For intervention in the right coronary arteries, Amplatz right is our first choice. If this does not succeed, a Judkins right or an Amplatz left catheter is used.

Note: At any stage during cannulation of the coronary ostium, do not push too much, or the assembly may prolapse into the descending aorta.

These steps may seem complicated, but arteria lusoria is very rare, and patience and perseverance can help you complete the procedure in the usual fashion. If the first few attempts to enter the ascending aorta are unsuccessful, switch to the left radial or the femoral route. Do not get discouraged. One day you will beat the learning curve and address this situation effortlessly.

■ SUMMARY

During one's journey to become a "committed radialist," one needs to go through a process known as "a new learning curve." A new interventionalist will take a longer time as compared to an experienced operator. One needs to understand normal vascular anatomy of the region, acquired variations, and congenital anomalies. If there are issues, they need to be resolved. In this chapter, we have done our best to resolve practically all important issues related to TRA. The tips and tricks discussed here shall help both beginners and experienced operators.

■ REFERENCES

1. Barbeau G. Radial loop and extreme vessel tortuosity in the transradial approach: advantage of hydrophilic-coated guidewires and catheters. *Catheter Cardiovasc Interv.* 2003;59(4):442–450.
2. Calviño-Santos R, Vázquez-Rodríguez J, Salgado-Fernández J, et al. Management of iatrogenic radial artery perforation. *Catheter Cardiovasc Interv.* 2004;61(1):74–78.
3. Coppola J, Patel T, Kwan T, Sanghvi K, Srivastava S, Shah S, Staniloae C. Nitroglycerin, nitroprusside,

or both, in preventing radial artery spasm during transradial artery catheterization. *J Invasive Cardiol.* 2006;18(4):155–158.

4. Gilchrist I. Transradial technical tips. *Catheter Cardiovasc Interv.* 2000;49(3):253–254.

5. Kiemeneij F. Prevention and management of radial artery spasm. *J Invasive Cardiol.* 2006;18(4): 159–160.

6. Lo T, Nolan J, Fountzopoulos E, et al. Radial artery anomaly and its influence on transradial coronary procedural outcome. *Heart.* 2009;95(5):410–415.

7. Louvard Y, Lefèvre T. Loops and transradial approach in coronary diagnosis and intervention. *Catheter Cardiovasc Interv.* 2000;51(2):250–252.

8. Patel T, Shah S, Sanghavi K, Pancholy S. Management of radial and brachial artery perforations during transradial procedures: a practical approach. *J Invasive Cardiol.* 2009;21(10):544–547.

9. Abhaichand R, Louvard Y, Gobeil J, et al. The problem of arteria lusoria in right transradial coronary angiography and angioplasty. *Catheter Cardiovasc Interv.* 2001;54(2):196–201.

10. Caputo R, Simons A, Giambartolomei A, et al. Transradial cardiac catheterization in elderly patients. *Catheter Cardiovasc Interv.* 2000;51(3): 287–290.

11. Cha K, Kim M, Kim H. Prevalence and clinical predictors of severe tortuosity of right subclavian artery in patients undergoing transradial coronary angiography. *Am J Cardiol.* 2003;92(10):1220–1222.

12. Dehghani P, Mohammad A, Bajaj R, et al. Mechanism and predictors of failed transradial approach for percutaneous coronary interventions. *JACC Cardiovasc Interv.* 2009; 2(11):1057–1064.

13. Grollman J Jr. The many faces of the anomalous left aortic arch. *Catheter Cardiovasc Interv.* 2001;54(2):202–203.

14. Patel T. Right trans-radial approach: working through arteria lusoria. *Indian Heart J.* 2006; 58(4):301.

15. Patel T, Shah S, Ranjan A. *Patel's Atlas of Transradial Intervention: The Basics.* Chapter 7, 62–102. Seattle: Sea Script Company; 2007.

16. Pancholy S, Coppola J, Patel T. Subcutaneous administration of nitroglycerin to facilitate radial artery cannulation. *Catheter Cardiovasc Interv.* 2006;68(3):389–391.

17. Valsecchi, O, Vassileva A, Musumeci G, et al. Failure of transradial approach during coronary interventions: anatomic considerations. *Catheter Cardiovasc Interv.* 2006;67(6):870–878.

18. Yiu K, Chan W, Jim M, et al. Arteria lusoria diagnosed by transradial coronary catheterization. *JACC Cardiovasc Interv.* 2010;3(8):880–881.

chapter 16

Complications of Transradial Access

Kirk N. Garratt, MD, MSc

■ SPECTRUM AND INCIDENCE OF COMPLICATIONS

The principal benefit of radial access over all alternatives is improved safety. This improvement is achieved primarily through reductions in vascular complications related to arterial access, but this is not to say that access-related complications do not occur. Furthermore, traversing the vasculature of the upper extremity and neck introduces opportunities for complications and injuries not usually expected with use of lower extremity access sites. Some complications, including bleeding complications, may be related to adjunctive pharmacology and other aspects of the procedure, and would not be reduced through use of radial access. So, as with all procedures, a certain tolerance for procedural complications is necessary with transradial intervention,

despite efforts to minimize them. In this chapter, complications of radial arterial access for percutaneous coronary intervention (PCI) are described and discussed.

■ COMMON COMPLICATIONS

Radial Artery Spasm

Spasm of the radial artery (and the more proximal arteries of the upper extremity) occurs commonly with radial artery trauma. This is understandable in a teleological sense: Upper extremities are at high risk of injury, and endogenous systems to attenuate bleeding in the event of serious trauma offer a survival advantage. Furthermore, a relationship exists between state of stress and vasospastic potential: Trauma and pain at the radial artery trigger significant catecholamine

Transradial Access: Techniques for Diagnostic Angiography and Percutaneous Intervention
©2013 Howard A. Cohen (Editor). Cardiotext Publishing, ISBN 978-1-935395-41-6.

release, which in turn causes or amplifies arterial spasm at the injury site. Radial artery spasm may be limited, such that catheterization may continue, but may be associated with significant patient discomfort. Spasm may also be severe, resulting in catheter entrapment, a potentially very serious problem. Radial artery spasm may be so severe that catheters or sheaths cannot be removed with force, and attempts may result in serious vascular injury.

The chief principle in management of radial artery spasm is prevention through administration of intra-arterial vasorelaxant drugs, given shortly after arterial entry. Without administration of vasorelaxant drugs, radial artery spasm has been reported to complicate more than one-fifth of transradial procedures.[1] With routine intra-arterial vasorelaxant medication, spasm should not complicate more than 5% of cases. Various medication cocktails used for this purpose are reviewed elsewhere in this textbook; although no clear front-runner drug combination has been accepted as having primacy over all others, the combination of a calcium antagonist and a nitrate or nitrate donor drug is popular owing to the ready availability of the drugs, their familiarity to interventional cardiologists, and at least some literature to support their use.[1,2] Addition of intra-arterial lidocaine, which will block arterial C-fiber pain receptors, has been useful as well. Of note, some of these drugs (notably lidocaine and verapamil) create a strong sensation of heat when administered to some patients. The discomfort of this can be minimized by diluting the drug with blood or saline (blood has greater buffering ability) and administering intra-arterial medication slowly. Early administration of sedative drugs intravenously is also helpful, but benzodiazepines and morphine analogues can lower systemic blood pressure, making arterial puncture harder. For this reason, many operators choose to withhold sedating drugs until after the arterial catheter is placed, counting on the retrograde amnestic properties of midazolam and similar drugs to block memory of sheath insertion.

Assessment of endothelial function along the radial artery route may be helpful in predicting spasm. A group from University of Athens Medical School reported measuring the hyperemic blood flow response to 5 minutes upper extremity ischemia using an occlusive sphygmomanometer, and found that an abnormal hyperemic response (an indicator of abnormal endothelial function) was highly correlated with spasm upon radial artery sheath withdrawal;[3] small arterial caliber and number of catheter exchanges also increased spasm risk.

Notably, longer sheaths have been generally avoided during radial artery procedures, over concerns that the longer sheath may provide greater resistance to removal if spasm occurs. Although this is logical, at least one study found that use of longer 25-cm hydrophilic sheaths was linked to less spasm than shorter 7-cm nonhydrophilic sheaths.[4]

Spasm may develop gradually, with catheters becoming increasingly difficult to manipulate during the course of the case, or can occur precipitously. Management of developing spasm follows three principles: (1) additional vasorelaxant medications, (2) sedation, and (3) time.

Mild to moderate vasospasm can be managed with additional nitrates, calcium antagonists, and perhaps lidocaine. If catheters become very difficult to manipulate, if the patient complains of significant pain during catheter movement, or if catheter entrapment occurs, alternative drugs should be considered. Intravenous nitroglycerin is available in all labs and may be given providing blood pressure is sufficient. Intra-arterial administration of papaverine, an opium alkaloid antispasmotic compound, has occasionally been pivotal in resolving spasm.[5] Intravenous labetalol can be of theoretical benefit, having both alpha and beta blocking properties, but any risk of unopposed alpha stimulation must be avoided. Nitroprusside should not be given, as its effects are chiefly on the microvasculature. The newer infusible dihydropyridine calcium antagonist, clevidipine, is untested for this application but likely will suffer from similar limitations; it has been used successfully to treat intraoperative spasm during coronary artery bypass surgery.[6]

For any serious vasospasm, pain relief is essential. The pain-spasm-pain cycle can only be broken when pain is abolished. Liberal use of conscious sedation drugs will usually suffice, but occasionally deeper anesthesia is needed. We have observed several cases of catheter entrapment that were overcome only when the patient was temporarily anesthetized with propofol; once the patient was asleep, radial artery relaxation was immediate. Although not available in many catheterization laboratories today, we have also found that the use of intra-arterial reserpine has succeeded in relieving spasm when other maneuvers failed. Stellate ganglion block has also been reported to be beneficial when all else failed.

Surgical removal of entrapped catheters is exceedingly rare.

Access Site Vascular Complications

Bleeding after sheath removal remains the most obvious complication of arterial cannulation, whether radial, femoral, or other arterial. Many reports in the literature, including randomized trials, attest to the reduction in bleeding complications when the radial artery is selected rather than the femoral artery,[7] even when patients undergo catheterization in the setting of full anticoagulation or intensive antiplatelet therapies.[8,9] A small randomized study from Greece found that transfemoral intervention in patients with international normalized ratio (INR) values between 1.8 and 3.5 (average about 2.6) is complicated by bleeding in more than one-third of patients, whereas transradial intervention can be performed with no increase in bleeding risk.[9] Reductions in bleeding events have been linked to reductions in procedural mortality in moderate population registries[10,11] although, interestingly, not in the large randomized RIVAL trial,[12] where rates of bleeding not related to CABG surgery were observed to be numerically less with transradial intervention but not statistically less. Several reasons might explain this finding, but a salient observation is that patients treated by those operators with abundant experience in transradial procedures did enjoy significantly lower bleeding rates and clinical complications compared with patients treated with transfemoral intervention, whereas those patients

treated by operators with less experience did not. This observation provides a compelling argument not just to use radial artery access when femoral access is problematic, but to use it always as your default technique. Operators committed to the use of the radial artery access route capture the benefits for their patients. A reassuring finding from RIVAL: The composite of all vascular complications were lower with radial artery use, even among those operators with least experience.

Bleeding from the radial arteriotomy site is usually superficial. Although a large, deep ecchymosis can occur, discoloring the forearm and distressing the patient for weeks, these events don't pose significant risk. Deep tissue bleeding into the forearm compartment is a different matter (see "Forearm Compartment Syndrome"). Superficial bleeding often arises when a radial hemostasis device is placed improperly, either misaligned with the arteriotomy or placed without sufficient compressive pressure. Adjusting the device should be the first step. If this fails to bring bleeding under prompt control, either manual compression should be used or a second compressive device may be applied, just proximal to the first. Pressure should not be excessive, and the duration of pressure should not be excessive: In our laboratories, pressure exceeding systemic blood pressure is only used in the event of significant superficial bleeding that cannot be controlled otherwise, and pressure is not left for more than 90 minutes in unanticoagulated patients.

If uncertainty exists about whether a bleed is superficial or deep, measures should be taken as outlined for forearm compartment syndromes.

Sterile Granulomas (Sterile Abscesses)

Sterile granulomas were first reported as an apparent complication of the use of silicon-coated vascular sheaths in 2003.[13] Such granulomas, in their acute phase, have the appearance of bacterial abscesses,[13-15] but are in fact sterile (hence they have been called sterile abscesses). Although some speculate that, despite their sterility, these granulomas may still have an underlying infectious etiology,[15] most believe they represent an inflammatory response to silicon or other lubricant material that becomes trapped in the dermis after sheath removal. A systematic review of this problem, evaluating the federal Manufacturer and User Facility Device (MAUDE) database that catalogues complications of medical devices, has found that only the sheaths manufactured by Cook, Inc., were reported to the Food and Drug Administration (FDA) as being linked to this complication.[16]

Sterile granulomas can be easily avoided by "stripping" the vascular sheath of excess lubricant material before insertion. Simply wiping the sheath with a saline-dampened gauze several times will suffice. If a granuloma develops, it may be managed conservatively. Local discomfort during the acute phase is improved if a tense granuloma is lanced and drained. Although antibiotic therapy is not indicated for sterile abscesses, acute phase granulomas may be indistinguishable from bacterial abscesses, so either a short course of antibiotic therapy aimed at common skin flora may be prescribed, or an aspiration sample of the lesion may be sent for culture. An untreated sterile granuloma will complete its acute phase within 2 weeks, and the resulting chronic granuloma will typically resolve completely (or nearly completely) within a year. Chronic granulomas may be associated with chronic pain and tenderness at the site; this also usually resolves with conservative management.

Radial Artery Narrowing and Occlusion

Occlusion of the radial artery is frequently reported to occur in 5% to 15% of patients following transradial arteriography or angioplasty,[4,17–21] although a recent prospective vascular ultrasound evaluation of 455 patients in Germany found early radial artery occlusion in 13.7% of patients after 5-Fr sheath use and in 30.5% of patients after 6-Fr sheath use.[20] Development of critical hand ischemia complicating transradial coronary intervention has never been reported[20] but is entirely possible if the integrity of the palmar arch has not been confirmed prior to cannulation. The forearm is relatively rich in collateral vessels too, which helps minimize the risk of severe hand ischemia. Nonetheless, the risk of hand ischemia should be borne in mind before any radial artery cannulation. Publications from the surgical literature suggest that radial artery thrombotic occlusion following placement of radial artery lines in critically ill patients is associated with a high prevalence of gangrenous digits requiring amputation. Moreover, surgical intervention is of limited help, perhaps because some of the damage is mediated through thrombotic emboli to the fingers.[22]

Although a patent palmar arch and abundant ipsilateral arterial collateral vessels in the forearm preclude significant consequences with radial artery occlusion, this complication is best avoided, if for no other reason than to facilitate use of the vessel during future procedures. This risk should also be kept in mind during patient evaluation: Patients who are expected to need a patent radial artery for use in planned vascular or coronary artery bypass surgery, as an arteriovenous shunt for hemodialysis, or for other reasons may not be good candidates for this approach.

Use of moderate-dose heparin (4,000 units or more) given after sheath insertion has been shown to lower the incidence of this complication,[23] but the very low doses of heparin (2,500 units or less), commonly used in diagnostic procedures, have not. Also, there is no apparent benefit with intra-arterial rather than intravenous heparin administration.[24] Bivalirudin given to patients having intervention did not produce meaningfully different late occlusion rates compared with patients given heparin alone following a diagnostic study.[23] Antithrombin therapy is not required to prevent thrombotic complications during diagnostic studies, although therapy should be considered if the study is prolonged.

A study from China using serial ultrasound studies found the medial-intimal thickness at the arteriotomy site increased by about 2.5-fold within 24 hours of cannulation, and was associated with 20% reduction in the mean vessel diameter and about 3% rate of vessel occlusion. However, by 30 days, the artery showed signs of healing, and the occlusion rate had fallen to less than 2%.[25]

Still, chronic evidence of vascular injury may persist, with chronically smaller radial arteries at the access site and distal to it; this may be especially prevalent in patients who undergo repeat transradial procedures.[26]

Occlusion likely occurs as a result of local arterial trauma, combined with external pressure and regional blood stasis during the period of compression after sheath removal. This combination may permit development of a significant thrombus resistant to absorption and resolution. If true, then minimizing the external pressure over the arteriotomy site and avoiding blood stasis is likely to be more effective in avoiding occlusion than any other maneuver. This has led to the practice of using much less compressive pressure than had been customary in the past, to achieve what has been called "patent hemostasis."[19] Patent hemostasis implies documentation of radial artery patency after application of a hemostatic device. Typically, this involves application of a compressive device after sheath removal, applying sufficient pressure to achieve complete hemostasis, then gradual reduction of the applied pressure until flow can be confirmed through the radial artery segment distal to the compression device while the ulnar artery is compressed manually. If the preoperative pulse was difficult to palpate, a Doppler probe can be used to confirm anterograde flow through the radial artery (this eliminates the need to compress the ulnar artery also, because a change in the flow signal direction can be easily appreciated). Use of the patent hemostasis technique has been reported to reduce acute and chronic radial artery occlusion significantly.[19] [*Editor's note:* See Chapter 6 on closure and hemostasis.]

Patients identified as having postprocedure radial artery occlusion before hospital dismissal may be considered for outpatient anticoagulant therapy. At least one study has shown that a 4-week course of heparin therapy led to restored patency of the vessel in nearly 90% of afflicted patients, while fewer than 20% of those not receiving heparin had patent radial arteries at 1 month.[17] It should be noted, however, that patients in this study were selected to receive heparin on the basis of hand symptoms, while asymptomatic patients with occlusion served as the control group.

■ RARE COMPLICATIONS

Forearm Compartment Syndrome

Forearm compartment syndrome may develop when bleeding into the forearm raises the intracompartmental pressure enough to cause ischemic injury to contained structures; nerves are most sensitive. [*Editor's note:* See Chapter 3 on anatomy.] Bleeding from the radial arteriotomy site may track deeply into the forearm and cause compartment syndrome, but this is quite rare. Most cases of compartment syndrome are related to bleeding from a vascular injury within the arm, often from around the olecranon fossa where the radial artery loops and other anatomic variants raise the risk of a perforation (Figure 16.1; ▶ Video 16.1). Hydrophilic guidewires can easily get trapped in small branches and perforate them, and cause profuse bleeding in the setting of vigorous anticoagulant therapy.

Forearm compartment syndrome should be suspected in any patient complaining of forearm pain, with an increase in forearm girth, diminished or absent hand pulses, and cool, pale hand or fingers. If doubt exists, place 2 fingers into the palm of the patient's hand and ask the patient to squeeze: Increased compartment pressure makes contraction of muscles intensely painful. If a patient is able to grip your fingers firmly without pain, he or she does not have compartment syndrome. Loss of sensation and pain on passive motion of the fingers are also consistent with the diagnosis of compartment syndrome.

Permanent neurologic injury can develop with high pressures sustained for more than 4 hours and can lead to Volkmann contracture of the hand.[27] Although this is undoubtedly the most serious vascular complication associated with transradial procedures, it is exceedingly uncommon. A review of all published literature on this topic between 1992 and 2007 found only 5 reports in the literature on this topic. A 2008 institutional

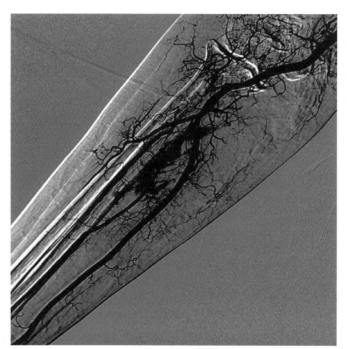

Figure 16.1 Forearm perforation occurring after transradial catheterization. *Source*: Al-Sekaiti R, Ali M, Sallam M. Radial artery perforation after coronary intervention: is there a role for covered coronary stent? *Cathet Cardiovasc Interv.* 2011;78:632–635.

review from one of the largest transradial practices in North America found 2 cases in more than 51,000 transradial procedures, yielding an incidence rate of 0.004%.[28] Small women may be at increased risk, and high doses of anticoagulants may contribute to the risk,[28] but the rarity of the event makes these observations suspect.

If forearm hemorrhage is suspected, certain steps are mandatory to minimize risk of permanent injury. All anticoagulants must be stopped; heparin should be reversed with protamine. Controlling pressure should be applied to the forearm to tamponade the bleeding area by applying circumferential forearm pressure equal to, or greater than, systemic blood pressure. Although standard sphygmomanometer cuffs are fine for this purpose, the inflatable pouches used for pressuring bags of saline are also suitable and typically available in catheterization laboratory environments (Figure 16.2). Protocols for applying pressure vary, but 2 consistent characteristics are (1) use of pressure sufficient to stanch arterial bleeding in the forearm and (2) intermittent release of this pressure to perfuse the hand. A sensible practice is to apply forearm pressure matching or exceeding

the systolic pressure, maintaining that pressure for 10 to 15 minutes, then releasing pressure to allow hand perfusion and venous outflow for about 2 to 5 minutes. Some operators advocate for use of external pressure that is slightly less than the systolic pressure.[28]

Between 2 and 4 cycles of external forearm pressure is typically enough to stop forearm hemorrhage, but continued bleeding may occur. Forearm fasciotomy may be required to prevent neurologic injury, even if bleeding has stopped. For these reasons, it is critical that an appropriate surgeon be called to assess the patient immediately. All radial operators should be aware of the best surgeon for this task: In many hospitals this would be a job for a vascular surgeon, but in some hospitals this may be the purview of a hand, an orthopedic, or even a general surgeon.

Delay in Delivery of Large-Caliber Devices

Among the rare complications that should be considered with transradial intervention is the possibility that reliance on the radial access route may limit emergency treatment options, particularly during high-risk procedures and circumstances. Although nearly all

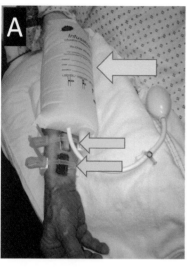
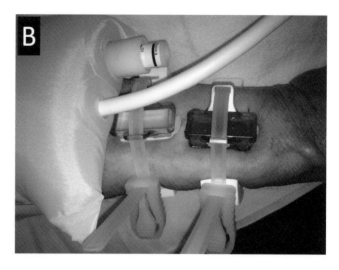

Figure 16.2 Management of forearm bleeding complications. (**A**) Inflatable pouch used to pressurize bags of saline (blue arrow) may be used to apply a broad band of pressure to a forearm with hematoma or perforation, and can be used while hemostatic bands are in place over the arteriotomy site. Note bleeding beneath the original hemostatic band (yellow arrow). Second hemostatic band (green arrow) placed proximal to original band often improves hemostatic control at arteriotomy. (**B**) Successful management of forearm hematoma with two hemostatic bands and a forearm pressure bag applied. Note that the integrated pressure gauge shows approximately 150 mm Hg pressure in the bag, exceeding systemic blood pressure temporarily.

interventional devices can be reliably used through the radial artery, placement of sheaths larger than 6 or 7 French can be difficult, especially in urgent circumstances. Placement of instruments requiring very large bore introducer sheaths, such as covered stents, may be problematic. For this reason, routine preparation of at least one femoral artery site for use if need arises is good practice.

Intra-aortic balloon pumps have been placed through upper extremity arteries, but these generally require surgical exposure of an axillary artery for safe application;[29] other upper extremity vessels are not of sufficient caliber to be suitable for this purpose. Therefore, all patients with an acute presentation in whom the potential need for hemodynamic support is judged to be significant should have a femoral artery site prepared and exposed for immediate use if needed.

Contrast-Induced Nephropathy

Some reports indicate that transradial access requires use of more contrast, owing to somewhat greater difficultly engaging coronary arteries and grafts.[30] However, acute kidney injury following catheterization may be related to atheroemboli arising from catheter manipulations within diseased aortae, and at least one group has reported less kidney disease developing within 6 months of catheterization when a radial, rather than femoral, approach is used;[31] although patients in the 2 groups were significantly different in many ways, logistic regression yielded a hazard ratio of greater than 4 for acute kidney injury with femoral rather than radial artery access.

Pseudoaneurysms and Arteriovenous Fistulae

Development of a radial artery pseudoaneurysm is rare,[21] while infected pseudoaneurysms are rarer still.[33] The scanty reports of such complications speak to the safety of the procedure, but also remind operators to be alert for these possibilities. Pseudoaneurysms are known to be the consequence of vascular injury such as perforations (Figure 16.3), but as these events are so uncommon, no procedural or clinical factors have been identified as being clearly linked to increased risk.

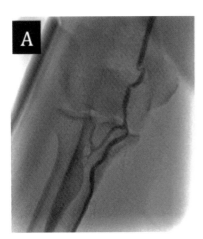
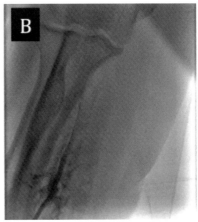
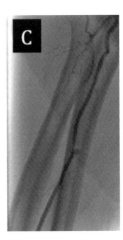

Figure 16.3 Perforation of radial artery and subsequent development of radial artery pseudoaneurysm. Catheter advancement through a tortuous radial artery (**A**) resulted in vascular injury and forearm bleeding (**B**). Despite successful management acutely, the patient returned 5 days later with pain and swelling of the forearm. Repeat study identified radial artery pseudoaneurysm development at the site of vascular injury (**C**). *Source*: Williams PD, Eccleshall S, *Heart*. 2009;95(13):1084.

Pseudoaneurysms may present as painful or painless pulsatile masses within days to months after transradial catheterization.[32] Ultrasound and Doppler imaging demonstrate classic narrow-based characteristics, often with relatively laminar flow into and out of the pseudoaneurysm.

Small pseudoaneurysms may be compressed, but best management of larger radial artery pseudoaneurysms is likely surgical.[34] Injection of thrombin or a sclerosing compound is possible,[35] but the smaller dimensions of the vessel and associated increased shear stress might increase the risk of distal embolization of sclerosis agent compared with femoral pseudoaneurysm therapy. The superficial nature of the artery lends itself well to open repair when needed.

Arteriovenous fistulae (AVF) develop following trauma to an artery and adjacent vein. This is thought to be rare with radial access because most forearm veins are of small caliber. Patients present with painless pulsatile masses having a thrill; diagnosis is with ultrasound and Doppler imaging (Figure 16.4). Repair is usually surgical[32] although magnetic resonance angiography (MRA) of the site may be helpful in assessing whether the AVF is due to a branch versus the main vessel. If only a small branch is involved, this may be amenable to percutaneous closure. Depending on location in the radial artery, percutaneous use of a covered stent has also been used with good success (R. Rosen, MD, personal communication, March 2012).

Cardiovocal (Ortner) Syndrome

An exceedingly rare complication results from injury to the recurrent laryngeal nerve that loops around the right innominate artery and innervates the right vocal cord.[36] This is usually a complication of disease or surgeries of the aorta of great neck vessels, but has been reported to occur after difficult catheter manipulations through tortuous innominate vessels during transradial procedures. Management is conservative.

■ SUMMARY

The principal benefit of radial artery access for angioplasty is the added safety it offers. Nearly all studies confirm that complications are less frequent than with femoral artery access, but they can still occur and can be very serious. Common complications include radial artery spasm, sterile granuloma development, and radial artery occlusion (transient or persistent), which are generally benign in nature; the risk of these complications can

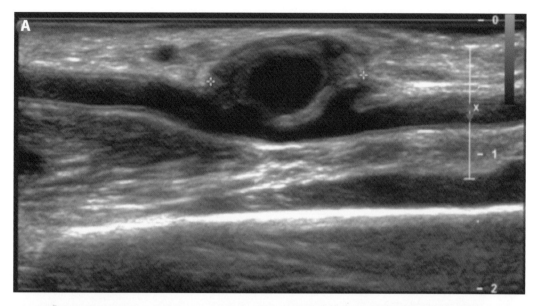

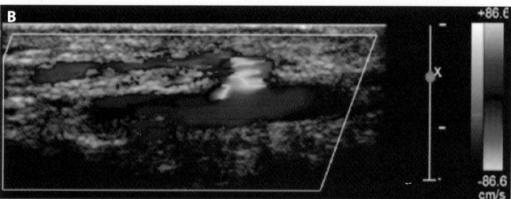

Figure 16.4 Ultrasound image of forearm of 59-year-old man 3 weeks after transradial intervention. (**A**) Image is consistent with radial artery pseudoaneurysm. (**B**) Ultrasound image of forearm of 61-year-old man one year after transradial intervention. Doppler images demonstrate presence of arteriovenous fistula. *Source*: Spence MS, Byrne J, Hargeli L, Mildenberger R, Kinloch D. Rare access site complications following transradial coronary intervention. *Can J Cardiol.* 2009;25(6):e206.

be readily diminished with simple measures easily incorporated into routine practice. More serious vascular complications include the development of a forearm hematoma with compartment syndrome, which stands as the most important to recognize quickly and manage correctly because it can lead quickly to permanent neurologic injury. Surgical decompression of the forearm compartment is the mainstay of therapy for this problem. Radial artery pseudoaneurysms and arteriovenous fistulae are rare but can cause forearm perfusion problems and discomfort and often require surgical intervention for repair. A very

rare but notable complication is Ortner's syndrome: damage to the recurrent laryngeal nerve caused by excessive deformation of a highly tortuous right innominate artery, avoidable by recognizing the anatomy most likely to place a patient at risk of this complication and using an alternative access route.

As with other aspects of medical practice, awareness of complication possibilities, knowledge of appropriate preventive and corrective actions, and recognition of actual adverse events are the keys to a transradial interventional practice characterized by a minimum of complications. It's also worth remembering that although transradial access has much to recommend it, there is no room for zealots in a transradial practice: failure to transition to another access route when circumstances place a patient at increased risk of complications related to radial artery use is not defensible. Conversion from radial to femoral access because of complication risk should be very uncommon, but is not an admission of technical ability; indeed, it is a measure of good medical judgment.

■ REFERENCES

1. Varenne O, Jegou A, Cohen R, et al. Prevention of arterial spasm during percutaneous coronary interventions through radial artery: the SPASM study. *Cathet Cardiovasc Interv.* 2006;68(2):231–235.

2. Kiemeneij F, Vajifdar BU, Eccleshall SC, Laarman G, Slagboom T, van der Wieken R. Evaluation of a spasmolytic cocktail to prevent radial artery spasm during coronary procedures. *Cathet Cardiovasc Interv.* 2003;58(3):281–284.

3. Deftereos S, Giannopoulos G, Kossyvakis C, et al. Radial artery flow-mediated dilation predicts arterial spasm during transradial coronary interventions. *Cathet Cardiovasc Interv.* 2011;77(5):649–654.

4. Caussin C, Gharbi M, Durier C, et al. Reduction in spasm with a long hydrophylic transradial sheath. *Cathet Cardiovasc Interv.* 2010;76(5):668–672.

5. Osman F, Buller N, Steeds R. Use of intra-arterial papaverine for severe arterial spasm during radial artery catheterization. *J Invasive Cardiol.* 2008;20(10):551–552.

6. Patel M, Meyer T, Tharakan A, Tobias JD. Intraoperative administration of clevidipine to prevent vasospasm after radial and internal mammary artery grafts during coronary artery bypass surgery. *Am J Ther.* Epub July 10 2010.

7. Jolly SS, Amlani S, Hamon M, Yusuf S, Mehta SR. Radial versus femoral access for coronary angiography or intervention and the impact on major bleeding and ischemic events: a systematic review and meta-analysis of randomized trials. *Am Heart J.* 2009;157:132–140.

8. Siudak Z, Zawislak B, Dziewierz A, et al. Transradial approach in patients with ST-elevation myocardial infarction treated with abciximab results in fewer bleeding complications: data from EUROTRANSFER registry. *Cor Art Dis.* 2010;21(5):292–297.

9. Ziakas AG, Koskinas KC, Gavrilidis S, et al. Radial versus femoral access for orally anticoagulated patients. *Cathet Cardiovasc Interv.* 2010;76(4):493–499.

10. Chase AJ, Fretz EB, Warburton WP, et al. Association of the arterial access site at angioplasty with transfusion and mortality: the M.O.R.T.A.L study (Mortality benefit Of Reduced Transfusion after percutaneous coronary intervention via the Arm or Leg). *Heart.* 2008;94:1019–1025.

11. Rao SV, Ou FS, Wang TY, et al. Trends in the prevalence and outcomes of radial and femoral approaches to percutaneous coronary intervention: a report from the National Cardiovascular Data Registry. *JACC Cardiovasc Interv.* 2008;1:379–386.

12. Jolly SS, Yusuf S, Carins J, et al. Radial versus femoral access for coronary angiography and intervention in patients with acute coronary syndromes (RIVAL: a randomized, parallel group, muticentre trial). *Lancet.* Epub April 4 2011.

13. Kozak M, Adams DR, Ioffreda MD, et al. Sterile inflammation associated with transradial catheterization and hydrophilic sheaths. *Cathet Cardiovasc Interv.* 2003;59(2):207–213.

14. Zellner C, Yeghiazarians Y, Ports TA, Ursell P, Boyle AJ. Sterile radial artery granuloma after transradial cardiac catheterization. *Cardioasc Revasc Med.* 2011;12(3):187–189.

15. Tharmaratnam D, Webber S, Owens P. Sterile abscess formation as a complication of hydrophilic radial artery cannulation. *Intl J Cardiol.* 2008;130(1):e52.

16. Zellner C, Ports TA, Yeghiazarians Y, Boyle AJ. Sterile radial artery granuloma after transradial procedures: a unique and avoidable complication. *Cathet Cardiovasc Interv.* 2010;76(5):673–676.

17. Zankl AR, Andrassy M, Volz C, et al. Radial artery thrombosis following transradial coronary angiography: incidence and rationale for treatment of symptomatic patients with low-molecular-weight heparins. *Clin Res Cardiol.* 2010;99(12):841–847.

18. Stella PR, Kiemeneij F, Laarman GJ, Odekerken D, Slagboom T, van der Wieken R. Incidence and outcome of radial artery occlusion following transradial artery coronary angioplasty. *Cathet Cardiovasc Interv.* 1997;40(2):156–158.

19. Pancholy S, Coppola J, Patel T, Roke-Thomas M. Prevention of radial artery occlusion-patent hemostasis evaluation trial (PROPHET study): a randomized comparison of traditional versus patency documented hemostasis after transradial catheterization. *Catheter Cardiovasc Interv.* 2008;72:335–340.

20. Uhlemann M, Mobius-Winkler S, Mende M, et al. The Leipzig vascular ultrasound registry in radial artery catheterization: impact of sheath size on vascular complications. *JACC Cardiovasc Interv.* 2012;5(1):44–46.

21. Kanei Y, Kwan T, Nakra NC, et al. Transradial cardiac catheterization: a review of access site complications. *Cathet Cardiovasc Interv.* 2011;78(6):840–846.

22. Valentine RJ, Modrall JG, Clagett GP. Hand ischemia after radial artery cannulation. *J Am Coll Surg.* 2005;201(1):18–22.

23. Plante S, Cantor WJ, Goldman L, et al. Comparison of bivalirudin versus heparin on radial artery occlusion after transradial catheterization. *Catheter Cardiovasc Interv.* 2010;76(5):654–658.

24. Pancholy SB. Comparison of the effect of intra-arterial versus intravenous heparin on radial artery occlusion after transradial catheterization. *Am J Cardiol.* 2009;104(8):1083–1085.

25. Zhenxian Y, Zhou Y, Zhao Y, Zhou Z, Yang S, Wang Z. Impact of transradial coronary procedures on radial artery. *Angiology.* 2010;61(1):8–13.

26. Wakeyama T, Ogawa H, Iida H, et al. Intima-media thickening of the radial artery after transradial intervention: an intravascular ultrasound study. *J Amer Coll Cardiol.* 2003;41(7):1109–1114.

27. Chandraprakasam T, Kumar RA. Acute compartment syndrome of the forearm and hand. *Indian J Plast Surg.* 2011;44(2):212–218.

28. Tizon-Marcos H, Barbeau GR. Incidence of compartment syndrome of the arm in a large series of transradial approach for coronary procedures. *J Interv Cardiol.* 2008;21(5):380–384.

29. McBride LR, Miller LW, Naunheim KS, Pennington DG. Axillary artery insertion of an intra-aortic balloon pump. *Ann Thorac Surg.* 1989;48(6):874–875.

30. Jaffe R, Hong T, Sharieff W, Chisholm RJ, et al. Comparison of radial versus femoral approach for percutaneous coronary interventions in octogenarians. *Cathet Cardiovasc Interv.* 2007;69(6):815–820.

31. Vuurmans T, Byrne J, Fretz, E, et al. Chronic kidney injury in patients after cardiac catheterisation or percutaneous coronary intervention: a comparison of radial and femoral approaches (from the British Columbia Cardiac and Renal registries). *Heart.* 2010;96(19):1538–1542.

32. Spence MS, Byrne J, Hargeli L, Mildenberger R, Kinloch D. Rare access site complications following transradial coronary intervention. *Can J Cardiol.* 2009;25(6):e206.

33. Tsao JW, Neymark E, Gooding GA. Radial artery mycotic pseudoaneurysm: an unusual complication of catheterization. *J Clin Ultrasound.* 2000;28(8):414–416.

34. Collins N, Wainstein R, Ward M, Bhagwandeen R, Dzavik V. Pseudoaneurysm after transradial cardiac catheterization: case series and review of the literature. *Cathet Cardiovasc Interv.* Epub July 6 2011.

35. Herold J, Brucks S, Boenigk H, Said SM, Braun-Dullaeus RC. Ultrasound guided thrombin injection of pseudoaneurysm of the radial artery after percutaneous coronary intervention. *Vasa.* 2011;40(1):78–81.

36. Plastiras SC, Pamboucas C, Zafiriou T, Lazaris N, Toumandis S. Ortner's syndrome: a multifactorial cardiovocal syndrome. *Clin Cardiol.* 2010;33:E99–E100.

■ VIDEO LEGENDS

Video 16.1 **Run 1:** Excessive tortuosity of upper extremity arteries below the olecranon fossa (videoclip label: Nadel Run 1). **Run 2:** Excessive tortuosity of upper extremity arteries above the olecranon fossa. Note pseudostenosis of forearm arteries as a result of forced straightening of tortuous vessels. Radial approach abandoned to avoid injury (videoclip label: Nadel Run 2). **Run 3:** Tortuous radial artery with forced straightening, perforated while attempting to advance diagnostic catheter. Perforation managed with external pressure (videoclip label: AJ radial art perf).

chapter 17

How to Start a Transradial Program at Your Hospital

Ankitkumar K. Patel, MD, MPH

Zoltan G. Turi, MD

■ INTRODUCTION

Although the catheterization laboratory staff may find the transition from a transfemoral to a transradial laboratory to be challenging, the knowledge base for starting a transradial program is incremental to the experience already at hand with the transfemoral approach. The resistance to transitioning to a transradial program has been high in the United States. Thus, although the introduction of transradial access by Campeau in 1989[1] for diagnostic catheterization and by Kiemeneij in 1993[2] for percutaneous coronary intervention (PCI) led to widespread adoption of the technique in much of the world, there has been relatively recent acceptance in the United States, with low-percentage (single-digit) utilization until the last several years.[3] Among the reasons cited for failure to adopt a technique that is generally recognized as safer have been the logistic difficulties of transitioning laboratories that perform virtually 100% femoral access. In general, the causes for inertia relate to several factors: training demands for both staff and operators, the perception (largely accurate) that there is a long learning curve, and the complexity of choosing and stocking disposables. Although the brachial approach was prevalent in much of the first decade after Sones[4] pioneered coronary angiography via a surgical cutdown, the catheters used in that era have little applicability to modern practice, and few practicing invasive cardiologists have extensive experiences with the nuances of the Sones technique. [*Editor's note:* Nonetheless, the radial approach has similarities with the Sones

Transradial Access: Techniques for Diagnostic Angiography and Percutaneous Intervention
©2013 Howard A. Cohen (Editor). Cardiotext Publishing, ISBN 978-1-935395-41-6.

technique, and those few remaining interventional cardiologists with experience in the Sones technique will find the radial technique is easier to master.] In addition, relatively few teaching laboratories prior to the past few years performed transradial procedures in sufficient volume to comprehensively train fellows. As a result, most operators and hospitals have had to initiate transradial programs without the benefit of in-house expertise.

In general, transitioning to radial access requires a significant commitment. The purpose of this chapter is to review the practical issues involved and to provide some suggestions for shortening the inherent learning curve. Indeed, one of the major purposes of this textbook is to shorten the learning curve for the new operator. In addition, some practical suggestions are provided for smoothing the transition. Table 17.1 is a summary of the salient issues to be considered and serves as an outline for this chapter.

1. Convincing the Femoralists

Longtime femoral access catheterizers, which include most invasive cardiologists in the United States, have a list of rationalizations for why femoral should remain the preferred approach. The list[5] includes *easier access* to both the femoral artery itself and to the coronaries and *better intubation of the coronaries* with more backup support for PCI. In practice, these concerns were confirmed by RIVAL[6] where crossover was required in 7% of radial cases but only 0.9% of femorals. An additional issue cited by dedicated femoral catheterizers is the *quality* of the angiography: Femoral access is likely to result in better catheter engagement and thus better visualization. The latter is also enhanced by predominantly 6-Fr catheter use via the femoral versus 5-Fr via the radial (in particular in laboratories that use manual dye injection). *Shorter time*[6] and *less radiation*[7] have been a consistent feature of femoral versus radial access studies, again modified by operator experience. Most radialists concede these points with the qualifier that operator experience ameliorates many of these differences: Once through the learning curve, the

Table 17.1 Requirements for Transitioning to Transradial Catheterization.

1.	Accept shortcomings of femoral access.
2.	Recognize benefits of radial access.
3.	Educate physician operators.
4.	Educate cath lab staff.
5.	Observe established radial operation.
6.	Choose and obtain proper equipment.
7.	Choose initial cases prudently.
8.	Avoid high-risk cases initially.
9.	Start slow.
10.	Select a project leader.
11.	Collect feedback from patients (especially those who have had prior femoral access) and staff.
12.	Stay the course.

This list is adapted from Pinak Shah, Transradial Intervention Program, Society of Cardiac Angiography and Interventions, January 15, 2011. http://www.cardiovascularbusiness.com/index.php?option=com_articles&view=article&id=25868:scai-a-12-step-program-for-femoral-aholics

issues above are at least partly addressed, although even the most experienced tercile of radialists in RIVAL had higher crossover incidence with radial than with the femoral approach.[6] [*Editor's note:* I suspect that there would be an insignificant (or at least a smaller) difference in crossover-rate transradial versus transfemoral access if switching from right to left transradial were compared to switching from right to left transfemoral access. In practice, when transradial access fails even in experienced hands, the switch is invariably to transfemoral as both femoral access sites are routinely prepared, and the contralateral radial access site is not.] One can concede the point that *large devices* are unlikely to be accommodated by the limited size of the radial artery. [*Editor's note:* In Europe and Asia, where hydrophilic glidesheaths are available, device size is not an issue. Even with routine 6-Fr guides, there is little that cannot be done except for simultaneous kissing stents or rotational atherectomy with large burrs.] In our laboratory, acceptance of radial by femoralists has followed a predictable course: One operator enthusiastically adopted radials and served as the point person, 2 operators followed gradually thereafter, with the fourth jumping on the bandwagon when the staff evinced enthusiasm and the trend was clearly apparent. The fifth and last convert switched over through peer pressure: Patients being referred specifically for radial access required readjustment of clinic schedules and other responsibilities to cover radial cases when that individual was in the cath lab.

2. Recognize the Benefits of Radial

The data for lower complication rates with radial access,[3,6,8] greater patient comfort, and simpler postprocedure management, including early ambulation and simpler and cheaper closure methodologies, are reasonably supported by the literature.[9] The argument that combining vascular closure devices with a femoral approach is the equivalent of performing the procedure via the radial route has not been compelling.[10] The cost benefits plus shorter length of stay for radials along with a mandate for same-day discharge of PCIs will draw the support of cath lab managers and hospital administrators. Patient preference lends a significant impetus and spreads fairly rapidly in the community, and lack of a strong radial operation eventually becomes a commercial disadvantage for many hospitals.

3. Educate Physician Operators

As with most procedures, physician education requires reviewing the evidence base as well as some "how to" literature.[11] An increasing number of courses are offered as well. Some particularly important elements to consider include the following:

- Develop a sophisticated knowledge of the subtleties and limitations of the Allen's test.

- Use an oximeter/plethysmography device along with the Barbeau classification[12] rather than a simple "positive/ negative" grade for the Allen's test.

- Develop a comprehensive understanding of the factors that cause, as well as the means to treat, spasm, intractable pain, hand ischemia, and perforation/ compartment syndrome.

- Understand and choose patient-specific periprocedure polypharmacy.

- Have a plan of action for challenges posed by arm, subclavian, aortic, and coronary anatomy.

Consider having a proctor on site for the first few days of radial procedures, and make certain that 1 or 2 operators who will lead the transition perform as many cases as possible with the proctor present.

4. Educate Cath Lab and Hospital Staff

Just as there will be recalcitrant physician operators, cardiac cath lab staff may exhibit reluctance to switch from the "tried and true" femoral approach, in particular because labs that perform radial catheterization uncommonly are likely to associate radial access with prolonged access times, high failure rate and crossover, extended procedure duration, and often a "messy" process in general, with patient pain, blood and fluids on the floor, and in general anything but the smooth and quick procedures associated with longtime femoral access operations. The substantial increase in failure and complications for the occasional operator have been well documented in the brachial literature;[13] many of the reasons for failure are identical to those seen with the occasional brachial as well as the occasional radial approach. Staff need to be exposed to the same evidence base that physician operators rely on to understand the rationale for transitioning to radials, and a lead nurse or technician should be sought to champion and oversee the transition. Having a dedicated radial team of technicians and nurses in the early phases of the transition may be helpful as well.

5. Take a Field Trip

Instead of "reinventing the wheel," it makes substantial sense to take physician operators and cath lab staff to visit a successful transradial laboratory. There are considerable bits of know-how involved in successful transradial catheterization that may not be found easily in the literature or on the Internet. This applies to mundane but important aspects such as preprocedure radial artery assessment, prepping and draping the patient, preparing the left radial, equipment selection, pre- and postprocedure management, management of the x-ray gantry, and working with the periprocedural polypharmacy distinct to the radial approach. Currently there are no accreditation standards and no training program standards in transradial catheterization. A number of academic courses coordinated by high-volume radialists provide an excellent initial exposure to the transradial approach. Beyond the lectures, these courses provide a unique opportunity to ask questions and network with individuals who have been practicing transradial catheterization.

After attending a course and visiting a high-volume radial center, the next step in the development of a transradial program is to plan a meeting of all interested parties. Practice partners and interventionalists will be interested in physician staffing needs. Catheterization laboratory staff will be vital in the preparation and troubleshooting of the new radial program. Cardiology fellows and physician assistants will need to be trained on preprocedural radial evaluation of patients. Nurses and technicians will need to be trained on radial site preparation, arm board placement, and catheter selection. The recovery room staff will need to be made aware of monitoring for radial complications and management of vascular closure methods. For patients who are admitted to the floors or intensive care units, nurses will need to be in-serviced. Hospital administration should be involved in some of these meetings to provide the infrastructural support.

6. Choose the Right Equipment

Individual aspects of equipment selection have already been covered in this book. It is important to appreciate that the evidence base for an optimal radial approach remains in evolution, and many recommendations are empiric rather than evidence based. Thus there is fervent support for both sides of several debates: hydrophilic versus nonhydrophilic wires to traverse the arm, short versus longer sheaths, short micropuncture versus longer-sheathed IV insertion-type needles, arm boards versus no arm boards, sheathed versus sheathless catheters, all-in-one versus dedicated right and left coronary diagnostic and guiding catheters, and so on.[14] The same applies for type and amount of anticoagulation.[15] A particularly vexing issue for cath lab staff is that individual operators tend to choose different "cocktails" and equipment, much more so than with routine femoral cases. In our laboratory, we finally had a meeting of operators and came up with a compromise that was acceptable to all radial catheterizers.

7. Pick Your First Cases Carefully

It is essential to start with a manageable group of patients who have a high chance of success and low risk of complications. As a rule, it is initially best to avoid elderly, thin, short or very tall, and diabetic patients. Similarly, patients who are known to require PCI, coronary artery bypass graft (CABG) patients, or procedures that will require larger than 5-Fr sheaths are less desirable for novices, although after the early learning curve all of these patients will be not only appropriate but in most cases desirable candidates for a transradial approach.

Initially, both the planned radial site and a backup femoral site should be prepared for catheterization. This will allow for minimal disruption in the event the radial access is unsuccessful. Some seasoned centers will transition to only preparing the radial site once an adequate learning curve has been achieved.

Many skilled operators facilitate a more rapid learning curve by working in conjunction with a partner in a dual-operator scenario. In academic centers, after this initial learning period, a cardiology fellow can be the first or second operator once the primary operator has developed adequate comfort with the procedure. As proficiency increases in the radial technique, it is reasonable to begin transitioning to more complex cases, including emergent PCIs.

8. Avoid High-Risk Cases

It is better for the patient, the operators, and the lab as a whole to have the basic methodology, early learning curve, and equipment issues resolved before beginning truly high-risk cases. Among the considerations, an important element of transition to the radial approach is the public relations element within the cath lab and the community. Ultimately, certain types of procedures, most prominently ST-elevation myocardial infarction (STEMI), should be done via the radial route given compelling evidence of superior outcomes.[3,6] These cases should be done, however, only when the operator is over the learning curve, as door-to-balloon time is of crucial importance to these patients.

9. Start Slow and Ramp Up

In our laboratory, I chose to start radial catheterizations by scheduling 5 cases on the first day. This is the worst possible way to introduce the radial technique. If even 1 case requires transition to femoral or has any major time delay or complication, it will likely set back the program substantially. A slow planned transition is much more preferable,[16] and with proper preparation the transition from a nearly all femoral to a nearly all radial operation can be accomplished in a reasonable time frame (see Figure 17.1).

10. Get Colleagues Onboard Including Project Leader

Having a single primary project leader will smooth the transition substantially. Meetings with administration regarding costs, with staff regarding methodologies, and with colleagues regarding clinical issues are best handled by a single committed catheterizer who keeps abreast of the literature and gets involved in all aspects of equipment selection and other logistics. A good technique to use for staff buy-in is to involve them early in quality improvement measures.[17] [*Editor's note:* The increased efficiency and decreased cost as well as patient satisfaction will be very attractive to administration; see Chapter 14.]

11. Get Feedback from Patients, Particularly Those with Prior Femoral Access

Patient satisfaction, and by inference staff satisfaction, is an essential element of promoting radial access. Most patients who have had prior femoral access and closure give glowing testimonials to their preference for the radial approach, which in general results in much greater comfort, particularly postprocedure, when the discomfort associated with lying flat or with compression or vascular closure devices does not apply.[18] Staff members will appreciate the simpler postprocedural management of radial access sites as compared to femoral access sites.

12. Stay Committed

Learning curves are not linear. As operators become more comfortable with the radial technique, they will invariably have periods of higher complications, more crossovers to femoral, and increased procedure times. This has been documented for a variety of methodologies related not just to radial artery access and closure[16] but to femoral vascular closure devices[19] and to medical procedures in general.[20] This is partly the result of including more complex and higher-risk cases in patients who were initially avoided. It is important to keep perspective and to persist long enough to allow a fair comparison between the lab's prior experience with femorals, including a variety of clinical, operational, and financial outcomes, and the radial experience once the learning curve is mature.

■ SUMMARY

Transradial catheterization is increasing throughout the world and now in the United States as well. Patient satisfaction and lower complication rates have driven the transition for many femoral access laboratories to primarily radial operations. With adequate preparation and perseverance through the learning curve, the radial approach can become the primary means of catheterization for all except large sheath and some limited

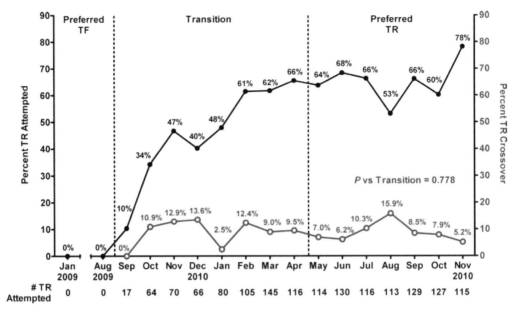

Figure 17.1 Transition from transfemoral (TF) preferred to transradial (TR) preferred in one high-volume laboratory. The red line demonstrates the percentage of cases that required crossover to femoral, peaking at 13.6% in the early learning curve, and again at 15.9% as volume and operator involvement increased and case selection liberalized. *Source*: Reproduced with permission. From Turner S, Sacrinty M, Manogue M, et al. Transitioning to the radial artery as the preferred access site for cardiac catheterization: an academic medical center experience. *Catheter Cardiovasc Interv.* 2011. doi:10.1002/ccd.23387.

peripheral access procedures. As newer technologies specifically designed for the transradial approach come to market, radialists will have an even greater range of procedures that they can perform. Careful introduction of the radial technique should make the transition relatively seamless.

■REFERENCES

1. Campeau L. Percutaneous radial artery approach for coronary angiography. *Cathet Cardiovasc Diagn.* 1989;16(1):3–7.
2. Kiemeneij F, Laarman GJ. Percutaneous transradial artery approach for coronary stent implantation. *Cathet Cardiovasc Diagn.* 1993;30:173–178.
3. Rao SV, Ou FS, Wang TY, et al. Trends in the prevalence and outcomes of radial and femoral approaches to percutaneous coronary intervention: a report from the National Cardiovascular Data Registry. *J Am Coll Cardiol Intv.* 2008;1:379–386.
4. Proudfit WL, Shirey EK, Sones FM Jr. Selective cine coronary arteriography: Correlation with clinical findings in 1,000 patients. *Circulation.* 1966;33(6):901–910.
5. Turi ZG, Wong SC. Perspective: femoral access is preferred or don't throw the femoral out with the bathwater. *J Am Coll Cardiol.* 2013 (In Press).
6. Jolly SS, Yusuf S, Cairns J, et al. Radial versus femoral access for coronary angiography and intervention in patients with acute coronary syndromes (RIVAL): a randomised, parallel group, multicentre trial. *Lancet.* 2011;377(9775):1409–1420.
7. Brasselet C, Blanpain T, Tassan-Mangina S, et al. Comparison of operator radiation exposure with optimized radiation protection devices during coronary angiograms and ad hoc percutaneous coronary interventions by radial and femoral routes. *Eur Heart J.* 2008;29(1):63–70.
8. Nadarasa K, Robertson MC, Wong CK, et al. Rapid cycle change to predominantly radial access coronary angiography and percutaneous coronary intervention: effect on vascular access site complications. *Catheter Cardiovasc Interv.* 2012;79(4):589–594.
9. Roussanov O, Wilson SJ, Henley K, et al. Cost-effectiveness of the radial versus femoral artery approach to diagnostic cardiac catheterization. *J Invasive Cardiol.* 2007;19(8):349–353.
10. Mann T, Cowper PA, Peterson ED, et al. Transradial coronary stenting: comparison with femoral access closed with an arterial suture device. *Catheter Cardiovasc Interv.* Feb 2000;49(2):150–156.

11. Patel T, Shah S, Ranjan A. *Puncture Technique: Patel's Atlas of Transradial Intervention*. Seattle, WA: Sea Script Company; 2007:17.

12. Barbeau GR, Arsenault F, Dugas L, Simard S, Lariviere MM. Evaluation of the ulnopalmar arterial arches with pulse oximetry and plethysmography: comparison with the Allen's test in 1010 patients. *Am Heart J*. 2004;147(3):489–493.

13. Hildick-Smith DJ, Khan ZI, Shapiro LM, Petch MC. Occasional-operator percutaneous brachial coronary angiography: first, do no arm. *Catheter Cardiovasc Interv*. 2002;57(2):161–165.

14. Bertrand OF, Rao SV, Pancholy S, et al. Transradial approach for coronary angiography and interventions: results of the first international transradial practice survey. *JACC Cardiovasc Interv*. 2010;3(10):1022–1031.

15. Plante S, Cantor WJ, Goldman L, et al. Comparison of bivalirudin versus heparin on radial artery occlusion after transradial catheterization. *Catheter Cardiovasc Interv*. 2010;76(5):654–658.

16. Turner S, Sacrinty M, Manogue M, et al. Transitioning to the radial artery as the preferred access site for cardiac catheterization: an academic medical center experience. *Catheter Cardiovasc Interv*. Aug 1 2012;80(2):247–257.

17. Steffenino G, Fabrizi MB, Baralis G, et al. Implementation of radial arterial access for cardiac interventions: a strong case for quality assurance protocols by the nursing staff. *J Cardiovasc Med*. (Hagerstown). 2011;12(2):116–121.

18. Sciahbasi A, Fischetti D, Picciolo A, et al. Transradial access compared with femoral puncture closure devices in percutaneous coronary procedures. *Int J Cardiol*. 2009;137(3):199–205.

19. Resnic FS, Wang TY, Arora N, et al. Quantifying the learning curve in the use of a novel vascular closure device: an analysis of the NCDR (National Cardiovascular Data Registry) CathPCI registry. *JACC Cardiovasc Interv*. 2012;5(1):82–89.

20. Ramsay CR, Grant AM, Wallace SA, Garthwaite PH, Monk AF, Russell IT. Assessment of the learning curve in health technologies: a systematic review. *Int J Technol Assess Health Care*. 2000;16(4): 1095–1108.

Appendix

Videos for use with this book can be found at **www.transradial.cardiotextpublishing.com**.

Chapter 5

Radial Artery Access Video

Video 5.1   Note the low angle of insertion and the bounce of the needle as it advances slowly toward the artery using gentle palpation of the artery with the tips of the first two fingers of the left hand. The needle should be bouncing up and down and not side to side. As you get closer to the artery, the bounce increases. If you press too hard with your left hand, you may obliterate the bounce. Apply just enough pressure to trap the needle between your fingertips and the artery. The flow may be pulsatile, but in many cases the flow may be slow. The bright red color of the blood will assure you that the artery has been entered. The wire should advance easily and without any pain. If there is any pain, it is likely that the wire is subintimal and should be withdrawn with the flow rechecked. If there is resistance to advancement of the wire, it is either subintimal or in a side branch. In this case, you can see that the wire can be torqued and advanced but then meets resistance. Finally, the wire should pass the side branch and advance easily. The needle is withdrawn, and a small nick in the skin is made with a #11 blade. (Some catheter and dilators do not require a dermatotomy with a #11 blade.) Once the sheath has been inserted, medications can be administered prophylactically to prevent spasm.

Brachial Loop

Video 5.2   The loop in the brachial artery above the elbow is overcome with an angled Glidewire gradually advanced through the loop. It is advisable to overcome the loop with

a soft-tipped angled or J-tipped guidewire followed by a catheter in order not to dissect the artery or cause spasm.

Video 5.3   Note that the loop is now straightened by the guidewire and is now safe to traverse with a catheter. All subsequent catheter exchanges should be made over an exchange-length guidewire.

Severe Tortuosity of the Radial Artery

Video 5.4   Note the severe tortuosity of the radial artery with the angled-tipped Glidewire entering a small branch at the top of the curve (recurrent radial artery). You can see how advancing a catheter into this vessel at the very least would cause severe spasm and at worst could cause perforation. This is why any resistance of a guidewire or a catheter should be interrogated with an angiogram through the sheath. The severe loop shown in this example may be overcome with a J-tipped guidewire (which will probably not enter the small branch) or, if this is unsuccessful, a transition-less 0.014 soft coronary guidewire can overcome the bend. Once the severe curve is overcome, a Glide Catheter can be passed over the guidewire and the coronary guidewire then exchanged for an 0.035 J-tipped Glidewire.

From Descending Aorta to Ascending Aorta

Video 5.5   Note tortuosity of the subclavian artery with the tip of the angled Glidewire appearing to be in the ascending aorta.

Video 5.6   Note how the guidewire and the following Judkins Left 3.5 diagnostic catheter have straightened out the tortuosity, but the tip of the guidewire is now in the descending aorta.

Video 5.7 With the tip of the diagnostic catheter at the aortic knob and the guidewire in the descending aorta, the patient is asked to take a deep breath, and the catheter is torqued toward the ascending aorta as the guidewire is retracted and then readvanced when the catheter is pointing toward the ascending aorta. Once the position in the ascending aorta is achieved, any catheter exchange should be made over a long guidewire to maintain position in the ascending aorta and to obviate the need of renegotiating the severe tortuosity.

Dilated and Tortuous Subclavian and Aorta

Video 5.8 Note extreme tortuosity of subclavian artery. This may be negotiated with a J-tipped guidewire advancing a catheter over the curves and ultimately into the ascending aorta.

Video 5.9 The left main coronary artery (LMCA) is engaged with a 110-cm-long multipurpose catheter with the guidewire in place in order to overcome the extreme tortuosity. The guidewire is carefully withdrawn once the LMCA is approached in the left coronary cusp with the adjustment of advancing or withdrawing the catheter until the LMCA is selectively engaged.

Severe Tortuosity Straightened Out by Guidewire

Video 5.10 Note the severe tortuosity of the subclavian artery that is negotiated with an angled Glidewire. A J-tipped Glidewire may be equally effective in negotiating the tortuosity. The advantage of the J-tipped Glidewire is that it may be helpful in avoiding side branches because it usually selects the large main branch and stays out of smaller side branches that can be perforated by the angled Glidewire. The disadvantage of the J-tipped Glidewire is that it has no steerability. The angled Glidewire can be "steered away" from unwanted branches.

Video 5.11 The tortuosity is overcome by the angled Glidewire that is now in the ascending aorta.

Chapter 7

Video 7.1 Left coronary cannulation technique using universal catheter. A 5-Fr RBLBT (Cordis, Bridgewater, NJ) is positioned in the left coronary cusp and advanced to engage the left coronary.

Video 7.2 Cannulation of the left coronary with a universal catheter using the superior approach with a 5-Fr RBLBT (Cordis, Bridgewater, NJ). The curve is opened from above using a J-wire, and the catheter is advanced into the left coronary.

Video 7.3 Right coronary cannulation technique using universal catheter. The right coronary cusp is usually inferior to the left coronary cusp. Thus, engagement of the right coronary involves counterclockwise rotation and forward advancement into the right coronary artery.

Chapter 16

Video 16.1 **Run 1:** Excessive tortuosity of upper extremity arteries below the olecranon fossa (videoclip label: Nadel Run 1).

Run 2: Excessive tortuosity of upper extremity arteries above the olecranon fossa. Note pseudostenosis of forearm arteries as a result of forced straightening of tortuous vessels. Radial approach abandoned to avoid injury (videoclip label: Nadel Run 2).

Run 3: Tortuous radial artery with forced straightening, perforated while attempting to advance diagnostic catheter. Perforation managed with external pressure (videoclip label: AJ radial art perf).

Index

CPSIA information can be obtained at www.ICGtesting.com
Printed in the USA
BVIW12n0457291217
503254BV00001B/1